Qualitative Research in Occupational Therapy:
Strategies and Experiences

Dedication

This book is dedicated to all the research participants who so generously shared their experiences with us.

Cover Credit:

The cover art symbolizes the circular, emergent nature of qualitative research designs and strategies.

"Used with permission. Copyright retained by the artist, Johnny Jaworski."

NISA

NISA stands for Northern Initiative for Social Action, and is a non-profit, incorporated charitable organization, located at the Kirkwood site of Network North in Sudbury, Ontario.

It is an alternative to traditional mental health services; and seeks to provide meaningful and safe working environments for individuals who are consumers/survivors of mental health services.

NISA believes in the overall wellness of the community and the individual's role in creating their own opportunities for good quality of life. This is achieved by the belief that consumers/ survivors can function well in society and make valuable contributions when given the opportunity to do so. NISA fulfills its mission and objectives through a variety of programs and initiatives; including a research unit, a journal, *Open Minds Quarterly*, The Artist's Loft, Warm Hearts/Warm Bodies, and a Computer Recycling Depot. NISA is grounded on the notion that meaningful occupation and leading a healthy lifestyle are key to optimum wellness.

For more information on NISA, visit their web site at www.nisa.on.ca

Qualitative Research in Occupational Therapy:
Strategies and Experiences

Edited by

Joanne Valiant Cook, Ph.D., OT(C)

Associate Professor

School of Occupational Therapy

The University of Western Ontario

DELMAR

THOMSON LEARNING ™

Australia Canada Mexico Singapore Spain United Kingdom United States

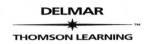

Qualitative Research in Occupational Therapy: Strategies and Experiences

Joanne Valiant Cook

Health Care Publishing Director:
William Brottmiller

Acquisitions Editor:
Candice Janco

Editorial Assistant:
Maria D'Angelico

Executive Marketing Manager:
Dawn F. Gerrain

Channel Manager:
Tara Carter

Executive Editor:
Cathy L. Esperti

Production Editor:
James Zayicek

Cover Image:
Johnny Jaworski

For permission to use material from this text or product, contact us by:
Tel   (800)730-2214
Fax   (800) 730-2215
www.thomsonrights.com

Library of Congress Cataloging-in-Publication Data

Qualitative research in occupational therapy: strategies and experiences / edited by Joanne Valiant Cook.
    p. cm
Includes bibliographical references and index.
ISBN 0-7693-0079-0
1. Occupational therapy—Research—
    Methodology.
2. Qualitative research. I. Cook, Joanne Valiant.

RM735.42 .Q355 2001
615.8'515'072—dc21

                                    00-065616

NOTICE TO THE READER

Publisher does not warrant or guarantee any of the products described herein or perform any independent analysis in connection with any of the product information contained herein. Publisher does not assume, and expressly disclaims, any obligation to obtain and include information other than that provided to it by the manufacturer.

The reader is expressly warned to consider and adopt all safety precautions that might be indicated by the activites herein and to avoid all potential hazards. By following the instructions contained herein, the reader willingly assumes all risks in connection with such instructions.

The Publisher makes no representation or warranties of any kind, including by not limited to, the warranties of fitness for particular purpose or merchantability, nor are any such representations implied with respect to the material set forth herein, and the publisher takes no reponsibility with respect to such material. The publsiher shall not be liable for any special, consequential, or exemplary damages resulting, in whole or part, from the readers' use of, or reliance upon, this material.

Contents

Preface

This book has been prepared by occupational therapists for occupational therapists interested in pursuing research. The book had its beginning in 1998 at the World Federation of Occupational Therapy conference in Montreal, Canada. I organized a panel presentation on qualitative studies of occupation in which the presenters were former and current graduate students in the Master of Science program in the School of Occupational Therapy at The University of Western Ontario. The panel was well received by a large audience. We were approached by a representative of Singular Publishing Inc. and invited to submit a book proposal on qualitative research in occupational therapy.

This book is the result of many discussions among the contributors. There are a great number of excellent qualitative texts and studies published in the past two decades. We did not strive to duplicate them, nor did we aim to be a comprehensive text. Our goal was to write a book that was complementary to the existing literature but unique in providing an occupational therapy perspective to the methods and interpretative analyses of qualitative inquiries.

We wanted to provide an overview and example of the value and usefulness of qualitative research studies of occupation, occupational therapists' practices, and the experiences of occupational therapy clients. Thus, this text is designed primarily for occupational therapy students and novice researchers. We believe, however, that it will also be of interest to students and researchers of health issues in other disciplines such as nursing, physical therapy, and sociology.

The book is organized into five parts. Part I, Introduction, provides an overview of the qualitative paradigm of research inquiry and its "fit" with the research issues and values of occupational therapy as a profession and an academic discipline.

Part II, Strategies of Design and Inquiry, explores the major strategies of research design and data collection. Each strategy is illustrated with examples from the author's research studies of occupational therapy issues.

Part III, Personal Research Journeys, offers five narratives of personal research experiences. These include descriptions of developing a research question, the successes and problems involved in data collection, the "agonies" of data analysis and interpretation, and the questioning of the competence of self in performing research. Two of the narratives chronicle the manner in which a single research study evolves into a program of research because one "answer" turns out, in reality, to be "more questions." These stories provide what most texts do not: a clearly detailed, very personal account of how qualitative research studies evolve, change, and emerge as the study proceeds.

Part IV, Qualitative Research Studies of Occupation, Occupational Therapists, and Client Experiences, reprints twelve previously published articles on studies of occupation, occupational therapists, and client experiences. These studies illustrate the utility of qualitative inquiry and its strategies of design and data collection to explore the issues of importance to the profession of occupational therapy.

Part V is an annotated bibliography of selected texts for further reading and elaboration of the issues raised in the previous parts of this book. The bibliography is not intended to be comprehensive nor inclusive of all the published literature. It does represent those works that the contributors to this book have found to be most useful in furthering their knowledge of the methods, designs, and principles of qualitative research.

Concluding Note

All the contributors to this book are strongly committed to the qualitative paradigm of research. At the same time, we recognize and value the contribution of quantitative studies to the expansion of our knowledge base. However, we also know that many of our questions, concerns, and issues cannot be studied only by testing hypotheses and counting survey questionnaire answers. We need to explore all the complexities of occupation through intimate, personal involvement with the persons who are engaged in occupation and with those who are deprived of chosen occupations due to disability or sociocultural handicap. We hope that you, the reader, will also become committed to research using qualitative strategies and join us in the exciting, rewarding, often frustrating, and always challenging journey that will enable us to be a research-based, knowledgeable, academic, and professional discipline.

Joanne Valiant Cook
London, Ontario, Canada

Acknowledgments

There are always numerous persons and organizations whose contributions to the completion of a book are appreciated. Those mentioned here are especially significant. They are not listed in order of importance but in what we hope is the logical chronological order.

1. Dr. Frank Stein, the editor of *Occupational Therapy International*, who suggested to Singular Publishing that our presentation at the World Federation of Occupational Therapy Conference (WFOT) in 1998 merited some consideration for future publication.
2. The Canadian Occupational Therapy Foundation (COTF), which supported the development of the manuscript with a publication grant.
3. Lynne Helwig, who worked her word processing magic on the COTF grant application and many of the early drafts of chapters.
4. Susan Buitinga, who was responsible for the "clean" final manuscript that went to the publisher. Her reworking of all the drafts into a coherent "whole" was remarkable.
5. Sandy Sargeant, who came out of the "bull pen" to lend her usual efficient and speedy expertise to last minute corrections and additions.
6. Helen Kerr, Administrative Assistant, Tina Czyzewski, Secretary to the Director and the Graduate Program, and Jackie Klee, Acting School Secretary of the School of Occupational Therapy, The University of Western Ontario. Without them, the process of preparing this work would have been much more difficult, time-consuming, and stressful.
7. The families and friends of the contributors, who lent both moral and practical support whenever it was needed.

They are:

Frank, Susan, and Jonathan Corring

Mary and Ted Landry, Dr. Trevor Birmingham, and Daisy, the "amazing chocolate brown dog"

Bill, Robert, and Matthew MacGregor

Frank, Zachary, and Daniel Moll

Norm and Nathan Williams (Nagle)

Lloyd, Lindsay, Zachary, Matthew, and Nicholas Rebeiro

Mark and Mitchell Rudman

Uzi, Sahar, and Yannai Segal

Stan, the one who is not here, but who is always there

None of the contributors to this book will receive royalties. All royalties have been assigned to the Canadian Occupational Therapy Foundation (COTF) to support research studies that use qualitative methods of inquiry.

Contributors

Deborah Corring, M.Sc., OT(C)
Program Co-Leader
London/St. Thomas Psychiatric Hospital
St. Thomas, Ontario, Canada

Deborah Laliberte-Rudman, M.Sc., OT(C)
Ph.D. Candidate
Lecturer
University of Toronto
Toronto, Ontario, Canada

Jennifer E. Landry, M.Sc., OT(C),
    O.T. Reg. (NS)
Assistant Professor
School of Occupational Therapy
Dalhousie University
Halifax, Nova Scotia, Canada

Laura MacGregor, M.Sc., OT(C)
Conestoga College
Kitchener, Ontario, Canada

Sandra Moll, M.Sc., OT(C)
Assistant Professor
School of Rehabilitation Science
McMaster University
Hamilton, Ontario, Canada

Susan Nagle, M.Sc. OT(C)
Clinical Supervisor
Occupational Therapy and Clinical
    Recreation Departments
Credit Valley Hospital
Mississauga, Ontario, Canada

Karen L. Rebeiro, M.Sc., OT(C)
Clinical Researcher
Northeast Mental Health Centre
Sudbury, Ontario, Canada

Ruth Segal, Ph.D., OT(C), OTR
Assistant Professor
Department of Occupational Therapy
School of Education
New York University
New York, New York

About the Authors

Joanne Valiant Cook (Editor)

Joanne Cook is a graduate of the former diploma program in physical and occupational therapy at The University of Toronto. She earned an honors B.A. in sociology from the University of Toronto and Trent University. Her master of arts and doctor of philosophy degrees in sociology were completed at York University, Toronto, Ontario, Canada. She taught in the Department of Sociology at Trent University before moving to the School of Occupational Therapy at The University of Western Ontario in 1990, where she currently holds the rank of associate professor. Her clinical, consulting, and research experiences are primarily in the field of mental health and illness with a particular focus on innovations in service programs. Her research strategies and designs have always been within the qualitative paradigm of inquiry.

Deborah Corring

Deborah Corring, M.Sc., OT is currently program coleader at London/St. Thomas Psychiatric Hospital, St. Thomas, Ontario, Canada, and also owner/operator of her own consulting business, Client Perspectives. Her research interests focus around the client definition of client-centred care, service evaluation by clients, and client perspectives of their needs in housing, employment, and other areas of recovery.

Deborah Laliberte-Rudman

Deborah Laliberte-Rudman is currently a lecturer in the Department of Occupational Therapy at the University of Toronto, Toronto, Ontario, Canada. She is also a Ph.D. candidate in the Department of Community Health, University of Toronto. Her interest in the application of qualitative methodology and methods to questions regarding occupation began while she was a masters student in the occupational therapy program at The University of Western Ontario. Her interest in conducting research of relevance to older adults stems from her clinical work. She has been involved in a number of studies that have used qualitative methods, including a study exploring the meaning of quality of life for persons with schizophrenia and a study examining the experiences of stroke survivors and their caregivers related to the use of wheeled mobility devices. In her doctoral work, she is applying qualitative methods to explore issues related to identity, occupation, cultural images, and aging.

Jennifer E. Landry

Jennifer E. Landry received her bachelors and masters degrees in occupational therapy at The University of Western Ontario. She is an assistant professor and community resources coordinator with the School of Occupational Therapy, Dalhousie University. Her research interests include the disability experience, occupational engagement, the sociocultural environment, and gender issues. She is currently pursuing Ph.D. studies at Dalhousie University.

Laura MacGregor

Laura MacGregor completed her undergraduate degree in occupational therapy at the University of Toronto in 1990. She completed a master of science degree at The University of Western Ontario in 1995. Currently, she divides her professional time between teaching part-time in the OTA/PTA program at Conestoga College and managing a small private practice working with people involved in motor vehicle accidents.

Sandra Moll

Sandra Moll is an assistant clinical professor at McMaster University in Hamilton, Ontario, Canada, and is a part-time instructor in the Psychosocial Rehabilitation Programme at Mohawk College. Her interest and commitment to the value of qualitative research developed through her masters thesis work studying the clinical reasoning of therapists working in psychosocial occupational therapy. Her ongoing research interests include qualitative approaches to program evaluation and exploring the perspective of individuals with a severe and persistent mental illness.

Susan Nagle

Susan Nagle received a bachelor of science degree in occupational therapy from Queen's University in Kingston, Ontario, Canada, and a master of science degree in occupational therapy from The University of Western Ontario in London, Ontario, Canada. She began her career working in the area of chronic care and geriatric psychiatry, but since 1989, she has worked exclusively with people with severe and persistent mental illness. She has shared her knowledge of working with people with schizophrenia through part-time teaching at the University of Toronto, McMaster University, The University of Western Ontario, Queen's University,

Mohawk College of Applied Arts and Technology, and Humber College of Applied Arts and Technology. Currently, she combines clinical practice with a supervisory role at the Credit Valley Hospital, a community hospital in Mississauga, Ontario, Canada. In this position, she is pursuing research as part of the quality management programs both in the Occupational Therapy Department and the Schizophrenia Program.

Karen L. Rebeiro

Karen L. Rebeiro is a clinical researcher at Northeast Mental Health Centre in Sudbury, Ontario, Canada. She completed her bachelor of science in occupational therapy at Queen's University and The University of Western Ontario in 1985, and her master of science in occupational therapy at The University of Western Ontario in 1997. Karen currently works in a consumer-run, occupation-based, mental health initiative called NISA/ Northern Initiative for Social Action. This program is based on her research and is the setting for current research studies.

Ruth Segal

Ruth Segal earned her occupational therapy degrees and her doctorate in occupational science at the University of Southern California. She has done research with families of children with special needs (attention deficit hyperactivity disorder, developmental coordination disorder, and physical disabilities). She is currently an assistant professor in the Department of Occupational Therapy at New York University.

PART

Introduction

CHAPTER

Qualitative Research in Occupational Therapy

Joanne Valiant Cook

> [S]cientists can no longer remain as external observers, measuring
> what they see; they must move to investigate from within the subject
> of study and employ research techniques appropriate to that task.
>
> —Morgan & Smircich (1980, p. 498)

In 1991, Elizabeth Yerxa, in a special issue of the *American Journal of Occupational Therapy*, called on therapists and researchers to seek "a relevant, ethical, and realistic way of knowing . . ." (p. 199). She proposed that the qualitative paradigm of inquiry was best suited to that task. What does it mean to be relevant, ethical, and realistic, and why are qualitative strategies of research appropriate for that challenge?

The following discussion examines the manner in which: the values, beliefs, and language of occupational therapy coincide with those of the qualitative paradigm of science; the domain of jurisdiction for occupational therapy—the enabling of chosen occupational engagement—requires an inquiry approach capable of capturing the complexity

and subjectivity of the phenomenon; the questions that occupation and persons engaged in occupation raise for research answers are those that can best be addressed through the use of qualitative strategies and designs.

Values, Beliefs, and Language

"[Q]ualitative researchers study things in their natural settings, attempting to make sense of or interpret phenomena in terms of the meanings people bring to them" (Denzin & Lincoln, 1994, p. 2). "Enabling occupation means collaborating with people to choose, organize and perform occupations which people find useful or meaningful in a given environment"(CAOT, 1997, p. 30) These two quotations reflect many of the values and beliefs that the profession of occupational therapy and adherents of qualitative inquiries hold in common. Both hold a view of reality in which the person's perspective and meanings attached to actions are central to understanding human behavior. Therefore, in order to make sense of the other's behavior, close, intimate interaction between the experiencer and the learner is essential.

In qualitative research, the aim is to gain *understanding* of phenomena rather than *predicting* the behavior of abstract populations. Similarly, occupational therapy practice aims to recognize the uniqueness of each occupational being and develop, in partnership with them, an understanding of their occupational performance issues in order to collaboratively engage in a program of interventions that suits that individual. Both occupational therapists and qualitative researchers recognize that the individual has the knowledge and expertise of the phenomenon of study and that we are often the learners, not the experts. Spradley expresses this value in these terms: "I want to understand the world from your point of view. I want to know what you know in the way you know it. I want to understand the meaning of your experience, to walk in your shoes, to feel things as you feel them, to explain things as you explain them. Will you become my teacher and help me understand?" (1979, p. 34).

Kielhofner summarizes the literature on the value of recognizing the client's perspective and states, "Occupational therapy holds that it is important to know and respect the unique perspective of the patient or client. . . . [T]his value includes the recognition that disability is a personal matter, experienced uniquely by each person. According to this value, the experiential world of the patient or client should be the focal point of the therapeutic process" (1997, p. 86). Similarly, the Canadian Association of Occupational

Therapists in a list of values and beliefs held by the profession states that "clients have experience and knowledge about their occupations" (1997, p. 31) that must be recognized in any therapeutic process.

This emphasis on the subjective or "emic" perspective rather than the "etic" or neutral, outside, observer perspective is one of the distinguishing features of qualitative research, and it appears to be shared by the profession of occupational therapy in its culture, if not always in its practice. Thus, qualitative strategies of research are apt for those who wish to develop understanding of persons as occupational beings. As Yerxa has stated, "[E]ngagement in occupations encompasses not only the observable performance of individuals, but also their subjective reactions to the activity and objects with which they are occupied" (1980, p. 529).

Qualitative researchers' purposes are to study people and process in their natural world, learn the person's perspective, understand people's worlds and their subjectively constructed realities, tell a story which shares that understanding, and make a difference through that understanding. Occupational therapists "affirm the value of occupation and emphasize a client centered practice and respect for the subjective perspectives of clients and patients. These themes also affirm that therapy is a process of active engagement and empowerment . . ." (Kielhofner, 1997, p. 88) Therapists also want to make a difference by enabling clients to engage in chosen occupations at the level of competence they desire. This sharing of values and in many ways the same language in expressing those values indicates a complementarity between the profession's research needs and the methods of the qualitative paradigm of inquiry.

In providing his definition of qualitative research, Cresswell reflects this complementarity in words that might have been written by an occupational therapist: "Qualitative research is an inquiry process of understanding based on distinct methodological traditions of inquiry that explore a social or human problem. The researcher builds a complex, holistic picture, analyzes words, reports detailed views of informants, and conducts the study in a natural setting" (Cresswell, 1998, p. 15). The importance of recognizing complexity and a holistic perspective is essential to research that seeks to understand the primary domain of occupational therapy, the study and enabling of occupation.

Understanding Occupation

One of the axioms of qualitative study is that "realities are multiple, constructed and holistic" (Lincoln & Guba, 1985, p. 37). Further, qualitative researchers believe that "[t]he *whole* phenomenon under study is understood as a complex system that is more than the sum of its parts; [the] focus [is] on complex interdependencies not meaningfully reduced to a few discrete variables and linear, cause-effect relationships" (Patton, 1990, p. 40). Likewise there is recognition of the complexity and multidimensional nature of occupation. "Occupation is a complex process in which persons fulfil needs and purposes as they interact in their environment. This complexity may not be visible *because the meanings, purposes, values and beliefs behind what people do are not directly observable*" [italics added] (CAOT, 1997, p. 34). "Occupations are the ordinary and familiar things that people do every day. This simple description reflects, but understates, the multidimensional and complex nature of daily occupation" (Christiansen et al. 1995, p. 1015). The Canadian Association of Occupational Therapy lists the following key features of occupation: "Occupation is a:

- basic human need
- determinant of health

- source of meaning
- source of purpose
- source of choice and control
- source of balance and satisfaction
- means of organizing time
- means of organizing materials and space
- means of generating income
- descriptor
- therapeutic medium" (1997, p. 34)

The American Association of Occupational Therapists state in a position paper that occupations have performance, contextual, temporal, psychological, social/symbolic, and meaning/spiritual dimensions (Christiansen et al. 1995, p. 1015). Kielhofner summarizes the literature on the characterization of occupations and states "that occupation:

- Comprises work, play/leisure, and daily activities
- Arises as a response to and fulfils a specific motive or need
- Involves doing or performance that calls upon specific capacities
- Entails completion of a specific form
- Interrelates with the sociocultural context
- Provides meaning
- Interweaves with the developmental process" (1997, p. 55).

Kielhofner asserts that "occupation can never be understood independent of the sociocultural, physical, and temporal context in which it takes place. Occupational behavior is always environmental behavior"(1997, p. 60).

Given the complex, multidimensional, subjective nature of engagement in occupation, the methods of qualitative research are the most suitable for developing understanding of this multifaceted phenomenon. The strategies of participant observation, in-depth interviewing, document analysis, introspection and reflection, and interpretation permit, in fact demand, prolonged engagement with the phenomena of study, a recognition of the importance of environ- mental and personal context, and the neces- sity of providing thick description of the experiences and perspectives of the individ- ual involved in the object of study. In order to capture complexity, our methods of inquiry must provide a moving picture, not snap- shots devoid of context and subjective per- spective. Isolating discrete variables, as done in quantitative studies, in order to measure the effect of one on the other will not capture the processual, idiosyncratic, subjective aspects of engagement in occupation. Complex, multidimensional phenomena require complex, multidimensional, flexible, emergent strategies to examine them.

Our values and beliefs about occupation and occupational beings are most compatible with the beliefs, values, and strategies of qualitative inquiry. "Our constructions of the world, our values, and our ideas about how to inquire into those constructions, are mutu- ally self-reinforcing. We conduct inquiry via a particular paradigm because it embodies assumptions about the world we believe and values that we hold, and because we hold those assumptions and values we conduct inquiry according to the precepts of that par- adigm" (Schwandt, 1989, p. 399). The inquiries we make—the questions we ask when we conduct research—are the kinds of questions that can only be answered with methods which are capable of capturing process and holistic understanding, rather than those which explore linear causality and variable relationships of discrete parts of the occupational person.

Research Questions and Studies

Why are splints more often found in bureau drawers rather than on a person's hands or wrists? Why are clients who are functionally fit through adaptations to disability unable to return to many of their preferred occupa- tions? Why do clients who appear to need and could benefit from adaptive devices refuse to use them or have them installed in their homes? These are questions I have heard therapists pose. They will not be answered by research that evaluates the effectiveness of the splint in reducing pain or deformity. They will not be answered by research that assesses function in terms of physical occupational performance compo- nents. Nor will they be answered by ques- tionnaires that evaluate client knowledge of safety issues. These are questions that require the input of the experts—the clients—to help us understand their life experiences and perceptions or meanings. They are what Maxwell (1996) defines as "process questions." Maxwell makes the dis- tinction between variance questions and process questions: "Quantitative researchers tend to be interested in whether and to what extent variance in x causes variance in y. Qualitative researchers, on the other hand, tend to *ask how* x plays a role in causing y, what the process is that connects x and y" (p. 20). "Variance questions focus on differ- ence and correlation. . . . Process questions, in contrast, focus on *how* things happen, rather than whether there is a particular relationship or how much it is explained by other variables. . . . Qualitative researchers thus tend to focus on two kinds of questions that are much better suited to process theory than to variance theory: questions about the *meaning* of events and activities to the peo- ple involved in these and questions about the influence of the physical and social *con- text* on these events and activities" (Maxwell, 1996, pp. 58, 59).

What does it mean in practical terms to focus on a process question? It means that we begin to develop understanding of the prob- lems rather than experimentally trying to test our predetermined solutions. Too often, in social and medical research we impose our theoretical knowledge to test preconceived notions of what should or ought to work before we really have any knowledge of what the issue is for the actor in the situation. That is, often, we do not know what we do not know. Even the National Aeronautics and Space Administration (NASA), known as a bastion of scientific inquiry, invited qualitative researchers to conduct participant observation and in-depth interviewing to augment their simulation studies. "NASA is developing a marked preference for naturalistic studies of human behavior in aeronautics . . . because the naturalistic studies translated better into the real world than the laboratory research. Although simulators remain as important training devices they are proving less effective in the discovery of problems" (SSSI, 1990, p. 17).

Why is the discovery of problems so important in understanding occupation and occupational engagement for occupational therapists? We cannot test or develop solutions until we have knowledge of exactly what the problems are. For example, in answering the questions in the beginning of this section, we need to know how and why clients use or do not use their splints. One answer I have heard from clients is that yes, the splints help to relieve pain and delay deformity, but they get in the way when performing everyday activities. That is, for some clients, occupational performance is the greater priority. When interviewing clients who refuse assistive devices, one learns that such devices are perceived as "stigma symbols" (Goffman, 1963). That is, they are indicators to the world and to the clients themselves that they have a disability or impairment, and clients are often unwilling to accept that designation of self. In Part IV of this text there are several studies that explore the consequences of sociocultural handicapping experiences for persons with impairments or disabilities who are "functionally" able but perceived as disabled in the physical and social environment and thus handicapped in the opportunities available to participate in those environments.

There are many research purposes of interest to occupational therapists for which qualitative studies are suitable. Maxwell (1996) lists these research purposes as:

1. Understanding the *meaning* for participants in the study of the events, situations, and actions they are involved with and of the accounts that they give of their lives and experiences. (p. 17)
2. Understanding the particular *context* within which the participants act and the influence that this context has on their actions. (p. 17)
3. Identifying *unanticipated* phenomena and influences and generating new grounded theories about the latter. (p. 19)
4. Understanding the *process* by which events and actions take place. (p. 19)

There are many types of studies that may be undertaken using qualitative methods that address the issues of concern for therapists. These include, but are not limited to:

1. Exploratory, descriptive, pilot studies which can help refine questions, discover what you did not know but thought you *did* know, and establish clearer definitions of "problems."
2. Health and illness experience narratives of clients, their families, and clinicians' perspectives. We know a great deal about signs and symptoms but considerably less about the experience of dealing with those signs and symptoms within everyday living. Also, explanations of illness vary from client to client and among health care providers, and how these varying explanations affect experience is a neglected area of research.
3. Chronological case studies of clients' experiences, interventions and programs, and clinicians' experiences in practice

and in developing innovations. Case studies can be a very effective means of building our research base as each case study contributes another brick to our understanding of the whole house which is occupation. "A man [sic] may learn a great deal of the general from studying the specific, whereas it is impossible to know the specific by studying the general" (Rawlings, 1942, p. 359).

4. Participant action research which involves clients and consumers of health services as active researchers in solving the issues of concern. Such research is particularly valuable for formative evaluation of programs of services.

5. Cultural ethnographies which examine the values, beliefs, and norms of behavior of professions, particular client groups who share a diagnosis or disability, and organizations that provide services to persons with disabilities.

6. Grounded theory studies which examine a specific aspect of experience in order to develop conceptual and theoretical understandings based on the data which can then be used to explain processes and direct further exploration of the phenomenon(a).

Part IV of this book contains several studies illustrating the types of research that can be conducted using qualitative methods. "Because occupation is an extremely complex phenomenon and has not been subjected to rigorous research until recently, many questions about its nature and its relationship to health and well being remain unanswered. This emphasizes the need for further study" (Christiansen et al. 1995, p. 1016). The authors of this book believe and have demonstrated by their own studies that the qualitative paradigm of research can be a guiding light in our search for understanding of the complexity of occupation and its role in a person's quality of life.

An Endnote on Ethics and Trust

As occupational therapists, we are committed to respecting and valuing the uniqueness of individuals and their rights to choose and manage their daily occupations. We are also committed to the recognition of their expertise about themselves and their disabilities (CAOT, 1997; Kielhofner, 1997). Qualitative inquiry also acknowledges the participants in research studies as the experts, having the right to share in research endeavors and their results. The establishment of the trustworthiness (Lincoln & Guba, 1985) of qualitative research is partially dependent on member checking with one's informants to ensure that the interpretations of their experiences reflect their perspective. Thus, qualitative research is consonant with the espoused values of occupational therapy. The canons of qualitative research demand that the researcher maintain a journal of his or her own involvement, biases, and predetermined conceptions in order to account for the influence these may have on the research report. Checking with the participants often highlights and corrects the interpretations we make that have been influenced by our own subjective perspectives. To engage in qualitative research, one engages in close interpersonal relationships with informants/parti- cipants. While "friendship is not an essential condition for conducting research . . . being accepted and trusted is" (Glesne & Peshkin, 1992, p. 106). Trust and acceptance depend on the adherence to the ethical canons of our profession and the qualitative paradigm of research which are constructed according to similar values and beliefs about people, the environment, and engagement in it. We can be "relevant, ethical and realistic" (Yerxa, 1991, p. 199) when our professional knowledge and practices are based on research evidence gathered through strategies that are based on and support those purposes.

References

Canadian Association of Occupational Therapists. (1997). *Enabling occupation.* Ottawa, Canada: CAOT Publications ACE.

Christiansen, C., Clark, F., Kielhofner, G., & Rogers, J. (1995). Position paper: Occupation. *The American Journal of Occupational Therapy* 49(10), 1015–1018.

Cresswell, J. (1998). *Qualitative inquiry and research design.* Thousand Oaks, CA: Sage.

Denzin, N., & Lincoln, Y. (Eds.). (1994). *Handbook of qualitative research.* Thousand Oaks, CA: Sage.

Glesne, C., & Peshkin, A. (1992). *Becoming qualitative researchers.* White Plains, NY: Longman.

Goffman, E. (1963). *Stigma: Notes on the management of spoiled identity.* Englewood Cliffs, NJ: Prentice-Hall.

Kielhofner, G. (1997). *Conceptual foundations of occupational therapy* (2nd ed.). Philadelphia: F. A. Davis Company.

Lincoln, Y., & Guba, E. (1985). *Naturalistic inquiry.* Newbury Park, CA: Sage.

Maxwell, J. (1996). *Qualitative research design: An interactive approach.* Thousand Oaks, CA: Sage.

Morgan, G., & Smircich, L. (1980). The case for qualitative research. *Academy of Management Review* 5(4), 491–500.

Patton, M. (1990). *Qualitative evaluation and research methods* (2nd ed.). Newbury Park, CA: Sage.

Rawlings, M. (1942). *Cross creek.* New York: Charles Scribner.

Schwandt, T. (1989). Solutions to the paradigm conflict: Coping with uncertainty. *Journal of Contemporary Ethnography* 17, 379–407.

Society for the Study of Social Interaction. (1990). NASA interested in qualitative inquiry. *SSSI Notes* 17(3) 17.

Spradley, J. (1979). *The ethnographic interview.* Fort Worth, TX: Harcourt Brace Jovanovich College Publishers.

Yerxa, E. (1980). Occupational therapy's role in creating a future climate of caring. *The American Journal of Occupational Therapy* 34, 529–534.

Yerxa, E. (1991). Seeking a relevant, ethical, and realistic way of knowing for occupational therapy. *The American Journal of Occupational Therapy* 45(3) 199–204.

PART

Strategies of Design and Inquiry

There are many types of research designs and data collection methods available to the qualitative researcher. The selection depends on the research purpose and research question. Often both design and data collection strategies are altered, as the research process unfolds and the researcher discovers new avenues of inquiry to pursue.

In this part of the text, the authors provide a description of some of the most common qualitative methods (interviewing, participant observation, and focus groups) and an increasingly common research design strategy (participant action research). In providing an overview of these methods and design, the authors illustrate their descriptions with anecdotes and examples from their own research studies. These chapters are intended to be introductory, and the reader who wishes to gain further detail and diverse perspectives on the methods is encouraged to consult other texts, some of which are listed in An Annotated Bibliography of Selected Further Reading contained in this book.

CHAPTER

2

Participant Action Research

Deborah Corring, M.Sc., OT(C)

> *Not everything that counts can be counted. Not everything that can be counted, counts.*
>
> —Albert Einstein

Time magazine recognized the author of this quote as the person of the century. Most everyone would describe him as intellectually gifted and a man of "hard science." For this man of "hard science" to recognize that "not everything that counts can be counted" gives me even greater confidence in suggesting that qualitative research has an important role to play in exploring those things that "cannot be counted, but count."

This chapter explores participant action research principles, the rationale for their use, examples of their use in health care, a description of personal experience with them, their fit and relevance to occupational therapy, philosophy, and values and the challenges of this approach. In addition, a discussion of the benefits and limitations of using this approach together with accompanying examples is provided.

Participant Action Research: What Is It?

"Science is not achieved by distancing oneself from the world; as generations of scientists know, the greatest conceptual and methodological challenges come from engagement with the world" (Whyte, 1991). In a very general sense, the purpose of naturalistic inquiry or qualitative research is to observe, understand, and come to know diverse phenomena so that one may describe, explain, and generate theory (DePoy & Gitlin, 1994, p. 135). "Coming to know" is a pretty tall order when one chooses to explore an area that is largely unexplored. For example, an exploration of the definition of client-centred care lacked any reported studies that examined a client definition of client-centred care until 1998, when Rebeiro and Allen published their article and then in 1999, when Corring and Cook reported their findings. Prior to those two studies, much had been written about client-centred care by professionals, but the absence of the client perspective on the subject was glaring by its omission (Corring, 1996).

Marshall and Rossman (1989) note the need to use qualitative techniques in the initial phase of an investigation that is largely exploratory. One style of qualitative inquiry is endogenous research. Endogenous research represents the most open-ended, nonstructured, approach to research. In this approach, researchers need to be "insiders." Endogenous research has also been referred to as "action research" and more recently as "participatory action research" or PAR (DePoy & Gitlin, 1994).

Participatory action research (PAR) is a powerful design strategy that can advise both science and practice. PAR is client-centred and focuses on practical problems of importance to its constituents (Whyte, 1991). This approach to inquiry and evaluation research should be welcomed by the profession of occupational therapy. As many know, Canadian occupational therapists have been guided by a client-centred approach to practice since 1983 (CAOT, 1983). Very recently, a position statement on evidence-based occupational therapy called for the integration of client information, critical review of relevant research, expert consensus, and past experience as a means of promoting evidence-based practice in occupational therapy (CAOT et al., 1999).

In participatory action research, people whose experience is being studied participate actively with the professional researcher throughout the research process from initial design to the final presentation of results and discussion of their action implications (Whyte, 1991, p. 20). As Rogers and Palmer-Erbs (1994) suggest, by involving individuals who have the most to gain from a research study, more relevant questions will be asked, and more relevant and acceptable intervention strategies will be developed. PAR is a result of pressure to make research more useful to the work of clinicians, directly benefit the participants, and involve them in guiding the research project (Stuart, 1998). Obviously this approach is very different from the traditional ways in which research studies usually have been conducted. There are some fundamental principles to which one must pay attention and some shifts in approach and attitudes that are critical. There are ethical concerns that also must be addressed.

Principles

As noted previously, PAR places a heavy emphasis on participation by those whose lives are being studied. Consequently, PAR means that the researcher must be willing to give up traditional unilateral control over the research process (Whyte, 1991). Mere involvement is not the same as participation says McTaggart (1991). According to McTaggart, to participate means to "share" or "take part" whereas involvement means to "include," "entangle," or "implicate"; involvement is not authentic participation (McTaggart, 1991; Rogers & Palmer-Erbs, 1994).

As Rogers and Palmer-Erbs (1994, p. 5) note, the general differences between PAR and traditional research are defined by the following factors:

- An emphasis on learning from and learning about subjects.
- Valuing subjective experiences of subjects.
- Researcher acting as a consultant not a professional.
- Research requiring input from insiders rather than being conducted by outsiders.
- Subjects are both subjects and researchers.
- Subjects are active and involved in all parts of research process rather than passive subjects only.

- PAR lends itself to qualitative studies and to studies of the disability experience rather than the traditional paradigm that lends itself to controlled, experimental research.
- Subjects act as change agents, converting results into new policy and programs.
- The research agenda is influenced directly by those under study rather than by professional and sociopolitical forces.

For example, the authors of the *Homeless Outreach Project for Employment* (H.O.P.E.), a four-month pilot study (Camerdese & Youngman, 1996), used participant action research strategies to examine whether homeless men and women in the study viewed themselves as educable and employable, what their educational and vocational histories and aspirations were, what motivated them to return to school or work, and what services and supports would best facilitate rehabilitation. The H.O.P.E. study assumed that "people who experience mental illness and/or homelessness possess an experiential authority and are thereby uniquely equipped to serve both as *interpretive listeners* to the experiences of others and as *spokespersons* for optimal service development" (Camerdese & Youngman, 1996, p. 46). This study is a fine example of the principles of PAR in action.

Giving up traditional control/authority or achieving a balance of authority that is more aligned to a participant/informant configuration (Mishler, 1986) is difficult. Researchers using PAR strategies need to negotiate, empower, and enter into dialogue with participants (Lindsey & Stajduhur, 1998). PAR enables marginalized groups to have a voice (Lindsey & Stajduhur, 1998). This approach fits well with a profession such as occupational therapy that seeks to empower clients, give them a voice, and understand their lived experience of illness and disability.

The Origin and Development of PAR

PAR first emerged in the 1940s in work done by Kurt Lewins around group dynamics and human relations (Stuart, 1998). PAR has been used in psychology, education, industrial and agricultural research, and more recently in health services research.

Whyte (1991) suggests that PAR evolved from three streams of intellectual development and action: social research methodology, participation in decision making by low-ranking people in organizations and communities, and sociotechnical systems thinking regarding organizational behavior (p. 7). A growing number of social scientists, he argues, have been emphasizing the principle that "good science must eventually lead to improved practice" (p. 8), and they have consequently supported strategies such as PAR in order to link research and action, and thus the advancement of science and the improvement of human welfare (p. 8).

Participation in decision making by low-ranking organizational members (Whyte, 1991) appeared in the 1970s in industry due to a growing management interest in worker participation in quality of work life programs and expanded into the field of agriculture in the late 1980s. Parallels in health care have occurred not only with the growth of consumerism (Chamberlin et al., 1989), but also with a changing health care paradigm. The health care system has shifted from a predominantly medical model focused on disease, impairment, and medical practitioners to a person-focused, recovery-focused model valuing the role of rehabilitation as well as rehabilitation professionals (Shackleton & Gage, 1995).

Whyte's (1991) third stream of intellectual development, the sociotechnical systems framework, first appeared in the literature in the 1950s in articles examining the "social systems of factories" (p. 11). The framework was based on the idea that in order to understand work behavior, researchers must look at the integration of social and technological factors. In order to look at the integration of factors, Whyte argues, one must go into the field to learn from those who are using the technology. To draw another parallel to health care, Whyte would agree that in order to understand "what works" for clients, therapists must ask their clients, the users of the technology (CAOT et al., 1999).

Other authors (Rogers & Palmer-Erbs, 1994) also describe the use of PAR in education and the solving of social problems. Its principles of assisting individuals to define the problem(s), analyze the problem(s), and formulate a plan of action to address the problem(s), have been credited with promoting mobilization and development at a local level that not only led to greater understanding of the issues, but enabled participants to use the findings to improve their circumstances.

Ethical Concerns

Stuart (1998) suggests that there are four basic principles for considering ethical issues when using PAR. These four principles are respect for persons, nonmaleficence, beneficence, and justice.

Respect for persons in PAR, Stuart argues, includes recognizing an individual's right to autonomous decision making, ensuring a process that includes participants in negotiating research procedures, and ensuring that participants are fully aware of potential implications of the research.

Nonmaleficence or "doing no harm" requires that the researcher assess the degree of risk to the participants simply by their being part of the project. Stuart argues that PAR's potential for creating positive change for participants often mitigates any potential negative effects.

Beneficence or duty to advance the good of others is the hallmark of the PAR approach, since PAR requires that the primary benefits of the research are for the participants (Stuart, 1998). Finally, Stuart argues that the principle of justice is also a natural fit with the PAR approach, since it focuses on promoting social action for marginalized groups.

The Use of PAR in Health Care: Some Examples

A search of two major health care databases, CINAHL (1982–February 1999) and Clin Psych (1989–March 1999), illustrated the increasing use of PAR in health care in a variety of ways.

PAR is being heralded as a new paradigm for research and program evaluation. It is being used to evaluate self-help programs (Chamberlin, Rogers, & Ellison, 1996; Chesler, 1991), for service evaluation by clients (Corring, 1998a), and for gaining a better understanding of the "revolving door phenomenon" in psychiatric hospitals (Davidson, Stayner, Lambert, Smith, & Sledge, 1997). PAR is being used to better understand the concepts of empowerment (Corrigan & Garman, 1997) and issues surrounding community integration for individuals with disabilities (Gallagher & Scott, 1997; Robinson & Miller, 1996). It is being used to examine clinical practices (Street & Robinson, 1995), facilitate changes in service delivery (Corring, 1996, 1998a), create and change health care policy (Clarke & Maas, 1998; Powell & Cameron, 1991), and capture the complexity and meaning of the illness experience from the individuals who experience the everyday realities of the illness (Davidson et al., 1997). PAR is also being used to add a client definition to client-centred care (Corring, 1996; Rebeiro & Allen, 1998), a client perspective to quality of life issues (Corring, 1998a; Lindsey & Stajduhur, 1998), and a client perspective on the benefits of collaborative research (Woodside, Cikalo, & Pawlick, 1995). Two of the previously noted references are described as follows to illustrate the use of PAR.

Davidson et al. (1997) used phenomenological and participatory action research methods in an attempt to understand the problem of recurrent inpatient admissions for individuals diagnosed with serious mental illness, an issue more commonly referred to as the "revolving door phenomenon." These researchers interviewed 12 recidivist patients following their most recent discharge from inpatient care and explored with them their experiences of rehospitalization, the circumstances leading to hospitalization, the functions it served in their lives, their experiences of the new relapse prevention interventions provided to them in the hospital, factors affecting their lack of participation in these interventions following discharge, and their thoughts on what they would find more useful in staying out of the hospital in the future. Analysis of the data was accomplished by using established data analysis procedures and also including the participants themselves in helping researchers to understand and interpret their responses. Once an initial draft of major themes was identified, a group of the original participants was convened and asked for their feedback on the tentative understanding of their responses. They were asked to identify any areas of importance that had been missed and comment on how well the researchers had represented their experiences and concerns. The final stage of the PAR strategy involved working collaboratively with the participants to translate the implications of these findings into designing new interventions to prevent their future readmissions.

The researchers stated that the conventional, clinical view of rehospitalization "missed the mark" by assuming that readmissions were caused primarily by the deficits and dysfunctions associated with the disorder. Efforts to prevent hospitalization also "missed the mark" by focusing on those same features of the disorder for early intervention. An alternative approach was developed using the participants' feedback. Instead of emphasizing the professional's need to prevent relapse and readmission, efforts were directed to restoring a decent quality of life for clients in the community and, as a consequence, making the hospital a place that was not as necessary to seek respite, privacy, safety, and social supports. Social isolation, loneliness, feelings of hopelessness about their illness, and treatment not focused on recovery all needed to be addressed. Program and service changes were made with the full involvement of the participants, and significant gains were made. Readmission rates were reduced by almost 70 percent, and days spent in the hospital were reduced by more than 90 percent for the first 15 clients who participated in the project. The researchers concluded that "for any method to be useful in identifying factors in recovery, it first needs to be grounded in understanding of the experiences and role of the person with the disorder" (Davidson et al., 1997, p. 780).

In a second study, Lindsey and Stajduhur (1998) used a PAR approach to ascertain the desirability and feasibility of a supported living/respite care community home for people with HIV/AIDS (PWA). The research came about as a result of an expressed need by the HIV/AIDS community to consider such a facility due to caregiver burnout issues and the lack of options other than hospital admission if care at home was not feasible. A stakeholder analysis resulted in invitations to individuals associated with AIDS care and housing and related others to participate. Key stakeholders became research participants (members of the research team), and others were research respondents (providers of data/validators of results).

The research team determined that focus group meetings and open-ended individual interviews would be the most effective methods to collect data. The researchers conducted focus groups with associated professionals, and street workers conducted groups and interviews with individuals uncomfortable with the researchers. All groups and interviews were audiotaped and transcribed. Field notes were also kept. Data analysis involved breaking the data down into segments, coding them, and identifying themes. Feedback was sought to ensure accuracy of results. Results of the study indicated support for the idea of a home that was cost-effective, provided options for PWAs, and had a homelike environment. In addition, participants expressed a need for consistency of care at each level of the illness experience and identified potential barriers such as stigma, cost, "turf wars," "red tape," and "not in my backyard" attitudes.

Fit between PAR and the Clinician's Role in Practice

PAR, by definition, requires data collection to occur in the field and involve those under study. Dr. Opler (1994), Clinical Professor of Psychiatry at Columbia University, stresses the necessity of research occurring in clinical settings. He argues that research within clinical settings fosters a rich alliance and collaboration between researchers, clinicians, and consumers, increasing the chances of producing knowledge that is relevant and informed by the real phenomenon that clinicians, consumers, and family members struggle with daily (p. 31). Vera Hassner (1994) notes that most major breakthroughs in psychiatry were discovered unexpectedly through clinical observation. PAR is a natural fit for those interested in understanding and promoting client-centred care, empowerment, and self-help while continuing to engage in clinical practice.

Using PAR in Research— A Personal Experience

My involvement in formal research started in 1994 when I began a part-time master's program in occupational therapy. The decision to pursue a graduate degree after many years as a clinician and administrator was a difficult one. I worried about being overwhelmed by the demands of study and felt that I might be just a little too old to be a student again. But I was tired of not being able to converse with my colleagues involved in research in a meaningful way, and so I ventured forth.

Course work focused on practice and research issues in occupational therapy, qualitative and quantitative research strategies, and designs and statistics. I became intrigued by concepts I had never really taken the time to explore in-depth before graduate school. The complexities of clinical reasoning, the tacit knowledge that clinicians develop with experience, the critical questions and dilemmas facing the profession of occupational therapy, and the many facets of the illness experience for individuals living with disabilities all fascinated me. It became very difficult to decide what the focus of my required thesis research would be, until I realized that there appeared to be a major gap in our profession's knowledge and understanding of our adopted approach to practice, that of client-centred care. The perspective of the client was missing from the literature on the concept and its application to our practice (Corring, 1996). The omission was somewhat puzzling when partnership, client involvement, and client empowerment were thought to be fundamental elements of this approach to practice (Law, Baptiste, & Mills, 1995).

Once my focus had been decided, I began to explore which research strategy might best address the question. I took an immediate liking to qualitative research. Qualitative inquiry was the only choice, in my opinion, to use in trying to achieve an understanding of how clients might define client-centred care. The next question was what type of qualitative inquiry would be most suitable.

I had been working as an occupational therapist for 22 years prior to entering graduate school. For most of those years, I had worked in mental health in different capacities and for 12 of those 22 years I worked in a local provincial psychiatric hospital. I worried about how I could gather this kind of data without influencing the results: first, because of my own attitudes and values; second, how respondents might be influenced by my professional credentials; and finally by my current position as an administrator of mental health services. My reading eventually led me to articles describing participatory action research strategies. They appeared to provide the answers to my dilemma.

I was fortunate to be associated with two individuals who acted as facilitators for our hospital's patient council. They had both been consumers of mental health services themselves, had acquired postsecondary education in social sciences and journalism, and were both delighted with the prospect of joining me as coresearchers. The project immediately became richer because of their involvement. We discussed issues of professional power, consumerism, stigma, and health care service delivery in-depth. We explored various ways of accessing client opinion on the topic, and with their able assistance and direction, a research project design began to emerge. Two local consumer/ survivor agencies agreed to support the project by encouraging their members to participate, providing input into the questions to be asked, and providing physical space within their agency to meet with consumers.

Still, I worried about my influence on the process. My coresearchers agreed to facilitate the data collection from consumers by meeting with the consumers directly. At first, I believed that I should not be part of the data

gathering, but at the encouragement of my thesis advisor, I participated as a passive observer in the data collection process. It was good advice, and I know now that I would have missed a very important part of the process had I not been involved. The role of the observer allowed me to experience the PAR data collection process. The warmth, tears, friendship, support, laughter, and deep sense of caring of participants added in a very real way to my ability to understand and appropriately analyze the results. The experience added a depth to the understanding of the data that might not be achieved in quantitative data collection.

After the data collection was completed, audiotapes transcribed, and an initial analysis of themes drafted, I returned with my coresearchers to present the preliminary findings to the group of respondents. They were asked to comment on the themes, categories, and elements chosen and whether they adequately represented what they had said, as well as to suggest other wording that might be a more accurate description from their perspective. I participated more directly in the conversation with respondents than previously. Their level of comfort with my participation in this part of the process was reflected in the suggestions for changes they wanted made. Changes in wording and elements were discussed and incorporated, and I achieved a sense of having done a relatively comprehensive job of representing their views. In addition, respondents commented on how positive the experience of being involved in the project had been for them. They were pleased that they had been asked for input and had great hopes for how the final report might be used to make a difference for mental health clients. We discussed strategies for action that their consumer/ senior agencies could implement, as well as individuals/agencies with whom they would share the report on its completion. I promised to provide each agency with a copy of the completed document. Requests for copies and feedback regarding results have since been received from several institutions and agencies.

My next foray into participation action research began in the summer of 1998. I had secured my first contract for my newly formed consulting business, Client Perspectives. I was contacted by the planner of a District Health Council and asked to contact their local mental health consumer/survivor agency for details about the project. I met with the executive director of the agency. We agreed that I would use focus groups and participatory action strategies to explore satisfaction with local mental health services. We agreed that I would run two groups at their agency and one on the inpatient unit at the local hospital. The director agreed to contact the local hospital to gain their cooperation in setting up the inpatient focus group. We agreed on the date for the first focus group, and the executive director agreed to contact agency members for volunteers to participate. We discussed possible individuals who could act as a cofacilitator of the group(s). A self-identified mental health consumer would, hopefully, offset any negative influences I might bring as a mental health professional conducting the group.

I arrived for the first group prepared to meet with my cofacilitator to discuss her role in the focus group and hold the first group. Eight volunteers were eager and willing to participate. They all signed consent forms after being duly informed of the purpose of the group and how the data would be used. Two of the volunteers had been involved in my thesis research and spontaneously shared with the group that I was a person who they knew would listen and accurately reflect their perceptions. This show of support was very helpful in establishing a relaxed atmosphere conducive to good discussion.

Following the first focus group, I received a telephone call from the executive director.

She was upset and relayed the news that the local hospital was not receptive to the idea of an inpatient group and was, in fact, questioning the entire project. The executive director asked that I attend a meeting the following week at the District Health Council offices. In attendance would be representatives from the local hospital and a community mental health agency, representatives from the local Family Network, and the District Health Council planner.

The meeting began with a very definite agenda. The hospital and community agency were definitely not interested in evaluation of their services by the consumer group. They spoke of other recent evaluations of services that had left their staff feeling rather bruised and battered and did not think that it would be productive for anyone to pursue yet another evaluation. The representatives of the Family Network expressed anger over not being included in the design of the project, since their understanding was that it was to be a shared project among the families and the consumer/survivor group. The executive director of the consumer/survivor group was becoming increasingly anxious and clearly felt pressured by others present at the meeting. Further discussion finally led to a potential focus for the study. All present agreed to a change in focus from service evaluation to the identification of quality of life issues for local mental health consumers and family members of mental health consumers. Although there was agreement on the focus, there were questions remaining regarding the data collection strategies to be used to collect the data. Some individuals preferred to see a quantitative approach used (i.e., surveys), and most did not fully appreciate the qualitative strategies being suggested. All present agreed to have a second meeting where I would present them with a choice of a possible quantitative approach and a possible qualitative approach.

At the second meeting, I presented both options. I spoke of the benefits, limitations, and costs. I was able to convince the group that the qualitative approach was the method of choice, since it provided them with the maximal opportunity for shaping of the results in a form that would assist them in their objectives for further development of both consumer and family support services. It was agreed that three focus groups would be held with members of each group (family members and consumer/survivors) to collect data. In keeping with PAR principles, each group would be cofacilitated by a peer of the participants, and each group would assist in development of focus group questions and the analysis of the results.

After a somewhat rocky start, we had the go-ahead. Data was collected over the next six weeks. Volunteers were recruited through the local groups and advertisement of the project in a local newspaper. Careful analysis of the data took place with the participation of representatives of both groups, and the preliminary themes and categories were evaluated by group participants. On receiving copies of the completed reports, both groups agreed that the results would be helpful in their discussions with the Ministry regarding funding of new services.

Challenges of PAR

Ensuring Participation

As noted previously, involvement is not the same as participation (McTaggart, 1991). Participatory action research calls for a significant change in the roles of clients and professionals (Corrigan & Garman, 1997; Woodside, Cikalo, & Pawlick, 1995). Some clients will come with the prerequisite skills and knowledge, but many may not. The organizers of the H.O.P.E. project

(Camerdese & Youngmen, 1996) anticipated that training would be required in basic social and communication skills, research techniques and policies, professional standards for interpersonal behavior, hygiene, and confidential data management. They spent the first two weeks of the project providing this training.

In PAR, the researcher must not only be cautious about the use of power, but must also actively work to redistribute power and create both dialogue and equality in decision making (Stuart, 1998, p. 305).

Role of the Facilitator

The researcher's understanding of the role of the facilitator in the PAR process is critical. The facilitator guides the process; provides a flexible structure for discussion; uses ordinary language to promote trust, respect, and empathy in the group; and strives to offer the participants ways of understanding how they view themselves (Soltis-Jarrett, 1997). The researcher with a clinical background must guard against acting as if he or she is conducting a clinical service. Participants are not there for therapy but to share their perspectives and opinions on the stated topics. Support, redirection, and refocusing may be necessary, but solely for the purposes of reaching full understanding of their words, not to provide therapy.

Ensuring Action

Occupational therapists, clients, administrators, regulators, the public at large, and the professional and academic community must assume an active role in advocating change (CAOT et al., 1999). Health care reform in all sectors is demanding change. Consumers and practitioners advocating client-centred care must work together to achieve change that is responsive to consumer need. PAR is an ideal strategy to support such a process.

References

Camerdese, M. B., & Youngman, D. (1996). H.O.P.E.: Education, employment and people who are homeless and mentally ill. *Psychiatric Rehabilitation Journal, 19*(4), 45–56.

Canadian Association of Occupational Therapists and Health and Welfare Canada. (1983). *Guidelines for the client-centred practice of occupational therapy.* Ottawa, Canada: Department of National Health and Welfare.

CAOT, ACOTUP, ACOTRO, PAC. (1999). Joint position statement on evidence-based occupational therapy. *Canadian Journal of Occupational Therapy, 66*(5), 267–269.

Chamberlin, J., Rogers, J. A., & Sneed, C. S. (1989). Consumer, families and community support systems. *Psychosocial Rehabilitation Journal, 12,* 93–106.

Chamberlin, J., Rogers, S. E., & Ellison, M. L. (1996). Self-help programs: A description of their characteristics and their members. *Psychiatric Rehabilitation Journal, 19*(3), 33–42.

Chesler, M. A. (1991). Participatory action research with self-help groups: An alternative paradigm for inquiry and action. *American Journal of Community Psychology, 19*(5), 757–766.

Clarke, H. F., & Maas, H. (1998). Comox Valley Nursing Centre: From collaboration to empowerment. *Public Health Nursing, 15*(3), 216–224.

Corrigan, P. W., & Garman, A. N. (1997). Considerations for research on consumer empowerment and psychosocial interventions. *Psychiatric Services, 48*(3), 347–352.

Corring, D. J. (1996). *Client-centred care means I am a valued human being.* Unpublished master's thesis, The University of Western Ontario.

Corring, D. J. (1998a). *A report on quality of life issues.* London, ON: Client Perspectives.

Corring, D. J., & Cook, J. V. (1999). Client-centred care means I am a valued human being. *Canadian Journal of Occupational Therapy, 66*(2), 71–82.

Davidson, L., Stayner, D. A., Lambert, S., Smith, P., & Sledge, W. H. (1997) Phenomenological and participatory research on schizophrenia: Recovering the person in theory and practice. *Journal of Social Issues, 53*(4), 767–784.

DePoy, E., & Gitlin, L. N. (1994). *Introduction to research: Multiple strategies for health and human services.* St. Louis, MO: Mosby.

Gallagher, E. M., & Scott, V. J. (1997). The STEPS project: Participatory action research to reduce falls in public places among seniors and persons with disabilities. *Canadian Journal of Public Health, 88*(2), 129–133.

Hassner, V. (1994). What is ethical? What is not? Where do you draw the line? *The Journal of the California Alliance for the Mentally Ill, 5*(1), 4–5.

Law, M., Baptiste, S., & Mills, J. (1995). Client-centred practice: What does it mean and does it make a difference? *Canadian Journal of Occupational Therapy, 62,* 250–257.

Lindsey, E., & Stajduhur, K. (1998). From rhetoric to action: Establishing community participation in AIDS-related research. *Canadian Journal of Nursing Research, 30*(17), 137–152.

Marshall, C., & Rossman, G. (1989). *Designing qualitative research.* Thousand Oaks, CA: Sage.

McTaggart, R. (1991). Principles for participatory action research. *Adult Education Quarterly, 41*(3), 168–187.

Mishler, E. G. (1986). *Research interviewing: Context and narrative.* Cambridge, MA: Harvard University Press.

Opler, L. A. (1994). Conducting clinical psychiatric research in "non-research" settings. *The Journal of the Californian Alliance for the Mentally Ill, 5*(1), 30–31.

Powell, T. J., & Cameron, M. J. (1991). Self-help research and the public mental health system. *American Journal of Community Psychology, 19*(5), 797–805.

Rebeiro, K. L., & Allen, J. (1998). Voluntarism as occupation. *Canadian Journal of Occupational Therapy, 65,* 279–285.

Robinson, A., & Miller, M. (1996). Making information accessible: Developing plain English discharge instructions. *Journal of Advanced Nursing, 24*(3), 528–535.

Rogers, S. E., & Palmer-Erbs, V. (1994). Participatory action research: Implications for research and evaluation in psychiatric rehabilitation. *Psychosocial Rehabilitation Journal, 18*(2), 3–12.

Shackleton, T. L., & Gage, M. (1995). Strategic planning: Positioning occupational therapy to be proactive in the new health care paradigm. *Canadian Journal of Occupational Therapy, 62*(4), 188–196

Soltis-Jarrett, V. (1997). The facilitator in participatory action research: Les raisons d'etre. *Advances in Nursing Science, 20*(2), 45–54.

Street, A., & Robinson, A. (1995). Advanced clinical roles: Investigating dilemmas and changing practice through action research. *Journal of Clinical Nursing, 4*(6), 349–357.

Stuart, C. A. (1998). Care and concern: An ethical journey in participatory action research. *Canadian Journal of Counselling, 32*(4), 298–313.

Whyte, W. F. (Ed.). (1991). *Participatory action research.* Newbury Park, CA: Sage

Woodside, H., Cikalo, P., & Pawlick, J. (1995). Collaborative research: Perspectives on consumer-professional partnerships. *Canada's Mental Health, 43*(1), 2–5.

CHAPTER

In-depth Interviewing

Deborah Laliberte-Rudman, M.Sc., OT(C) and Sandra Moll, M. Sc., OT(C)

> *To understand other persons' constructions of reality we would do well to ask them (rather than assume we can know merely by observing their overt behaviour) and to ask them in such a way that they can tell us in their terms (rather than those imposed rigidly and a priori by ourselves) and in a depth which addresses the rich context that is the substance of their meanings (rather than through isolated segments squeezed into a few lines of paper).*
>
> —Jones, 1985, p. 46

The word *interviewing* covers a wide range of practices, from structured survey interviews composed of close-ended questions to unstructured interviews resembling conversations. Even within the qualitative research paradigm there are numerous types of interviews, such as life history interviews and ethnographic interviews. This chapter focuses on one general type of qualitative interview, specifically the in-depth interview. The in-depth interview can be broadly defined as a relatively unstructured interview that is utilized to capture informants' perspectives on topics or issues of relevance in their lives (Kaufman, 1994; Seidman, 1991). A key characteristic of the in-depth interview is that its purpose is not to test hypotheses or

obtain facts, but rather to learn about "what is important in the mind of informants: their meanings, perspectives, and definitions; how they view, categorize, and experience the world" (Taylor & Bogdan, 1984, p. 88). The philosophy underlying the in-depth interview is succinctly and effectively captured by Jones in the preceding quote. That is, we need to openly talk to people in their own terms to truly understand how they view and experience the world.

Given the nature of in-depth interviewing, this research strategy is particularly suitable to use when one is interested in how informants understand and construct meaning regarding experiences and events in their lives. As in-depth interviewing can be used to explore almost any issue that is related to subjective human experience, the range of topics that can be explored with in-depth interviewing is wide (Seidman, 1991). Of special relevance to occupational therapists is the use of in-depth interviewing to further our understanding of occupation. Within the occupational therapy literature, a growing awareness of the complexity of occupation and the need for research methods that address this complexity is evident (Canadian Association of Occupational Therapists, 1998; Polatajko, 1994; Yerxa et al., 1990). One element of this complexity is the individualized nature of occupation, that is, the meaning of any occupation and its contribution to quality of life varies from individual to individual (Christiansen, 1994; Yerxa, 1993). This individualized nature of occupation means that to advance our understanding of occupation and its contribution to health we need to examine individuals' perceptions and experiences of occupation. Qualitative in-depth interviews are ideal for exploring the "meanings people hold for their everyday activities" (Marshall & Rossman, 1989, p. 81), how people view their own behavior, and how people experience their environments and occupation (Jones, 1985; Seidman, 1991; Taylor & Bogdan, 1984). In the context of occupational therapy practice, the in-depth interview can be used to address a variety of questions relating to therapists' and clients' experiences and perceptions of the process and outcome of practice.

This chapter describes the nature of in-depth interviewing. In addition, steps to take and issues to consider when preparing for and conducting in-depth interviews are addressed. Throughout the chapter, examples from two studies (included in this book) conducted by the authors will be used as illustrations. One of these studies explored occupational therapists' beliefs about the therapeutic value of activity in mental health practice (Moll & Cook, 1997). The other study explored seniors' perspectives on the importance and role of occupation in their lives (Laliberte-Rudman, Cook, & Polatajko, 1997). Hereafter, each study will be identified by the participants—"occupational therapists" or "seniors"—rather than citing the reference each time an example is used.

The Nature of In-depth Interviewing

One useful way to understand the philosophy underlying and the nature of in-depth interviewing is to contrast the role of the interviewer in structured, quantitative interviews with that of the interviewer in in-depth, qualitative interviews. In the traditional quantitative approach, the interviewer can be compared to a detective, who objectively gathers facts about the interviewee. The detective asks focused, often close-ended questions to arrive at a final conclusion. A process of deductive reasoning is employed. In the quantitative approach, the interviewer tries to avoid contaminating the data by maintaining a very neutral, detached tone. The questions are typically predetermined and have a standardized format. In-depth interviewing, in contrast, can be compared to a journey of discovery for both participants. The interviewee, or informant, guides the process, sharing experiences and ideas with the interviewer. The interviewer may have a general guide of areas to explore but follows the lead of the informant, rather than using a predetermined set of questions. The process is collaborative and inductive, rather than deductive. The interviewer is *not* a detached, passive observer, but a traveling partner on the journey of exploration. It is recognized that the direction of the interview is shaped by the interaction between the two parties. The in-depth interview process has been described as an "unfolding dialogue" (Beer, 1997) and an "interchange of views" between two persons conversing about a theme of mutual interest (Kvale, 1996).

Another important distinction to make in understanding the nature of in-depth interviewing is to differentiate it from clinical or therapeutic interviewing. One fundamental difference, for example, concerns the relationship between the interviewer and interviewee. In a clinical encounter, the interviewer or clinician is in a position of power. The person being interviewed usually comes to the clinician for help, and the clinician is perceived as an expert with specialized knowledge and training. In qualitative interviewing, the power differential is reversed. The interviewee or informant is the expert who has valuable information to impart to the interviewer. It is the interviewer who approaches the potential informant for assistance in understanding a particular area of interest. The interviewee, who agrees to help, has specialized knowledge to impart and during the course of the interview enhances the interviewer's knowledge base about the area of interest.

Although the shift in role from clinician to researcher may sound fairly straightforward, it may not be as easy as it sounds. Shifting from an expert to learner role may be particularly difficult if you are interviewing individuals who are members of your clinical population. The following quotations from two occupational therapists who have taken on the role of in-depth interviewer attest to some of the difficulties that may be experienced (Segal, Landry, & Rebeiro, 1998). One of these therapists reported that she felt "not really having the right to be asking these questions, as these people were not in the position of asking for help." She also reported, "I was hesitant to give up my list of questions, and my control over the situation." The other therapist found that she "was ever cognizant of not being a therapist and when the individual cried or made self-depreciatory comments . . . I found it very hard to remain neutral." The interviewees, too, may find it difficult to shift

from a client or patient role to one of an "expert" informant. They may have expectations of you and respond to you as a clinician rather than a learner.

In addition to the change in roles, the content and process of the clinical versus in-depth interviews are different. In clinical interviews, the clinician, as the authority, typically guides the direction of the interview to gather information about the specific needs of the client. The therapist may direct the focus of the interview by thinking ahead to particular assessment issues or intervention strategies for the client. The information gathered from the clinical interview is then synthesized by the expert clinician and translated for a therapeutic purpose. In the qualitative research interview, the interviewer may come with some general questions or topic areas, but it is the expertise of the interviewee that guides the direction and flow of the interview. The focus is much broader. Although you start with exploring the unique perspective of the interviewee, the interview is actually a strategy to understand the collective experience of individuals in the population of interest. Rather than trying to obtain a person-specific understanding, the goal is to see how that person's perspective fits within the "collective" understanding of the issue or topic area. Some of the differences between clinical and qualitative in-depth interviews are explored further in the section on conducting interviews.

Although the underlying philosophy of in-depth interviewing is constant, there is some variability in how in-depth interviews are designed. There can, for example, be differences in the amount of formality and structure. Types of interviews range from informal conversational interviews to guided interviews, to semistructured approaches (Grbich, 1999; Morse & Field, 1995; Patton, 1990). Interviews may be focused narrowly on a specific topic or broadly on general areas (Rubinstein, 1988). A researcher may conduct a series of interviews with one informant or may conduct a series of interviews with a range of informants. Regardless of the specific format, the focus is on enabling informants to tell their stories and share their experiences with minimal interruption from the interviewer (Morse & Field, 1995).

Rationale for Selection of the Strategy of In-depth Interviewing

In-depth interviews can be a very effective research method. However, selection of this method should be consistent with the nature of the research question. In-depth interviews can be very useful if you want to gain a window into subjective human experience or develop insight into how individuals think about the world (Seidman, 1991; Taylor & Bogdan, 1984). They are not the best choice, however, if you want to obtain an accurate description of current or past events or if you want to predict future behavior. The reason for this limitation is that responses to interview questions are based on the informant's constructions of reality and, therefore, are not necessarily an account of accurate reality. There can be a big difference between what people say and what they actually do (Taylor & Bogdan, 1984). Taylor and Bogdan (1984) caution that "through interviewing, the skillful researcher can usually learn how informants view themselves and their world, sometimes obtain an accurate account of past events and current activities, and almost never predict exactly how an informant will act in a new situation" (p. 83).

Another drawback to interviewing is that it is based solely on verbal interaction. Interviewing begins with the assumption that the perspective of others is meaningful, knowable, and able to be made explicit (Patton, 1990). It is important to consider the ability of your informants to articulate their ideas and experiences. Impairments in memory, concentration, or attention and problems with digressive or tangential thinking, for example, may make it difficult to conduct in-depth interviews with potential informants. Other potential barriers include hearing problems, language barriers, and other communication impairments. In addition, some informants may be uncomfortable or unwilling to share all that the interviewer hopes to explore (Marshall & Rossman, 1989). Strategies for overcoming some of these barriers will be addressed later in this chapter, but communication issues should be an important consideration when selecting a research method.

Some authors believe that participant observation is the ideal method for getting a detailed understanding of an issue or topic, since observations are conducted within the context that events and experiences occur (Taylor & Bogdan, 1984). Observation, however, is not always possible or practical. One of the advantages of interviewing over other qualitative research methods is that it provides an opportunity to explore past events or hard-to-access settings that would be difficult to observe (Marshall & Rossman, 1989; Taylor & Bogdan, 1984). Interviewing can be less time-consuming than participant observation if you want to explore the perspectives of a number of individuals (Marshall & Rossman, 1989). One must account, however, for the number of planned interviews and time to transcribe audiotapes of interview sessions (Seidman, 1991).

It is important to note that in-depth interviewing can be combined with other research methods. In the study conducted with mental health occupational therapists, participant observation of therapist treatment sessions was combined with in-depth interviews with each therapist. Utilizing more than one data method is a strategy called triangulation, which can be used to enhance trustworthiness of the study data (Lincoln & Guba, 1985). Therapists' comments about the value of a particular treatment activity, for example, could be compared to the researcher's observations of the impact of the activity on the clients and, therefore, lend support to the credibility of the findings.

Preparing for In-depth Interviewing

Once a researcher has decided to use in-depth interviewing and made some general design decisions, such as whether to use this method in combination with other information-gathering methods, there are a number of issues to consider and decisions to be made in planning interviews. Important issues to consider include: whether to use an interview guide; question design; informant selection; recording and transcription method; pilot testing; and ongoing analysis. When preparing a research proposal, it is essential to address these issues and provide a rationale for decisions made in designing an in-depth interview study. The overall goal is that a researcher should be able to demonstrate that interviews were carried out in a way that allowed him or her to maximize the extent to which the information reflects informants' perspectives.

Constructing and Using Interview Guides

A central issue in designing in-depth interviews is the degree to which the researcher structures the interview. The issue of how much structure is permissible and helpful is not straightforward. As pointed out by Jones (1985), there really is no such thing as a totally unstructured interview, as researchers always have some presuppositions and ideas regarding the questions they want to ask. Within the context of interviewing, a researcher is always making choices, partially influenced by his or her own interests, experiences, and knowledge, about what questions to ask and what issues to explore further and, in this way, is imposing a degree of structure. The challenge is to find a balance between having enough structure to enable the collection of relevant information and enough flexibility to enable unexpected information to emerge. Whatever degree of structure is built into an in-depth interview, it is essential that the interview format is flexible enough to allow informants to express their perspectives on the issue or issues being discussed (Marshall & Rossman, 1989; Patton, 1990).

A number of authors suggest that an interview guide be utilized to establish a loose framework for in-depth interviews (Grbich, 1999; Kaufman, 1994; Marshall & Rossman, 1989; McCracken, 1988; Chenitz & Swanson, 1986; Taylor & Bogdan, 1984). The degree of detail included in the guide is dependent on the extent to which a researcher feels able to identify important issues in advance, whether on the basis of fieldwork, preliminary interviews, other direct experience, or a theoretical framework (Morse & Field, 1995; Patton, 1990; Taylor & Bogdan, 1984). For example, an interview guide may consist of a list of topics to be explored with each informant with no predetermination of order of topics and no prewording of questions. At the other end of the spectrum, the guide may consist of a list of topics along with corresponding open-ended questions and potential probes (Kaufman, 1994; Morse & Field, 1995; Patton, 1990; Chenitz & Swanson, 1986).

There are both advantages and disadvantages associated with utilizing an interview guide for in-depth interviews. The most commonly mentioned advantage is that having some structure with respect to the issues being discussed and the questions being asked facilitates comparison of data across interviews in studies involving interviews with a number of informants (Grbich, 1999; Marshall & Rossman, 1989; Patton, 1990). As well, an interview guide can help a researcher maintain the conceptual focus of his or her study. An interview guide can also provide granting agencies and ethical review boards with a sense of the types of issues that will be discussed with informants (Morse & Field, 1995; Taylor & Bogdan, 1984). With respect to disadvantages, the interviewer may have less flexibility to respond to individual differences in responses and situational changes (Patton, 1990). The more structured the interview becomes, the less opportunity there may be for unanticipated material to emerge (Bauman & Adair, 1992).

Sample interview guides from the study conducted with seniors are included in Appendices A and B (see end of chapter). These appendices include both the initial guide that was used to begin the study and the final guide that resulted after revisions throughout the course of the study. There were two central research objectives to be addressed through the guide: to explore seniors' perspectives regarding the meaning they attach to daily occupations and to explore seniors' viewpoints regarding the factors that influence well-being. Following suggestions from several authors (Kaufman, 1994; McCracken, 1988), the guide consisted of topic areas, possible open-ended questions, and a list of potential areas to probe. In constructing the initial interview guide (see Appendix A), the first step was to identify broad topic areas. Five topics areas were derived based on a literature review and clinical and personal experiences with seniors. Within each topic area, one to three open-ended questions were developed and possible areas to be probed were outlined. The number of questions per topic area essentially depended on a judgment regarding how to best cover all potential aspects of the topic.

When you are new to the process of designing an interview guide, there may be a temptation to make the guide too detailed and structured. In the authors' experience it can be difficult to trust the process of simply following the informant's lead. In the study involving occupational therapists, for example, the researcher identified a number of topic areas to explore, based on an initial review of the literature. Considerable time was spent developing questions that would explore each area in detail, and the initial interview guide had five different sections with up to six to seven questions in each section. Unfortunately, this amount of detail meant that the interviewer relied too heavily on the interview guide at the expense of listening to cues from the informants about what issues to explore. Several sections were subsequently removed to facilitate a more natural flow of information.

In order to combat the potential disadvantages associated with an interview guide, we followed several suggestions in the literature regarding how a guide should be used. First, we attempted to use the guide not as a script, but rather as a minimally directive framework that enabled both researchers and informants to identify key areas (Grbich, 1999). McCracken (1988) describes the interview guide as a "rough travel itinerary with which to negotiate the interview. It does not specify precisely what will happen at every stage of the journey, how long each lay-over will last or where the investigator will be at any given moment, but it does establish a clear sense of the direction of the journey and the ground it will eventually cover" (p. 37).

Second, we modified the interview guides over the course of our studies so that informant-initiated topics that emerged in earlier interviews were incorporated into later interviews. Such modification is essential to ensure that topics viewed as important by informants are explored in depth (Rowles & Reinharz, 1988; Strauss & Corbin, 1990). For example, in the study conducted with seniors, questions about images and beliefs regarding aging were incorporated when many of the early informants spontaneously asserted that they neither felt old nor perceived themselves to fit negative societal images of aging. Probes were added to various sections of the interview guide (see Appendix B) to facilitate exploration of issues related to societal images of older people and the potential restrictions this might impose on available occupations.

Third, we also modified our interview guides after pilot testing and throughout the course of our studies to ensure questions were worded in ways that would maximize the extent to which informants were able to respond according to their own frameworks and in their own terms. For example, in the study conducted with seniors, it was found during the pilot testing phase that questions 4a and 4b, which asked how satisfied people were with the amount and variety of things they did, were often answered either with a yes or no response or a brief response indicating one's degree of satisfaction. These questions were revised, as can be seen in the final interview guide (see Appendix B). The new questions 4a and 4b, which asked informants to create a satisfying day, led to more detailed answers, composed of long descriptions of activities and reasons why these activities were found to be satisfying or not satisfying.

Overall, when using an interview guide, it is the responsibility of the interviewer to ensure that the interview does not become a vehicle for his or her agenda, but rather provides a way to explore informants' perspectives and experiences. When an interview guide is used, it should serve as a reminder of topics to discuss, and the interviewer must avoid forcing informants to rigidly follow the interviewer's agenda (Seidman,

1991). The interviewer needs to respect how informants choose to structure their responses and should always be responsive to concerns or topics raised by informants, even if these do not fall within the interview guide (Marshall & Rossman, 1989; Chenitz & Swanson, 1986). The interviewer needs to be flexible within the context of the interview, adapting the wording and sequence of questions and probes to suit the informant and the ongoing conversation. The interviewer needs to establish a dialogue with informants, which means that his or her questions will often follow from informants' responses, rather than from what is written in the interview guide. At the same time, throughout the interview, the interviewer needs to check back to the interview guide to ensure key topic areas are being covered and, when necessary, to introduce new topics in ways that fit within the flow of the interview (Jones, 1985; Kaufman, 1994; Patton, 1990; Seidman, 1991). When trends are noticed in the way informants are responding to questions, changes can be made to the interview guide so that it is best suited to the way in which informants choose to talk about issues. For example, in the study conducted with occupational therapists, the interview guide was structured so that questions pertaining to general beliefs about practice were asked prior to questions about specific clinical sessions that had been observed. The order of these sections was reversed when it was discovered that therapists found it easier to reflect on their specific experiences prior to more general perceptions and beliefs.

A final issue to consider is when and how to collect descriptive information regarding your informants. To maximize the extent to which the transferability of your study's findings can be assessed, it is important to collect descriptive information regarding informants, such as their age, marital status, and any other information that may be relevant to the topic of your study (Lincoln & Guba, 1985). Often, questions related to descriptive characteristics are close-ended. In our experience, it is best to place such questions at the end of one's interview guide. In this way, the close-ended nature of the questions will not interfere with the work you have done to encourage informants to speak in detail and depth in response to your open-ended questions. Questions about descriptive characteristics can be asked verbally or informants can fill out a written questionnaire.

Question Design

Whether or not an interviewer utilizes an interview guide, it is important to think about the ways in which he or she intends to ask questions. When an interview guide is used, the researcher can design potential questions that may or may not be asked in the exact way they are written. Thinking about and designing potential questions will help the interviewer ensure that questions are phrased in an open and nondirective manner (McCracken, 1988). When designing questions, it is essential that each question should establish "the territory to be explored while allowing the participant to take any direction he or she wants. It does not presume an answer" (Seidman, 1991, p. 62).

There are numerous manuals about question design for qualitative interviews to which the reader can refer for detailed information. Such manuals may be helpful if you find yourself struggling with how to word and order questions. For example, Spradley (1979) identifies three main types of questions: descriptive, structural, and contrast. Patton (1990) identifies six types of questions: experience/behavior, opinion/values, feeling, knowledge, sensory, and background.

Whatever types of questions are asked, five characteristics are important for wording (Patton, 1990).

Questions Should Be Open-ended

A truly open-ended question allows an informant to respond in his or her own terms. Thus, leading questions, which influence the direction that a response will take, should be avoided (Patton, 1990; Seidman, 1991). For example, in the initial interview guide used in the study with seniors (see Appendix A), question 4a, which asked if a person was satisfied with the variety of things he or she did, was a leading question that required revision. This question assumed two things: that satisfaction was the salient dimension informants should discuss and that variety was essential in determining satisfaction. Thus, it is not surprising that this question resulted in very brief answers that were often ratings of satisfaction. As well, some informants clearly expressed that "variety" really was not as important to them as other dimensions of activity. The revised questions 4a and 4b were designed to be more open-ended (see Appendix B). Question 4a invited informants to describe activities that they found satisfying, rather than asking about how satisfied they were with their activities. Question 4b asked about good and bad days, rather than satisfying days, so informants had the freedom to talk about all relevant dimensions of their feelings and thoughts.

Questions Should Be Singular

As with questions in all situations, no more than one idea should be contained in any question. The inclusion of more than one idea in a question can lead to confusion and tension, as an informant will not really know what to answer and the interviewer will not really know how to interpret an informant's response (Grbich, 1999; Patton, 1990).

Questions Should Be Clear

The clarity of questions largely depends on utilizing terms that are appropriate and meaningful to informants. To some extent, the choice of words needs to occur during the context of the interview as the interviewer comes to be familiar with the language a specific informant uses. However, some broad decisions about choice of words can be made in advance (Chenitz & Swanson, 1986; Grbich, 1999). For example, in the study conducted with seniors, the author defined *occupation* as anything people do in their everyday lives. As the term *activity* is usually used to express this concept outside the occupational therapy profession, it was decided to ask seniors about their activities rather than their occupations.

Questions Should Be Neutral

Questions should be worded in ways that convey that any response is acceptable (Patton, 1990). For example, if an occupational therapist is asking questions about how informants feel about a therapy program, questions need to be worded to allow informants to express both positive and negative opinions of the program.

Some Questions Should Ask for Description

One general type of question that is important to include in in-depth interviews is the descriptive question (Bauman & Adair, 1992; Grbich, 1999; Taylor & Bogdan, 1984). A descriptive question is one that asks an informant to describe an experience or event with which he or she is intimately familiar or an area of knowledge he or she knows well. For example, in Appendix B, question 1a, which asks informants to describe the things they do during a typical day, is a descriptive question aimed at eliciting detailed information regarding informants' daily lives and activities. Descriptive questions, used in combination with probes to elicit further examples and obtain clarification, prompt informants to provide detailed, rich descriptions of their experiences and perspectives. It is often recommended that an in-depth interview begin with a descriptive question in order to set the tone of the interview and provide informants with a sense of the type of responses an interviewer hopes to obtain. In some cases, especially with very verbal informants, an interviewer may only need to ask descriptive questions, along with probes, to collect the information required (McCracken, 1988; Morse & Field, 1995; Patton, 1990).

Informant Selection

Both issues of sampling and informant ability need to be considered when preparing an in-depth study. As with other qualitative research methods, a degree of flexibility needs to be built into the research design. The researcher needs to start out with a general idea of what kinds of people to interview and how to find them, but needs to remain willing to change his or her plan after the initial interviews. For instance, as a result of initial interviews, a researcher may discover that he or she neglected consideration of a whole class or category of informants in his or her initial research design (Taylor & Bogdan, 1984). For example, in conducting a program evaluation, one may have decided to interview clients and formal care providers, but may discover that it is important to also interview clients' family members.

Theoretical, or purposive, sampling is often recommended as the strategy of choice for qualitative interviewing studies (Lincoln

& Guba, 1985; Taylor & Bogdan, 1984). When using theoretical sampling, the researcher selects each informant according to his or her potential to aid the researcher in developing insights into the area being explored. After interviews are completed with several informants, the researcher consciously varies the type of informants interviewed in order to cover the full range of perspectives held by the group of people to which informants belong. The goal is to obtain a range of perspectives. For example, when interviewing seniors, an attempt was made to interview males and females; people who were widowed, divorced, single, and married; and people of varying economic and educational status. Ideally, interviews continue until the researcher believes that no new insights are emerging, that is, when theoretical saturation is achieved (Lincoln & Guba, 1985; Taylor & Bogdan, 1984). Deciding when theoretical saturation is achieved can be difficult. Sometimes, practical factors, such as time and the availability of informants, may make further interviews difficult, if not impossible. In our experience, as an interviewer, especially if you are conducting analysis as the interviews are occurring, there does come a point when you begin to sense that major issues are being repeated by new informants and very few new ideas are emerging.

Recording and Transcription Method

Interviews can be either manually or mechanically recorded (on audiotape or videotape). One of the advantages of mechanically recording interviews is that it is likely to be a more accurate method of data recording than handwritten notes. Considering that informants' words are the essential raw data for analysis and report writing, the accuracy with which informants' words are captured is an important consideration. At the same time, it

is always essential to check the accuracy of transcripts of recorded interviews rather than assuming a typist is able to understand and reproduce all that is said on the audiotape. Moreover, the use of a recording device permits the interviewer to be more attentive to the informant. It would be extremely challenging for an interviewer to both write down an informant's words and respond to an informant's comments and cues.

Researchers often hesitate to tape-record or videotape an interview believing that the existence of the recording device will interfere with the informant's ability to be open and honest. However, in our experience and in the experience of many other researchers (Jones, 1985; Patton, 1990), the existence of a recording device is quickly forgotten by both interviewer and informant. This is especially true if steps are taken to minimize the recorder's presence, such as placing the recorder out of an informant's direct line of sight.

One of the disadvantages of choosing to mechanically record interviews is that it will mean that a study will cost more to conduct. In addition to the costs associated with obtaining the recording equipment and tapes, there is the cost associated with having the recorded material transcribed. On average, it takes approximately four hours to transcribe one hour of audiotape (Patton, 1990). In those cases where it is not possible to mechanically record an interview, perhaps because of an informant's preference or the environment in which the interview is being conducted, it is essential that the interviewer take comprehensive notes both during the interview and immediately after the interview (Patton, 1990).

In those cases where interviews are recorded, a verbatim transcript should be created, as this will facilitate the process of data analysis. One issue to consider is who should do the transcription. Chenitz & Swanson (1986) suggests that transcripts should be completed by the interviewer, as shortly as possible after each interview, both to maximize accuracy of the transcripts and to begin the data analysis process. On the other hand, McCracken (1988) proposes that transcripts should be produced by a professional typist because interviewers may find the process frustrating and that overfamiliarity with the data may interfere with analysis.

The authors of this chapter differed in their decision regarding transcription. In the study dealing with seniors, the researcher was both the interviewer and the transcriber. When transcribing, this researcher began the process of data analysis by writing memos on index cards regarding possible units of meaning in the interviews. In addition, while transcribing, the researcher wrote memos regarding changes to make to future interview questions and about her performance in the interviews. It was found that transcribing the data did increase familiarity with the data, but that this familiarity assisted with data analysis. Thus, when an issue or area of meaning arose in an interview being transcribed, the researcher could often remember if and when that issue had arisen in previous interviews. At the same time, transcribing was a very time-consuming process, especially in the beginning. The process became less time consuming with experience and also with the rental of a transcription machine. The researcher who conducted the study with occupational therapists hired a transcriber, funding the expense through a research grant. This researcher obtained a familiarity with the data through reading the transcripts and making notes regarding initial observations and nuances of meaning. The quality of the transcriber's work was carefully monitored. Importantly, due to the confidential and often intimate nature of qualitative data, the researcher had the transcriber sign a consent form and agree to maintain confidentiality.

Whether transcription is done by the interviewer or by another person, several practical decisions should be made prior to the beginning of transcription to ensure consistency across transcripts and set up transcripts in a way that will facilitate data analysis. For example, there should be a system of notation set up to capture aspects of interviews, such as laughter or periods of silence, that are not words. Such notes will help the analyst understand the context in which words were spoken. There should also be a system of notation to capture when there are instances where the typist cannot understand what is being said and is, therefore, unable to transcribe a passage. To facilitate data analysis, which often involves writing notes on the actual transcripts, a large margin should be left on one side of the text, and the script should be at least double-spaced. As well, the researcher may want to create a face sheet to attach to each transcript that provides a description of the context in which the interview occurred, notes regarding conversations that occurred while the tape recorder was not on, and any other significant events or issues that arose during an interview (Patton, 1990). In cases where one is using computer software to assist in data analysis, steps should be taken to ensure transcripts are formatted so that they are compatible with the analysis software.

Pilot Testing

While a researcher may carefully prepare for a study, it is difficult to fully predict how informants will respond to one's topic and questions and how one will perform as a qualitative interviewer. Thus, it is essential to conduct pilot testing with persons who are similar to the intended study informants in order to assess the quality of the interviews. In addition, pilot testing helps with practical issues. It can help to gauge the amount of time interviews are likely to take, and it enables the interviewer to become increasingly comfortable with conducting qualitative interviews. During pilot testing, one begins a process of assessing interview quality and conducting data analysis that will continue throughout one's study.

With respect to the quality of interviews, pilot testing can be used to assess the relevance of questions, check if questions move informants to talk from their own perspectives, and examine whether the terms being used by the interviewer fit with the language used by informants. In the study conducted with seniors, three pilot test interviews were completed. As a result of these interviews, changes were made to all five sections of the interview guide. For example, it was found that the initial question 1a (see Appendix A), which asked informants to describe what they did during a typical day, could be somewhat overwhelming. Pilot test informants struggled with how to begin and organize their answers. The revised question 1a (see Appendix B) broke the day down into three time segments, which were asked about separately. This reframing of the question helped informants by providing an organizational framework for their responses.

Assessment of the quality of interviews also involves examining the interviewer. As occupational therapists and students, many of us have been through a process of reflection on our performance, as well as analysis by others, when we learned to conduct clinical interviews. A similar process of reflection and perhaps analysis by others such as a research advisor or a coinvestigator should occur as one is developing qualitative interviewing skills. While listening to audiotapes and reading transcriptions, an interviewer can consider several aspects of his or her performance such as: the extent to which his or her questions flow from what an informant has said; the degree to which he or she is unintentionally providing cues to informants regarding what he or she wants to hear; whether he or she is allowing times of silence during which informants can reflect on a question; and the extent to which questions are asked in an open-ended manner (Morse & Field, 1995; Patton, 1990). For example, when one of the researchers examined her pilot test interviews, she discovered that she tended to finish informants' sentences when they struggled with finding the right words and interjected too frequently with words like "right," which influenced the direction of informants' responses. Both of these behaviors were carefully monitored by the researcher over the course of the study to try to ensure that she was not imposing her perspective onto informants.

Overall, in the ideal transcript, the comments of the interviewer should make up a much smaller amount of text than those of the informant. One clear sign that an interviewer is being too leading and is likely imposing his or her own perspective is that the interviewer is talking more than the informant. The majority of the text should consist of an informant's descriptions and explanations, indicating the informant has the freedom to share his or her perspective (Morse & Field, 1995; Patton, 1990; Seidman, 1991).

Ongoing Analysis

In qualitative studies, the processes of data collection and data analysis should occur simultaneously to ensure that viewpoints of informants are thoroughly explored (Marshall & Rossman, 1989). Ongoing analysis throughout a study, beginning in the pilot testing phase, allows for emerging insights arising from the data to be fed back into the interview questions and research goals. It is likely that beginning analysis with the first interview conducted will allow interviews to become richer and fuller as the study progresses (Chenitz & Swanson, 1986; Kaufman, 1994).

Conducting Interviews

The process of conducting in-depth interviews involves establishing a conversational partnership that fosters an open interchange of information. The nature of the interchange is significantly influenced by the relationship that develops between the interviewer and informant. The interviewer should be sensitive to the stages of development of the relationship and match the intensity and emotional and intellectual challenge of the questions to the depth of the relationship that has developed (Rubin & Rubin, 1995).

Starting the Interview

The early stages of the interview are critical in establishing rapport with the informant and establishing an atmosphere of acceptance and trust. Werner and Schoepfle (1987) describe the first stage of the interview as one of apprehension. There is typically a degree of uncertainty. Informants do not know what to expect, are not sure how the interviewer will evaluate responses, and may be afraid that they will not meet the interviewer's expectations. The informants' responses to the interviewer will affect how they respond to questions and their decisions as to what aspects of their identities and lives to present (Kaufman, 1994). They may strive to please the interviewer rather than present their own beliefs or may try to present a front due to fears that they may be judged by others. Since the quality of the interview depends on full, honest, and thoughtful answers, it is

critical to spend time establishing a relationship of trust and rapport with each informant.

Responses to the interviewer may be affected by the informants' perception of their role and social status. Rubin and Rubin (1995) suggest that part of negotiating a relationship with the informant involves working together to define a mutually acceptable research role. Informants may respond differently, for example, if they perceive the researcher to be of higher social status or in an authority position. Some informants are flattered by being interviewed by a well-known person with established credentials, but others may be intimidated by being questioned by someone who has more education or experience (Rubin & Rubin, 1995). In the study of occupational therapists, some of the informants perceived the researcher to be an "expert" and felt intimidated by having the researcher observe their sessions and ask them about their beliefs. It was important to be sensitive to this issue and try to address these concerns early in the process. Presenting oneself as a student or novice can be an advantage, since it indicates that the informant is the expert who has some knowledge to impart. McCracken (1988) reports that it is better to appear "slightly dim and too agreeable," rather than show any sign of a critical or sardonic attitude.

In addition, differences between the interviewer and informant in terms of sex, age, ethnicity, and social status will have an impact on the informant's response to the interviewer and the type of information that is shared. There are differing opinions, however, as to whether these differences can have a positive or negative impact on the interview process. It has been noted that informants may initially be wary of individuals who are different from themselves and that it may take time to build trust and rapport (Grbich, 1999; Seidman, 1991). It can be important to have at least a basic familiarity with the cultural background of the informants so that relevant language can be used and pertinent questions asked (Grbich, 1999; Holstein & Gubrium, 1995). On the other hand, if the interviewer and informant are quite similar, assumptions may be made about areas of shared knowledge that would limit the extent of the information shared. If informants, for example, feel that the interviewer knows quite a bit about their experiences, they are less likely to provide detailed explanations and examples than if they feel that the interviewer knows very little (Rubin & Rubin, 1995). The interviewer may frame questions differently if there are a lot of similarities between himself or herself and the informant. The interviewer, for example, may overlook important aspects of informants' experiences or take information for granted and not seek out the depth and detail required from the informants (Chenitz & Swanson, 1986). Regardless of whether the differences are considered positive or negative, the interviewer should make note of these differences and the potential impact that they might have on the manner in which the questions are asked and responses are framed. If the interviewer is sensitive to these issues, he or she can modify the approach or use the differences to his or her advantage in the interview process. In the study of occupational therapists, the researcher was similar to the informants in terms of her clinical area of practice. Considering these similarities, the interviewer made an extra effort to try to explore the perspective of informants, to get the informants to define terms and describe their experiences. In the study with seniors, the researcher was much younger than her informants. Indeed, informants, on first meeting the researcher, often noted how young she appeared. This difference in age enabled the researcher to take on the role of student, as someone who was there to learn about life, and many of the informants eagerly took on

the role of teacher, willing to share both their positive and negative life experiences.

When starting the interview, it is recommended that you begin by conversing about general matters to establish a relaxed, conversational atmosphere (Chenitz & Swanson, 1986; McCracken, 1988; Taylor & Bogdan, 1984). Introductions and social "chatting" can help to set the informant at ease. Through casual conversation, you can also build connections and, therefore, seem less like a stranger. You may, for example, discover that you attended the same school, are interested in the same television programs, or share an interest in the topic of the interview. Rubin and Rubin (1995) suggest that since you are asking for a lot of openness from the informants, you are more likely to achieve this by being open and personal yourself. Balance is important, however, so that the interviewer shares enough to be alive and responsive to the informant, but not so much that the focus is taken away from the informant's words and experiences (Seidman, 1991). It may be better to err on the side of formality rather than familiarity at the start of the interview, recognizing that rapport needs to develop over time.

Interviewers should present themselves as courteous, respectful, friendly, supportive, and genuinely interested (Chenitz & Swanson, 1986; Jones, 1985; Seidman, 1991). McCracken (1988) states that in the opening minutes of the interview, the interviewer should portray an image as a person who is "benign, accepting and curious, but not inquisitive," and that he or she should be prepared and eager to listen to virtually any story with interest. Nonverbal communication can be just as important as verbal communication. Eye contact, facial expression, body posture, and tone of voice, for example, should be congruent with your expression of warmth, interest, and acceptance (Jones, 1985). The way you dress can also be important in creating a positive impression. It is suggested that your attire should be appropriate to the interview setting and convey respect to the informants.

At the outset of the interview, it is also important to provide an overview of what the study is about, what participants can expect from the interview process, and why their contributions are important (Kaufman, 1994). This information is important in relieving any anxiety that informants may have about not knowing what to expect and doubts about the value of what they have to say. Informants should be encouraged to answer questions freely, with reassurance that there are no right or wrong answers (Rubin & Rubin, 1995). They should also be assured of the confidentiality of their responses. If you are taping the interview or taking notes, it is important to discuss this with informants in advance. Most informants appreciate knowing that their words in spoken, written, and recorded form are considered to be confidential by the researcher and appreciate knowing how the data will be used once it is collected (Kaufman, 1994). Establishing procedures for informed consent and confidentiality will be discussed further in the section on ethical issues but is identified here as a crucial foundation for establishing a relationship of trust with informants.

In addition to factors related to the interviewer, there are a number of environmental factors that need to be considered when setting up interviews. Interviews may be conducted in a variety of places, including the researcher's office, a clinical setting, public places such as parks, or in the informant's home. Morse and Field (1995) suggest that the informant should choose the setting as long as it is private with little opportunity for interruption. If the informant is comfortable with the surroundings, this can facilitate a relaxed atmosphere and open sharing of information. The issue of privacy is very important, since interruptions can significantly disrupt the interchange of information. It is also important to schedule enough time to conduct the interview. If either participant feels rushed, this could have a detrimental effect on the quality of information gathered. At least one to two hours should be scheduled for each interview (Chenitz & Swanson, 1986; Taylor & Bogdan, 1984). Try not to schedule more than one or two interviews per week, since the intensity of listening involved in interviewing can be exhausting. Time for reflection is also needed between interviews, as well as time for transcribing and analysis.

Exploring Informants' Perspectives

After overcoming the initial period of uncertainty in the interview and initiating the process of rapport building, the next stage in the process has been identified as one of exploration (Werner & Schoepfle, 1987). In this stage, both parties try to discover what the other person is like and what he or she wants from the interview. It is a time of listening, observing, and testing. The role of the interviewer in conducting the interview has been described in different ways. Holstein and Gubrium (1995) talk about the "active interviewer," whose job it is to set general parameters for responses and facilitate responses that are relevant to the interviewer's area of interest. Rubin and Rubin (1995) describe the interviewer and informants as "conversational partners" who share the task of maintaining the flow of dialogue, creating a frame in which discussion takes place, and identifying issues to explore. In general, however, the interviewer should follow the informant's lead. It is important to let informants talk, to be patient, and to find out what they feel is relevant to share. As mentioned previously, a good interview is characterized by long detailed answers from informants with little or no interruption by the interviewer (Morse & Field, 1995; Werner & Schoepfle, 1987).

The overall goal of the interview is to get the informant talking in as much detailed description as possible. A range of responses from informants, however, is possible (Rubin & Rubin, 1995). Some informants may be eager to share ideas and do so very easily. Others may be more restrained and formal. Some may need prodding to elaborate, whereas others will not stop talking. Some informants may be very well informed, whereas others may know very little, and informants may vary considerably in their ability to reflect. The ideal informant in a qualitative in-depth interview is one who can find his or her place when off track, clarify misunderstandings, reflect on what he or she means, articulate feelings and thoughts, and interpret the verbal and nonverbal cues provided by an interviewer (Beer, 1997; Rowles & Reinharz, 1988; Taylor & Bogdan, 1984). Since many people do not meet the criteria of an ideal informant, modifications or adaptations must be made by the interviewer to accommodate the informant's unique needs or communication style. As occupational therapists, we often adapt our ways of clinical interviewing and interaction to suit the needs and abilities of our clients.

Individuals with disabilities that affect cognition, perception, hearing, and/or language may need specific accommodations to facilitate the interview and information sharing process. Some individuals, for example, may respond better to shorter, more frequent interviews or need frequent redirection to stay focused. Environmental distractions should be minimized. One's approach to asking questions may need to be modified to accommodate individual response styles (for example, pacing of questions, simplifying language). Impediments to memory can also be a problem. Therefore, it is better to ask informants to reconstruct a past experience, rather than asking them to remember a particular event. For example, an interviewer can ask "What was that experience like for you?" rather than "Do you remember what that experience was like?" Incorporating caregivers or other trained individuals as interpreters may be needed in some cases. When using interpreters, however, they should be coached on how to encourage the informants to share their ideas and how to translate verbatim responses, that is, to state exactly what the informant said, not a summary or interpretation.

Interviewing children can present some unique challenges as well, since they may have little experience in articulating their feelings, have inadequate autobiographical memory, or may find it difficult to overcome the sense that they should provide the "correct" answers to questions (Grbich, 1999; Seidman, 1991). Children (and others who may experience similar problems) may converse more easily when they are simultaneously engaged in an activity, such as drawing a situation that they are explaining, rather than being interviewed face to face (Grbich, 1999). It is also suggested that questions for younger children should be related to actions rather than feelings (Grbich, 1999).

Active, intense listening is a critical component of conducting in-depth interviews. Active listening may involve nonverbal behaviors such as nodding, pausing, waiting for a response, and letting the informant decide the direction of the next exchange of information. Neutral prompts, such as "I see," "hmm," or even repeating the main words that the informant presented, may be used to convey to the informant that he or she has been heard (Chenitz & Swanson, 1986; Kvale, 1996). At the same time, the interviewer should always monitor the impact of such prompts, as they may not always be perceived as neutral. For example, a phrase such as "I see" may lead an informant to believe the interviewer completely understands and no further elaboration is required. In the beginning stages of the interview, counseling techniques such as reflective listening or summarizing should be minimized (Morse & Field, 1995). Reflective listening includes statements such as "That made you angry" or "It seems like. . . ." The problem with reflective or summary statements is that they may lead the participant in a particular direction and inhibit the flow of the interview. The informant may find it easier to agree with the interviewer than explain how it really is, and any preliminary analysis may lead to premature closure of the topic area (Morse & Field, 1995). Instead, the interviewer should try to enhance his or her understanding, encourage reflection, and probe for details.

Although the interview guide may provide a general framework for the interview, probes and follow-up questions are very important to enhance the quality of the information that is gathered. Probes are used to deepen the response to a question, increase the richness of the data being gathered, and give cues to the interviewee about the level of response that is desired (Patton, 1990). Many different types of probes have been described in the literature (Chenitz & Swanson, 1986; Patton, 1990; Schatzman & Strauss, 1973). One common type of probe involves exploring details of the informant's response. The interviewer may ask for information about "who," "what," "where," "when," and "how" in order to get a more complete and detailed picture of an activity or experience. When interviewing occupational therapists, for example, some informants mentioned that they thought activities were valuable in group settings. In order to get details, the interviewer asked them to provide specific examples of when they used activities and with whom. Another type of probe may be used to encourage the informant to elaborate on a particular subject. Elaboration probes

can range from nonverbal cues such as head nodding to a direct verbal request to talk more about the issue of interest (for example, "Tell me more about. . . ."). Probing for clarification is another critical component of in-depth interviewing. The interviewer should probe for clarification, rather than taking for granted what may seem to be commonsense assumptions and understandings that others share (Taylor & Bogdan, 1984). Sometimes words that seem to be common can have very different cultural meanings. In the therapist study, for example, the therapists had different conceptualizations of the nature of "activity" and at the outset of the interview, were asked to elaborate on their definitions of the term. It can be useful to rephrase and ask for confirmation, asking for examples and telling the informant when something is not clear for you. When asking for clarification, however, the interviewer should be careful to indicate that the failure to understand is on the part of the interviewer and not the fault of the person being interviewed. Patton (1990) suggests that clarification probes should be used "naturally and gently." If two or more attempts at clarification are necessary, it might be best to leave the topic and return at a later point in the interview. The hallmark of a skilled interviewer is knowing when and how to probe. Insufficient probing indicates boredom or inattention, whereas too much probing turns the interviewer into an inquisitor (Rubin & Rubin, 1995). Probes provide an opportunity to communicate with the informant about what the interviewer is looking for, but should not dictate the direction and flow of the interview.

Rubin and Rubin (1995) describe ideal interviews as ones that capture "depth, detail, vividness and nuance." Depth involves obtaining layers of meaning, different angles on the subjects and broader understanding of the topic area. Asking follow-up questions, clarifying issues in subsequent interviews, tracking answers over time, and obtaining thoughtful responses can all contribute to interview depth. Detail is needed to provide clarity and solid evidence through examples. Detail can be achieved by asking for specific information, getting informants to describe experiences or tasks, and asking informants to share examples. Anecdotes or examples can also be used to enhance vividness of data collection. Vividness involves asking questions to evoke responses that will convey a range of feelings among readers. Nuance involves exploring complexity of meaning and illustrating the shades of gray that exist, rather than settling for "black and white" responses.

At times, the informant may talk at length but the information that is shared may not be relevant to the topic being discussed. There are many reasons why an informant might get off track or on a tangent when sharing information. The informant may, for example, feel that a particular issue is more important to discuss and want to share this with you first, or the informant may be avoiding a particular topic area. Some informants may simply lose track of the initial question or have a thought disorder that interferes with their ability to provide organized coherent responses. Initially, you want to encourage the informant to talk, note when he or she gets off track, and try to assess why this is occurring. Over time, it may be important to redirect the informant so that he or she focuses on pertinent issues and examples. Redirection may be in the form of subtle cues such as decreasing the number of verbal or nonverbal prompts, asking more focussed questions, or reminding the informant of the original question that was asked. Part of the role of the interviewer is to be sensitive to the nature and relevance of the information being shared and to focus the informant when needed.

Listening involves not only picking up on key words and ideas, but also trying to understand the meaning that this has for the informant. It takes effort to really hear and understand what people tell you. At times, you may suspect that the informant is holding back or providing superficial responses. The content of what an informant says, for example, may not be consistent with nonverbal behaviors. You may notice important omissions or contradictions in responses. The informant may avoid a topic or deliberately distort what he or she is saying. There are many potential reasons for these behaviors and strategies to deal with them outlined in the literature (McCracken, 1988; Rubin & Rubin, 1995; Taylor & Bogdan, 1984). Some informants, for example, may want to impress the interviewer and exaggerate success or downplay failure. They might avoid answering particular questions for fear that they will reveal their own ignorance or that you will expose their rationalizations and question their achievements. Others may find that they are saying more than they anticipated and shut down when they start to feel exposed or vulnerable. In some situations, a particular topic may be very uncomfortable for them to address, and as soon as they get close to talking about it, they change the subject in order to cope with their emotions. It is important to be aware of these behaviors and potential reasons for them. At times, you may need to be patient and give the informant time to develop a sense of trust. If you suspect that the informant is avoiding a topic, you may want to approach it less directly or in a less threatening way. If the informant jumps topics, he or she may need gentle redirection to the topic at hand. If you suspect that the informant is clearly distorting the information that he or she presents, you may need to gently confront the informant with the evidence and raise the issue directly.

In the case of exploring sensitive, personal, or emotionally charged topic areas, informants may need encouragement to respond. Chenitz and Swanson (1986) identify a number of facilitative strategies that the interviewer could try. "Door opening" statements such as "it must be hard to go through . . ." and "Others have had similar experiences, what was it like for you?" can give informants permission to share their experiences. Making general statements about the common experiences of others can reassure the informant that his or her concerns are acceptable and shared by others. You can talk about the universality of experiences, yet the range of behaviors that are possible. It is important as an interviewer to be comfortable with the nature of the topics being explored and the potential emotion that may accompany these experiences. When telling stories, participants may relive their experiences, including their emotional responses. In fact, a resurgence of emotions is a sign that the interview is tapping important areas of their experience (Morse & Field, 1995). Demonstrate emotional understanding through your nonverbal behaviors and verbally communicate your sympathy when warranted. Depending on the context, it may be appropriate to turn off taping devices and take a brief break during an interview if the situation becomes very emotionally charged for an informant or the interviewer. For some informants, the cathartic experience of sharing emotions can be a very positive experience. Others, however, may not be ready or willing to relive these experiences. The interviewer should be sensitive to the needs of each informant and know when to probe sensitive areas and when to leave them alone. Remember that if you push too hard for information before they are willing to share it, they may shut down, tell you nothing, lie, or distort their answer (Rubin & Rubin, 1995). Listen to see when questions are evoking stress and try to back off when levels get too high. To understand the issue, however, it is important to try to come back to it later.

Through the process of conducting interviews, you may develop a close relationship with the informant, particularly if you conduct repeated interviews with the same informant. At times, a quasi-therapeutic relationship may emerge, particularly if very personal and emotional issues have been discussed. The process may bring forth deeper personal problems that need therapeutic assistance. When designing the study, it is important to have a procedure for dealing with this potential problem. Kvale (1996) recommends having a therapist as a "backup" when needed. At the time of the interview, the interviewer may need to "lower the emotional tone" of a particularly emotional or stressful interview by refocusing on practical, nonthreatening topics.

Concluding the Interview

There are a number of issues to consider when concluding the interview. A period of debriefing at the end of the interview is recommended (Kvale, 1996; Rubin & Rubin, 1995). During the course of the interview, the informant may have shared some very personal or emotional experiences and may wonder how the information will be used. The informant may have a feeling of emptiness from revealing so much information about himself or herself and receiving little in return. On the other hand, some informants may have enjoyed the experience and gained new insights. The interviewer may want to spend some time summarizing the main points that were discussed and reviewing procedures that will be put in place to ensure confidentiality of responses. The informant should then be given an opportunity to ask any questions that he or she might have. Rather than terminating the relationship at this time, the interviewer should leave the door open for a follow-up interview if issues emerge through the process of data analysis

(Chenitz & Swanson, 1986; Rubin & Rubin, 1995). To enhance trustworthiness of the study, the interviewer may also want to discuss procedures for checking back with participants to confirm themes that emerge from the analysis process (member checking). Finally, informants should be thanked for their time and willingness to participate.

After you have finished with the formal closing and have turned off the tape recorder, the informant may resume the more casual chatting that marked the opening of the interview. Rubin and Rubin (1995) point out that this can be not only a way of winding down the intensity of the interview, but also a very informal and indirect way of passing on additional information. It is important to pay close attention, make notes as soon as you leave, and look them over in conjunction with the interview. Once the interview is complete, it is recommended that the interviewer spend a few minutes in a quiet room recording reflections on what he or she learned in the interview and observations regarding the interview process. Immediate impressions can provide a valuable context for later analysis of the transcripts (Kvale, 1996).

The Need for Reflection

The interview experience can be characterized as an evolving relationship between the researcher and participant. Participation in the interview process not only affects the informant but also can have a significant impact on the interviewer as well (see Chapter 6). Much of the content of the interview and the process of analysis is influenced by the researcher's own subjective experiences, biases, and beliefs (Hasselkus, 1997; Lincoln & Guba, 1985). The researcher is the primary data-gathering instrument and analytic tool and, as such, can have a significant influence on the study findings. One of the fundamental tenets of qualitative research is

that it is not possible to be purely objective in collecting information and that a "single, tangible reality" does not exist (Lincoln & Guba, 1985). Potential biases that the researcher brings to the process, however, must be identified.

Rather than trying to strive for objectivity, the interviewer should reflect on the ways in which he or she influences the process and document his or her thoughts in the form of a reflexive journal. Some authors argue that disciplined self-reflection can enrich the study findings (Banning, 1997; Frank, 1997). Through systematic examination of one's own experiences and reactions, new insights and deeper understandings can emerge (Frank, 1997).

The nature of the reflexive journal can take many forms. The researcher involved in the study with occupational therapists maintained a reflexive journal in a three-ring binder divided into three sections: methods log, personal log or daily diary, and "theoretical notes." The methods log was used to keep track of appointments, noting the dates and times of each contact. Arrangements for pilot testing the interview guide were outlined, including feedback that was received and changes that were made to the interview guide as a result of the feedback. Details were also documented regarding the process of negotiating access to facilities and recruiting informants. When a decision was made to add an additional informant to the study or changes were made to the interview schedule, the reasons for this were recorded in the methods log section. Lincoln and Guba (1985) recommend including a methods log as a trustworthiness strategy, since changes can be tracked through an audit by another individual.

The second section of the reflexive journal was identified as a personal log or daily diary. This was a place to record impressions of people and places that the researcher had visited. Some entries included comments about the nature of the developing relationship: "[name of therapist] seemed very pleasant and open to participating . . . not reserved," "I feel that some initial rapport was established today," or "her nervous laughter seemed to indicate that she was anxious about the questions I was asking and she seemed to be trying to give me the answers that I wanted to hear." At times, the researcher commented on her reactions to informants, "something about [name of therapist] really irked me," and then reflected on potential barriers to developing rapport. If circumstances prevented optimal performance of either participant, this was noted as well. One entry, for example, indicated that one of the informants had just quit smoking the day prior to the interview and had just received news that her vacation plans were canceled. Another entry commented on the fatigue of the interviewer resulting from observing several sessions in a row, then conducting two interviews in one day. All of these notations provided important contextual information for interpreting and analyzing the information that was shared in the interview. In addition, Lincoln and Guba (1985) note that writing about frustrations or other emotional responses to interviews can have a positive cathartic affect. Other types of information that might be included in this section are reconstructions of informal conversations that occur outside of the interview situation and notes about ways to improve one's approach in future interviews (Taylor & Bogdan, 1984).

The third section of the journal, entitled "theoretical notes," was used to facilitate and track the process of ongoing analysis. Initial entries in this section involved reflecting on personal beliefs and biases about the topic area and predictions about what might emerge from the study. As the study progressed, emerging insights were compared to these initial beliefs to see whether the process

of analysis was based more on the researcher's preconceived ideas or whether it was a true reflection of the informants' beliefs. Some entries involved attempts to link the study findings with themes identified in the literature. An example of an entry is as follows: "I read an article on . . . and it really inspired me to think about the therapists' responses in a different way." Other entries involved identifying unanswered questions and hypotheses about patterns that were emerging.

Maintaining a reflexive journal takes time and dedication to the process of self-reflection. Entries should be made after every contact with an informant or even more frequently as needed (Lincoln & Guba, 1985; Taylor & Bogdan, 1984). It is difficult to be disciplined in making entries when there are many other things to be done, but it can significantly enhance the analysis process. Data within the journal should be considered as important as data from interview transcripts when reviewing and analyzing research findings.

Ethical Issues

Throughout the process of the study, there are a number of important ethical issues to consider. Qualitative in-depth interviewing requires a high level of trust from participants in order to facilitate honest and open sharing of personal beliefs and experiences. It is a privilege to be able to get a glimpse into the perspectives of others, and the nature of the information may be deeply emotional and intimate for them to share. The researcher has a moral and ethical obligation to ensure that this trusting relationship is respected, not betrayed. Some of the major issues that the researcher needs to consider include: informed consent, ensuring confidentiality, balancing benefits and risks, issues of reciprocity, and responsibility in reporting study results.

Letters of Information and Informed Consent

Outlining procedures for informed consent is a standard part of most research protocols. Details regarding how informed consent will be obtained must be included in any proposal submitted for ethical approval and should be considered in all studies. Informed consent means letting the participants know about the overall purpose of the study, its general design, procedures to ensure confidentiality, and the potential risks and benefits of participation. Participants should be assured that their involvement in the study is voluntary and that they can withdraw at any time without any adverse effects. If you are, for example, interviewing individuals who are receiving occupational therapy services, it is important to clarify that participation in the study will not have any impact on services that they are currently receiving or may be receiving in the future. The researcher usually obtains written consent from participants. Formal, written consent involves providing participants with a letter of information about the study and then asking them to sign a form that verifies that they have been informed about the study, they understand the nature of what is required of them, and they agree to participate. Samples of a letter of information and a consent form are provided in Appendices C and D, found at the end of this Chapter.

One of the challenges in obtaining informed consent is that it may be difficult to specify details of the study requirements in advance. Fundamental to the nature of in-depth interviewing is that the design of the study may change over time in response to the data gathered and the analysis that emerges. Interview questions may change, the number of interviews required may change, and the number and nature of informants may change over time as well. Since analysis is an ongoing process, new categories may emerge which the researcher may want to explore through additional interviews. It is difficult to predict in advance the number of interviews that may be required for "theoretical saturation." As outlined earlier, interviews should continue until the researcher reaches a point where no new patterns in the data are emerging.

It can also be difficult to know how much information about the study to specify on the letter of information. It is important not to lead informants in a particular direction, but rather to keep the focus very broad and follow the themes and issues that the informants raise within the interviews. Some facilities may have specific requirements regarding the amount of information that must be included in the letter of information. If the researcher is concerned that the letter might be too restrictive and lead informants to respond in a certain way, negotiation may be required to develop a mutually acceptable letter.

Another potential problem with obtaining written consent from participants is that it creates a level of formality that may not be conducive to open, intimate sharing of ideas and experiences. It sets up a power differential where the participant is more a passive participant than an active participant in the research process (Rubin & Rubin, 1995). It also may be awkward to assure the informant of confidentiality, then ask him or her to sign a legal form stating that he or she is participating in the study. A decision needs to be made about who should be giving the consent to participate. Should consent be from the informants themselves, their supervisors, or their caregivers? In the study of occupational therapists, for example, several levels of consent were obtained. First, the therapists' supervisors were sent a letter of request about the study, followed by written consent from each therapist who agreed to participate and verbal and/or written consent of clients who were observed in sessions with the therapist.

In order to get around some of the concerns that have been raised regarding informed consent, some authors have proposed that consent to participate is implied by engaging in the interview process and that the main issues regarding consent and confidentiality emerge later when decisions are made regarding making the information public (Kvale, 1996; Lincoln, 1990). Lincoln (1990) talked about replacing the concept of informed consent with the view that consent should be more of a dialogue that runs throughout the process with "negotiation of research processes and products with one's respondents, so that there is a mutual shaping of the final research results" (p. 286). Kvale (1996) suggested that written agreement could be obtained after the interviews were completed regarding how the interview data would be used.

Confidentiality

A related issue to consider concerns protecting the confidentiality of informants. The researcher needs to be clear with potential informants about what information will be available to whom. Procedures should be in place to ensure that any data that could be used to identify informants (for example, consent forms, audiotapes, coding sheets) will be kept in a locked storage area. Plans should also be outlined for what will happen to this information once the study is completed. Transcribed data can be coded to ensure the anonymity of the informant. In writing up results of the study, descriptors of the participants can be altered to protect their identity. It can be a challenge, however, to alter descriptors without changing the meaning of the results. Applicability of the

research findings can be determined only if details are provided about who participated in the study and where and when it took place (Kvale, 1996). In the study of occupational therapists, for example, it was a challenge to protect the identity of participants, yet give important details regarding their level of experience, their area of clinical practice, and the settings in which they worked. In the final report, general descriptive data were provided to provide an overview of the sample group, but care was taken not to include identifying information within individual quotations.

There are a number of potential limitations to confidentiality that you may want to consider in advance. Informants, for example, might share information that reveals that they are a danger to themselves or others. Your ethical responsibility to protect confidentiality may be outweighed by your legal and moral responsibility to protect the individual from harm or to prevent the individual from harming others. In this situation, you need to consider whom you would contact and what information you would be obligated to share. You should discuss your intentions with the informant whenever legally possible before acting on them so that the relationship of trust is not jeopardized. In situations involving child abuse, one's legal responsibility is to report any suspicion to child protection agencies. In such a case, discussing one's intention may not be wise. Also, in such a case, the participant should probably no longer be included in the study. Another situation that may compromise your ability to protect confidentiality concerns the potential involvement of the legal system. How might you handle the situation if your interview data was subpoenaed? One author describes a situation where he destroyed the interview data to protect informant confidentiality rather than turning it over to the courts (Rubin & Rubin,

1995). Although these difficult situations may never occur, anticipating potential situations in advance and developing a plan of action can help the process flow more smoothly if the situation does arise.

Participating in a qualitative study that involves in-depth interviews has a number of potential "risks" to the participants. At the outset of the interview, informants should be made aware of the potential risks involved in participating, as well as the potential benefits, either to themselves or others. The overall benefits of participating in the study should outweigh the risks.

At the outset of the interview, the potential risks may not be immediately obvious to informants and should be discussed with them. The interview process itself, for example, is not only time-consuming, but also may be intellectually and emotionally challenging (McCracken, 1988; Patton, 1990). The nature of what is shared can be highly personal and may expose sensitive areas of a person's life. As such, interviews can be more intrusive and can endanger privacy more than other quantitative approaches. In some cases, the openness and intimacy of the interview may lead the informants to disclose information that they never intended to reveal and may later regret revealing (Kvale, 1996; Patton, 1990). As a researcher, you are obligated to try to get past superficial answers, but you need to be sensitive to the vulnerability of informants and not violate their trust.

Although interviews pose some inherent risks, there are also a number of benefits that informants may gain from the interview process. McCracken (1988) describes the process as an opportunity to engage in conversation with the "perfect conversational partner." Informants, for example, might enjoy being the center of attention, with the interviewer listening eagerly to everything they have to say. They can share their ideas

without interruption and without having to take turns with another. Informants may have an opportunity to state an opinion that might otherwise go unheard. Although they may share some painful and personal experiences, the process of doing so can be cathartic, and the reflection involved can be stimulating and intellectually challenging. In some cases, the benefits may be not directly for the individual but to "enhance the human condition" (Kvale, 1996, p. 119). Informants may feel that it is worth sharing their stories if it could help someone else in a similar situation. By teaching others, they may be able to translate their suffering into something meaningful (Rubin & Rubin, 1995). The chapters in Part III, Personal Research Journeys, of this book include descriptions of the perceptions of "benefit" by many participants in the research.

Reciprocity and Responsibility

In addition to balancing study benefits and risks, the issue of reciprocity should be considered. The researcher should be sensitive to the vulnerability of informants and strive to make the process as equitable as possible. Although the interview process has been described as a "partnership," it is the informants who do the bulk of the talking and sharing of their personal experiences, for what may be very little in return. Strategies for building equity include obtaining explicit consent to participate, considering informant's needs when scheduling the time and place for the interviews, valuing the words of the informant, and never promising something that you cannot deliver (Siedman, 1991). Some informants will ask questions of the interviewer, in which case the interviewer should try to answer as openly and honestly as possible (Kaufman, 1994). Doing small favors for informants (for example, treating them to coffee, sending a thank-you note) may be part of your relationship development and can communicate your sincere appreciation of what they have been willing to share. There are limits, however, to the principle of reciprocity. Some favors such as lending money, offering advice, or providing a service that is outside of the interview context may strain the boundaries of your relationship.

One final but important ethical issue concerns communication of the study findings. Since quotations from the informants are often used to support the themes generated from the study, the researcher has an obligation to ensure that the presentation of their words is not only accurate, but also prevents the informants from being hurt. Typically, the informants are afforded an opportunity to review and comment on the findings prior to publication (Rubin & Rubin, 1995; Taylor & Bogdan, 1984). The interviewer may want to get permission from the informants to use particular quotations. Some authors stress that the researcher's first responsibility is to the participant and that the participant has a right to retract information or request that information not be included in a report (Morse & Field, 1995; Siedman, 1991). Even if the participants agree to presentation of the information, the researcher should consider the potential for any negative impact or political consequences of the study findings. Rubin and Rubin (1995) emphasize that the informants should not be hurt "emotionally, physically or financially because they have agreed to talk to you."

At times, the findings may not be flattering to the participants but may present an important perspective on the topic of interest. In the study of occupational therapists, for example, the author discovered that the therapists made many claims about the value of what they were doing with little evidence to back up their beliefs. When presenting the study findings, the author had to consider how the struggles of the therapists could be highlighted without discrediting their beliefs. The way in which the information is presented can be important in balancing the need to highlight potentially painful realities without violating the vulnerability of informants.

In presenting the study findings to the participants, the researcher needs to carefully consider the level of interpretation that will be reviewed. At times, the themes that emerge are at a level that goes beyond the direct experiences of individual informants. It may be difficult for informants to comment on interpretations that go beyond their own self-understanding (Kvale, 1996). If the researcher's interpretations are different from those of the study participants, it may not be clear how this disagreement should be handled. Disagreements regarding direct experiences may be handled differently than disagreements regarding higher level interpretations. If there is disagreement, however, this should probably be reported in the published article.

Data Analysis

Once data collection has begun, the question then becomes how to begin qualitative data analysis of in-depth interviews. In general, qualitative data analysis techniques are inductive. That is, the techniques involve searching for meaning in the data rather than imposing a previously defined coding system (Berg, 1989). There are many suggested specific methods for data analysis, and the reader should refer to texts that focus on qualitative analysis for further detail. Several of them are included in An Annotated Bibliography of Selected Further Reading in this book. A brief description of the analysis strategies we have used follows.

One needs to also consider whether one will conduct the analysis manually, using handwritten notes and a system of index cards or another notation system, or whether one will use a computer program, such as Ethnograph or Nudist. Again, there are numerous references discussing the advantages and disadvantages of both manual and computer analysis, for example, *Using Computers in Qualitative Research* by Fielding and Lee (1991). It must be kept in mind that all these techniques are used to code and retrieve data. They are part of the analytic process, but the coded data requires further analysis and interpretation.

Beginning data analysis in the pilot testing phase provides the researcher with some time to experiment with different methods of analysis and find one that fits with both the researcher's style and the data being collected. In the study conducted with seniors, the researcher decided to utilize the constant comparative analysis method outlined by Lincoln and Guba (1985). The first step of the analysis involved reading each transcript and writing down general impressions about issues or concepts that appeared important. This step allowed the researcher to obtain an overall sense of the data and helped her become aware of some the assumptions and biases she was bringing to the analysis process. The second step involved what Lincoln and Guba refer to as "unitizing." In this step, each transcript was again analyzed separately. Codes, which could be a single word or phrase, were written into the margins of transcripts to indicate chunks of meaning. These codes sometimes referred to one word in the transcript, a couple of words, a sentence, or a paragraph. While unitizing was the second step, it was also carried out throughout the analysis process as interviews were reviewed many times and new units of information were discovered. In the third step, which Lincoln and Guba label categorizing, the codes assigned to individual interviews were brought together. The researcher searched for trends in the codes used across interviews and grouped similar codes together into categories. As provisional categories were formed, memos were kept on index cards proposing a name for the category, rules of inclusion, and delineating properties and dimensions. Memos were also kept to record where quotes belonging to each category could be found within the transcripts. With each new interview and with several repeat readings of all interviews, these categories and their definitions went through several transformations. The fourth step of analysis involved forming themes. In order to prepare for this step, the researcher created computer-generated documents for each category containing all of the quotes thought to belong to that category. This final step involved searching for relationships among categories in order to subsume a number of categories under a larger theme. Several frameworks of relationships among the categories were tested against the data to obtain the framework offering the best reconstruction and interpretation of informants' perspectives.

Final Thoughts

This chapter has covered many details regarding in-depth interviewing. Although these are certainly important to keep in mind as one is planning and conducting in-depth interviews, it is also important to allow oneself to enjoy and learn from doing in-depth interviews. In our experience, conducting an in-depth study is like taking a journey, a journey into the world of informants that is filled with insights and interesting paths. It is hard, if not impossible, to predict all of the paths you will follow in your study and what your ultimate findings will be. While at times you may experience anxiety because you are not sure where you are heading, this uncertainty is often part of the process of doing in-depth interviews and likely means you are heading toward discoveries you never anticipated.

We have also found that talking with informants is a process that has changed us in many ways, for example, as therapists and learners.

Overall, there is a good fit between in-depth interviewing and occupational therapy. The philosophy behind both emphasizes the importance of understanding the perspective of the individual and the centrality of meaning for understanding behavior. As well, in our experience, most people enjoy talking about themselves, their lives, and their occupations. Similarly, we have enjoyed reflecting on, discussing, and writing about our experiences in learning to conduct in-depth qualitative interviews. Our learning continues.

References

Banning, J. H. (1997). Comment on researcher's subjectivity: From "coming clean" to analytic tool. *The Occupational Therapy Journal of Research, 17*(2), 130–132.

Bauman, L. J., & Adair, E. G. (1992). The use of ethnographic interviewing to inform questionnaire construction. *Health Education Quarterly, 19*(1), 9–23.

Beer, D. W. (1997). "There's a certain slant of light": The experience of discovery in qualitative interviewing. *Occupational Therapy Journal of Research, 17*(2), 110–129.

Berg, B. L. (1989). *Qualitative research methods for the social sciences.* Boston, MA: Allyn & Bacon.

Canadian Association of Occupational Therapists. (1998). *Enabling occupation.* Ottawa, Canada: Author.

Chenitz, W. C., & Swanson, J. M. (1986). *From practice to grounded theory, qualitative research in nursing.* Menlo Park, CA: Addison-Wesley.

Christiansen, C. (1994.) Classification and study in occupation, a review and discussion of taxonomies. *Journal of Occupational Science, 1,* 3–21.

Fielding, N. G., & Lee, R. M. (Eds.). (1991). *Using computers in qualitative research.* Newbury Park, CA: Sage.

Frank, G. (1997). Is there life after categories? Reflexivity in qualitative research. *The Occupational Therapy Journal of Research, 17*(2), 84.

Grbich, C. (1999). *Qualitative research in health: An introduction.* Thousand Oaks, CA: Sage.

Hasselkus, B. R. (1997). In the eye of the beholder: The researcher in qualitative research. *The Occupational Therapy Journal of Research, 17*(2), 81–83.

Holstein, J. A., & Gubrium, J. F. (1995). *The active interview.* Thousand Oaks, CA: Sage.

Jones, S. (1985). Depth interviewing. In R. Walker (Ed.), *Applied qualitative research* (pp. 45–55). London, England: Gower Publishing.

Kaufman, S. R. (1994). In-depth interviewing. In J. F. Gubrium & A. Sankar (Eds.), *Qualitative methods in aging research* (pp. 123–136). Thousand Oaks, CA: Sage.

Kvale, S. (1996). *InterViews: An introduction to qualitative research interviewing.* Thousand Oaks, CA: Sage.

Laliberte-Rudman, D., Cook, J. V., & Polatajko, H. (1997). Understanding the potential of occupation: A qualitative exploration of seniors' perspectives on activity. *American Journal of Occupational Therapy, 51*(8), 640–650.

Lincoln, Y. S. (1990). Toward a categorical imperative for qualitative research. In E. W. Eisner & A. Peskin (Eds.), *Qualitative inquiry in education* (pp. 277–295). New York: Teachers College Press.

Lincoln, Y. S., & Guba, E. G. (1985). *Naturalistic inquiry.* Newbury Park, CA: Sage.

Marshall, C., & Rossman, G. R. (1989). *Designing qualitative research.* Thousand Oaks, CA: Sage.

McCracken, G. (1988). *The long interview.* Newbury Park, CA: Sage.

Moll, S., & Cook, J. V. (1997). "Doing" in mental health practice: Therapists' beliefs about why it works. *American Journal of Occupational Therapy, 51*(8), 662–670.

Morse, J. M., & Field, P. A. (1995). *Qualitative research methods for health professionals* (2nd ed.). Thousand Oaks, CA: Sage.

Patton, M. Q. (1990). *Qualitative evaluation and research process.* Thousand Oaks, CA: Sage.

Polatajko, H. J. (1994). Dreams, dilemmas, and decisions for occupational therapy practice in a new millennium: A Canadian perspective. *American Journal of Occupational Therapy, 48,* 590–594.

Rowles, G. D., & Reinharz, S. (1988). Qualitative gerontology: Themes and challenges. In S. Reinharz & G. D. Rowles (Eds.), *Qualitative gerontology* (pp. 3–33). New York: Springer.

Rubin, H. J., & Rubin, I. S. (1995). *Qualitative interviewing: The art of hearing data.* Thousand Oaks, CA: Sage.

Rubinstein, R. L. (1988). Stories told: In-depth interviewing and the structure of its insights. In S. Reinharz & G. D. Rowles (Eds.), *Qualitative gerontology* (pp. 128–146). New York: Springer.

Schatzman, L., & Strauss, A. (1973). *Field research.* Englewood Cliffs, NJ: Prentice-Hall.

Segal, R., Landry, J., & Rebeiro, K. (1998). *The development of occupational therapy practitioner–researchers.* American Occupational Therapy Association Annual Conference (April).

Seidman, I. E. (1991). *Interviewing as qualitative research: A guide for researchers in education and the social sciences.* New York: Teachers College Press.

Spradley, J. P. (1979). *The ethnographic interview.* Fort Worth, TX: Harcourt Brace Jovanovich College Publishers.

Strauss, A., & Corbin, J. A. (1990). *Basics of qualitative research: Grounded theory procedures and techniques.* Newbury Park, CA: Sage.

Taylor, S. J., & Bogdan, R. (1984). *Introduction to qualitative research methods: The search for meanings* (2nd ed.). New York: John Wiley.

Werner, O., & Schoepfle, G. (1987). *Systematic fieldwork.* Newbury Park, CA: Sage.

Yerxa, E. J. (1993). Occupational science: A new source of power for participants in occupational therapy. *Journal of Occupational Science, 1,* 3–10.

Yerxa, E. J., Clark, F., Frank, G., Jackson, J., Parham, D., Pierce, D., Stein, C., & Zemke, R. (1990). An introduction to occupational science: A foundation for occupational therapy in the 21st century. In J. Johnson & B. Yerxa (Eds.), *Occupational science: The foundation for new models of practice* (pp. 1–18). New York: Haworth.

Appendix A

Initial Interview Guide for Study Conducted with Seniors

1. Description of Activities

(a) To begin with, I'd like to gain a general picture of the sorts of things you do. Could you describe to me what you do during a typical day?
Probes
   • Further description of specific activities
   • Social context of activities
   • Environmental context of activities

(b) If you could create for yourself the most satisfying day, what sorts of things would you do on that day?
Probes
   • As in 1(a)

2. Preferences for Activities

(a) What do you like doing?
Why do you like doing these things?
Probe
   • Discuss each activity mentioned with respect to outcome and opportunity.

Do you believe that doing these things influences how you feel?
Probe
   • In what way?

(b) What do you do that you do not like doing?
Why do you dislike doing these things?
Probe
   • As in 2(a)

Do you think that doing these things influences how you feel?
Probe
   • In what way?

3. Personal Relevance of Activities

(a) Of all of the things that you do, which are the most important for you to continue doing?
Probe
   • How come?

(b) What would it mean if you could no longer do the things that you consider important?
Probe
- Possible emotional, social, and instrumental effects

4. Satisfaction with Activities

(a) Do you feel satisfied with the variety of things that you do?
Probes
- Why/why not?
- What contributes to satisfaction?
- What limits satisfaction?
- How could you become more satisfied?

(b) Do you feel satisfied with the amount of things that you do?
Probes
- Why/why not?
- What contributes to satisfaction?
- What limits satisfaction?
- How could you become more satisfied?

(c) Are there things that you would like to be doing that you are not doing?
Probes
- Why do you want to do these things?
- What are the reasons for you not doing these things?

5. The Relationship between Activity and Well-Being

(a) What do you think contributes most to your well-being?
How do these things contribute to your well-being?

(b) If you were to give advice to a person about what can help a person be healthy as he or she ages, what would you say?

Appendix B

Final Interview Guide for Study Conducted with Seniors

1. Description of Activities

(a) To begin with, I want to gain a general picture of the sorts of things that you do. Could you describe to me what you do during a typical morning . . . typical afternoon . . . typical evening?
Probes
   - Further description of specific activities
   - Social context of activities
   - Environmental context of activities
   - *Feelings/opinions regarding activities
   - *Why they started/continue to do the activity
   - *Changes in the way they do an activity/how much they do an activity

2. Preferences for Activities

(a) What are your favorite things to do?
Why do you like doing these things?
Probes
   - Could discuss each activity mentioned above with respect to: feelings (during and after), outcome, opportunity for, *who with, *degree of choice, *reasons for doing.

(b) What are your least favorite things to do?
Why do you dislike doing these things?
Probes
   - As in 2a
   - *Do they avoid doing these things?

3. Personal Relevance of Activities

(a) Of all of the things that you do, which are the most important for you to continue doing?
Probe
   - How come?

(b) What would it mean to you if you could no longer do the things that you consider important?
Probes
   - Break it down into specific activities mentioned in 3(a)
   - Possible emotional, social, and instrumental effects
   - If person talks about health restrictions only: What would you do if a circumstance other than a health problem, such as a change in where you lived or a lack of money, was the reason that you couldn't do the things that are important to you?

4. Satisfaction with Activities

(a) If you could create for yourself the most satisfying day possible, what sorts of things would you do on that day?
Probe
   • *Why they chose specific activities

(b) When you look back at a day, what makes you feel that it was a good day?
When you look back at a day, what makes you feel that it was a not so good day?
Probes
   • *If person responds that they do not look back at a day, then ask them what makes up a good day; what makes up a not so good day?
   • Does having a variety of things to do during a day affect how you feel? How?
   • Is it important that you have enough things to do? Why?

(c) What are the things that are limiting how satisfied you are with the things that you do?
How could you become more satisfied with the things that you do?

(d) What are the things that you would like to be doing that you are not doing?
Probes
   • For what reasons do you want to do these things?
   • What are the reasons for you not doing these things?
   • *Discuss things that person used to do and is not doing anymore.

5. The Relationship between Activity and Well-Being

(a) What do you think contributes most to your well-being?
How do these things contribute to your well-being?

(b) If you were to give advice to a person about what can help someone be healthy as he or she ages, what would you say?
Probe
   • Both things to do and things to avoid

Final: Are there any other comments that you would like to make about the things that you do?

Appendix C

Letter of Information—Occupational Therapist Study

A research study is being conducted by a graduate student in the Masters of Science programme in Occupational Therapy at The University of Western Ontario, examining the ways in which therapists select and use treatment activities. Information gathered in this study may help to advance knowledge within the profession regarding how activities are actually used in practice.

If you decide to participate in the study, the investigator will consult with you to arrange a suitable time for data collection. The study will be conducted in two phases; observation of treatment sessions, followed by one or two interviews.

The first phase of the study involves observation of five of your therapy sessions, which will help the investigator understand how activities are actually selected and used in your day-to-day practice. Pending client consent, the sessions will be audiotaped, and the investigator will be in the room, recording observational notes. The investigator will endeavor to be as unobtrusive as possible so that your regular treatment sessions are not disrupted.

Since the investigator will be observing treatment sessions, informed consent of clients is required. You will be asked to approach the clients involved in your scheduled treatment sessions to see whether they would be willing to participate. A letter of information about the study and consent form will be provided and the investigator will be available to answer any questions that the client might have. If you feel that the client will not be able to tolerate the observation or audiotaping, treatment sessions with this client will not be included in the study. In addition, treatment sessions which include clients who are under 18, who are certified incompetent under the Mental Health Act, or who are otherwise unwilling or unable to provide consent will not be included. Within these limitations, the investigator would like to be able to observe consecutive treatment sessions wherever possible. Scheduling of observations will be negotiated with each therapist.

The second phase of the study involves an interview (approximately one hour in length) with the investigator. The interview is intended to supplement information gathered through observations and to provide an opportunity to explore issues that relate to activity selection and use. Occasionally, a short follow-up interview may be required for further clarification. You are not obliged to answer any questions that you find objectionable or that might make you feel uncomfortable.

All research data will be kept in confidence by the investigator. Notes and tapes will be kept in a locked storage area. Tapes will be transcribed by a professional typist who is aware of the importance of maintaining confidentiality and who has signed an oath to confirm her knowledge of procedures to maintain this. All names will be coded upon transcription and will not be used in the written data analysis. Following completion of the study, data, including audiotapes, will be maintained in a locked storage area and may be used for future research. You will not be identified in any publication or presentations of the results of the study.

Your participation in the study is voluntary. If you agree to participate, you may withdraw your consent and discontinue your participation at any time. This in no way will affect your performance record or conditions of employment.

If you have any questions either before or after the study, you may contact [researcher's name and telephone number]. Results of the study will be presented to participating therapists.

Appendix D

Consent Form—Occupational Therapist Study

I, _____, agree to participate in this research study investigating activity selection by occupational therapists. I have received a letter of information about the study, the nature of it has been explained to me and questions have been answered to my satisfaction.

_____   _____

Date   Signature

                                        _____

                                        Witness

CHAPTER

4

Participant Observation as a Research Strategy

Karen L. Rebeiro M.Sc., OT(C)

> [P]articipation entails the need to develop empathic understandings
> that come about only through close involvement with people. In these
> circumstances . . . research easily becomes an enjoyable experience.
>
> —Ernest T. Stringer, 1996, p. 56

The profession of occupational therapy is increasingly recognizing the necessity of research evidence as the basis for professional practice. In the last decade, there has been considerable debate among academics and practitioners as to which research methods are most appropriate to the study of human occupation. Advocates of qualitative strategies argue that the study of human occupation requires research methods capable of capturing the complexity and idiosyncrasies of the experience of engaging in occupation. The study of human occupation requires methods that can tap into, explore, and build knowledge of a phenomenon that, until recently, has lacked rigorous scientific inquiry.

Participant observation is both an overall approach to inquiry and a method of data collection. Participant observation is a qualitative method that is well suited to the study of human occupation. Yerxa (1991) observed that understanding human occupation requires that we as a profession understand the experience of direct engagement in it. Participant observation is direct involvement in "the here and now of people's lives [that] provides both a point of reference for the logic and process of participant observational inquiry, and a means for gaining access to phenomena that commonly are obscured from the standpoint of a nonparticipant" (Jorgenson, 1989, p. 9). Participant observation requires that the researcher have firsthand involvement in the setting. This immersion allows the researcher to hear, see, feel, and begin to experience reality as the participants do. Ideally, the researcher spends a prolonged period of time in the setting in order to accurately describe the social world actions and perspectives of the participants under study. The product of participant observation is a description of the insider's perspective from the researcher's experience of inside. "The world of everyday life as viewed from the standpoint of insider is the fundamental reality to be described by participant observation" (Jorgenson, 1989, p. 14). Further, participant observation aims to gain access to the subjective reality of everyday life. "The world as it is experienced and defined by insiders is required for accurate and truthful findings" (Jorgenson, 1989, p. 28).

The methods of participant observation aim to provide practical and theoretical truths about human existence. From this standpoint, "theory" may be defined as a set of concepts and generalizations. "Theories" provide an interpretation aimed at understanding some phenomenon. Participant observation stresses the logic of discovery and aims to build theories grounded in concrete human realities. The challenge of participant observation is "to combine participation and observation so as to become capable of understanding the experience as an insider, while describing the experience for outsiders" (Patton, 1990, p. 75).

The profession of occupational therapy recognizes that in its quest to be a client-centred and evidenced-based profession, therapists need to engage in research that better explains the experience of engagement in occupations and any related benefits to the clients. This has become crucial in order for occupational therapy to defend and support its jurisdictional claim to the use of occupation as therapy and active participation in occupations of choice as the desired outcome of occupational therapy intervention. Participant observation appears to be well suited to both the methods and process of occupational therapy practice.

Further, it is a data collection method that recognizes the importance of the client's perspective and seeks to understand experiences and phenomena from the client's worldview. According to Jorgenson (1989), "participant observation is especially appropriate for scholarly problems when little is known about the phenomenon and the phenomenon is somewhat obscured from the view of outsiders" (p. 12). Additionally, participant observation is especially appropriate for "exploratory studies, descriptive studies, and studies aimed at generating theoretical interpretations" and "to generate practical truths formulated as interpretative theories" (Jorgenson, 1989, p. 23).

Participant observation is very similar to participatory action research (PAR) (Whyte, 1991). According to Whyte (1991), PAR is a process "in which some of the people in the organization or community being studied actively participate with the professional researcher throughout the research process from the initial design to the final presentation of results and discussion of the action implications" (p. 147). PAR seeks to find solutions to problems defined by insiders, gain an inside perspective and understanding of the problem, and formulate a plan of action to solve the problem.

This chapter explores how participant observation was used as a research strategy to better understand the experience of occupational engagement and, in particular, to study the importance of human occupation for persons with a mental illness. I have completed four separate research projects utilizing different levels and intensities of participant observation as a method of data collection. In this chapter, excerpts from the field journals and methods logs from two of these studies are used to illustrate the process of conducting participant observation as a data collection technique. Excerpts from interview transcripts are also used to highlight discrepancies identified between participant observation findings and those of the in-depth interviews. Pseudonyms are used to conceal the identities of the participants.

The first study utilized observation as the primary data-gathering strategy. This strategy was then followed by in-depth interviewing. The second study utilized participant observation as a concurrent and complementary strategy to a series of in-depth interviews.

In each study, participant observation yielded important information about the client's experiences. In later studies, wherein participatory action research was employed and participant observation was the primary method for data gathering, the insights gleaned proved additionally useful to the therapist for program development, evaluation, and clinical intervention. The strategy of participant observation was the most influential in contributing to my understanding of the mental health system, the role of human occupation, and the enablement of participation in occupations within the community for persons with a mental illness.

Features of Participant Observation

According to Jorgenson (1989, p. 13), there are seven basic features of the method of participant observation.

1. A special interest in human meaning and interaction as viewed from the perspective of people who are insiders or members of particular situations and settings
2. Location in the here and now of everyday life situations and settings as the foundation of inquiry and method
3. A form of theory and theorizing stressing interpretation and understanding of human existence
4. A logic and process of inquiry that is open-minded, flexible, opportunistic, and

requires constant redefinition of what is problematic, based on facts gathered in concrete settings of human existence
5. An in-depth, qualitative, case study approach and design
6. The performance of a participant role or roles that involve establishing and maintaining relationships with natives in the field
7. The use of direct observation along with other methods of gathering information

In short, participant observation provides "direct experiential and observational access to the insider's world and meaning" (Jorgenson, 1989, p. 15). The here and now of everyday life is important to the method of participant observation for two reasons. First, this is where the researcher begins the process of defining and refining the research questions to be asked and answered. The researcher may enter the research setting with a predetermined set of questions to be answered based on observation or experiential knowledge but may find that the important questions to be asked are different. Second, this is the setting where the researcher participates. It is in the natural environment of the participants in which the research is conducted where the researcher will observe and participate as unobtrusively as possible and, hopefully, where answers will begin to emerge. Being an active participant in the natural setting where the research participants carry on as they would every day is a tremendous advantage to understanding their everyday life.

The Participant–Observer Continuum

The extent of participation is a continuum that varies from "complete immersion in the program as a full participant to complete separation from the activities observed, taking on a role as spectator; there is a great deal of variation along the continuum between these two extremes" (Patton, 1990, p. 74). This variation affords the researcher the opportunity to define the degree of participation that will yield the most meaningful information given the questions being asked, the participants being studied, the context of the research setting, and the amount of access the researcher is granted. According to Bogdan and Biklen (1992), "questions concerning how much [participation], with whom, and how you participate tend to work out as the research develops focus" (p. 89).

Research Questions Appropriate to the Method of Participant Observation

Since I am a firm believer in participant observation as a research method for studying issues related to mental health and human occupation, and because participant observation is such a versatile method, ranging from total observation to total immersion and everything in between, I see participant observation methods as appropriate methods for many of the research questions that occupational therapists ask. The educational backgrounds and training in the area of observation make participant observation a method that is well suited to occupational therapists. Further, participant observation is quite complementary to a client-centred approach to care.

Exploratory studies that seek to better understand phenomena of interest to occupational therapists and their clients begin with good observational methods and techniques. Research questions that seek specific information about the experiences of clients can best be answered by full participation in similar activities or by directly coparticipating with research participants. I have never used

participant observation as the sole strategy of inquiry. I have always followed participant observation with an in-depth interview or followed a series of in-depth interviews with a period of participation or have participated with clients in between a series of in-depth interviews. I am always observing, watching, and listening. I believe this to be a good practice for two reasons. First, it is always preferable in qualitative research to have more than one source or type of information on which to base your results. This improves the credibility of your findings (Lincoln & Guba, 1985). Second, I never found that I learned the whole picture from any single source or method. Most of my findings were based on information learned from in-depth interviews, participant observation, and other data-gathering strategies (i.e., observation, surveys, questionnaires, and written records).

The researcher is offered a great deal of flexibility in utilizing participant observation as a data-gathering method, especially in evolving qualitative studies that can change dramatically if informants decide not to talk to you or if the setting suddenly denies you access. As therapists, we all know that any clinical picture is one part "said," one part "observed," and one part "performed." The same can be said about qualitative research. Participant observation offers the researcher the flexibility, methods, and rigor required to conduct thorough studies that are capable of tapping into many perspectives of human experience. According to McCracken (1988), if some form of participant observation is possible in the research setting, the researcher should capitalize on this opportunity. Participant observation "can deliver data that are beyond the conscious understanding or implicit grasp of even the best intentioned respondent . . . and in many situations may be the only way to obtain reliable data" (McCracken, 1988, p. 28).

The following sections highlight and describe the practical steps involved in employing participant observation as a research method from gaining access to the setting, to pure observation and describing the setting, to more in-depth involvement or participation with clients. I have used examples from my own research to illustrate the steps and provide some practical suggestions for the reader.

Steps in Participant Observation

Gaining Access to the Setting: It Is Not as Easy as You Think

Gaining access to the desired research setting takes a bit of preparation and work ahead of time. Do not ever assume that access is going to be easy. In my study (Rebeiro & Allen, 1998) of the volunteer experience of a man with schizophrenia, I incorrectly assumed that I would be granted easy access to the setting because this was a clinic of my employer and because I had permission from John, the volunteer, to study his experiences. What I did not think about ahead of time and did not know was that John hid his schizophrenia illness from all of the employees in the clinic, including his immediate supervisor. So when the acting director of the clinic asked me why I wanted access and why I wanted to study John, I told him it was because I had a class project due that required me to observe one aspect of a volunteer setting and John had volunteered to help me out. The clinic director hesitated in granting me access and most likely allowed it only because he knew me and I was an employee who could be trusted to keep the confidentiality of the clients whom I would likely see in the setting. A second person, an administrative assistant, was very curious about why I was at the clinic and asked many questions that put me in a position of having to omit some of my reasons for being there and also conceal John's

identity. For me, going into the setting as a semicovert researcher was uncomfortable. However, it was required to gain access to John's experiences as a volunteer in this setting.

My precarious and somewhat covert access to the setting was not what I thought it would be. However, I think it worked to my advantage in that I did not spend a great deal of time with John on my first visit but, instead, paid more attention to the other staff, the physical layout of the building, and the official documents and records available at the clinic. This allowed me the opportunity to learn information that would contribute to my understanding of John's experiences. This perspective would not have been possible had I spent the majority of time doing in-depth interviews with John in his small and somewhat isolated corner of the clinic.

I also falsely assumed an easy access to the setting of another research study on a women's craft group because of my earlier involvement in establishing the group in 1990. I thought the participants would be happy to help me. I was wrong. It was only after spending a great deal of time (16 weeks) in and around the group and casually talking with the members that they began to trust me. It was only after I had secured their trust that I was then offered an opportunity to participate in the group. It was only after participating in the group for a period of nine weeks that I was able to secure my requisite number of interview informants.

Do not ever assume that you will be easily granted access to a setting or a group of informants, especially if the group you wish to study is a closed or private group of individuals. Plan ahead, make several visits to the research setting, and make contact with persons who can grant access. Prepare a list of benefits to be had by the organization or individuals by their granting access to you. Unfortunately, I was unable to share the findings of the study of John's volunteer experiences with the setting due to his request for confidentiality. Thus, I think it is best, if possible, to be open about your reasons for being in the research setting.

The Observer Role

On one end of the far continuum of participant observation are the methods and roles of being solely an observer. To be an observer means to place yourself, with permission of course, in a setting that you as a researcher are interested in learning more about or in a setting in which the informants participate. Observation is a method of data collection that is common to all qualitative studies. Observation can range from observing in a group meeting to being an observer in the community. To observe means to watch, listen, and to pay attention to everything that is said and done and not said or done in the setting. Observing means paying attention to people and things that you might deem unimportant or irrelevant to your research question. Jorgenson (1989) refers to these features as the mundane facts of the setting and those aspects that are by and large taken for granted or go unnoticed. In qualitative studies, you cannot presume what you need to know. Assume you might need to know everything and that you are entering the setting knowing nothing. The opportunity to gain access to a setting can be revoked or cut short, so it is very important to learn all that you can while you are there.

Notetaking

It is important to observe the physical environment of the fieldwork setting. This can be documented as a narrative, using a lot of adjectives to describe what you see from the moment you enter the setting until you exit it. It is imperative to be able to fully describe the setting to your advisors or audience (if you are going to publish your research). According to Jorgenson (1989), "making notes, keeping records, and creating data files are among the most important aspects of participant observation" (p. 96). Jorgenson suggests that one's notes should provide the reader with a literal record of everything that has taken place in the fieldwork. This allows them to partially enter the world you are researching.

With respect to notetaking, Spradley (1979) refers to both condensed and expanded accounts. Condensed accounts are observational field notes that are taken or jotted down while in the field. They are often abbreviated, serve as reminders or prompts to the researcher, and include "phrases, single words, and unconnected sentences" (p. 75). The expanded accounts are, quite simply, an expansion of the condensed accounts. This is the opportunity for the researcher to fill in the holes and details that were not possible to record in the field. For example, the condensed version of my field notes in a study that looked at volunteering might have included the following key words or phrases:

Brick building/nice out front/ugly out back/Fancy interior, especially by reception. Small 4 x 6 lobby/Library way at the back. Fancy decor.

In the expanded version of the notes, the fieldwork session might read as:

At 9:00 a.m., I approached the addictions building which is located in the west end of town, in close proximity to the downtown sector. The building is a two-story, red brick building and has two entrances: The first a beautiful steel, storm door with print curtains and a sign which reads "Break-Free Addictions Services"; the other, a back entrance which has a plain black and white sign which reads

"Women's Detox." As I entered the building, I noted that there was an extra steel door separating the entrance and the main reception lobby. Also, there was a Plexiglas wall partition separating the lobby from the receptionist. I had to stand on my toes in order to announce my arrival and ask for directions through a small round hole in the Plexiglas. In the small 4' by 6' lobby directly inside the front door to the right of the reception, there were two chairs, separated by a low coffee table on which were several magazines and pamphlets describing addictions services provided by the Break-Free clinic. The interior decor was set in peach and rose hues, with many walls.

The role of the observer requires one to come prepared. You will need paper, pencil (always better than a pen because it can be erased), and clipboard, which makes jotting down quick notes easier. If you are straightforward in declaring your role as an observer, then most places will be comfortable about letting you write notes. If not, you might keep either a miniature dictating machine or journal notepad in the car and speak or write as quickly as possible on exiting an observation session. I found the miniature dictating machine to be a good investment because I could never get all my thoughts down in writing as fast or efficiently as I could by speaking them into a microphone. I also found that I could not pay sufficient attention to the setting if I was always busy writing notes. The notetaking was distracting and got in the way of establishing and developing field relations. Writing a lot of notes can be equally intrusive in conducting in-depth interviews. People get distracted with notetaking and become curious about the notes. Even though, if I got stuck in an interview, I could refer to my notes to get back on track, I never felt terribly comfortable writing my notes in front of others. My personal prefer-

ence is audiotaping, then later transcribing the audiotape and adding my personal reflections on the computer.

Always date your notes and include the times you entered and exited the setting, the location and address of the research setting, and the full names and titles of all personal contacts. You will need this for accurate and trustworthy findings. I also carry business cards with me so that people in the setting know that I have a legitimate affiliation, and I take their business cards when these people offer them.

"Grand Tour" Positioning and Observations

On entering the setting, the observer should first conduct a general observation of the setting and the people in the setting. General observations involve a great deal of looking and listening. Do not go in to the setting looking for anything in particular on the first round. It is surprising what you can learn when you are not looking for anything in particular. Good observation also lends itself to other questions to ask once you are further immersed in the setting. For example, in the volunteer study, I came out of the grand tour observation wanting to ask why the library was located in the back of the building with limited access. I also wanted to ask why John felt that he had to conceal information about his schizophrenia in a mental health and addictions clinic.

General observation and documentation might later yield clues that can help explain certain findings derived from other sources. Conducting a general grand tour (Spradley, 1979) of the setting and the people helps the observer to be able to describe the setting in sufficient detail for later documentation and also for verifying the dependability of the research by providing a thick description of methods. Once a general overview of the setting has been documented, the observer can go back and focus in on one or two areas within the setting for the purposes of the study. The reader is referred to either Spradley's (1979, 1980) The Ethnographic Interview or Participant Observation for a good description of conducting grand tour observations of the setting.

Grand Tour Questions

A grand tour question is a question that seeks to gain large amounts of information about a particular cultural scene. Spradley (1979) identified four types of grand tour questions: typical grand tour questions, specific grand tour questions, guided grand tour questions, and task-related grand tour questions. Typical grand tour questions "ask the informant to generalize, to talk about a pattern of events" (p. 87). A typical grand tour question might be, "Can you tell me a bit about a typical day's activities for you?" A specific grand tour question asks information about a recent series of events or recent day. An example of a specific grand tour question would be, "Can you tell me a bit about how you spent your time at the clubhouse yesterday afternoon?" A guided grand tour question asks the informant to actually give a grand tour. An example is, "Can you show me around the addictions service and the library where you work?" Finally, a task-related grand tour question asks the informant to perform some simple task, such as making a diagram, that aids in the description of the setting of study. An example might be, "Can you draw me a map of the inside of the addictions building to help explain to me what it is like?"

Steps in the Observations

In this particular study, I made a point to first observe the setting and then John's actual volunteer experience on my second and sub-sequent visits. During the first visit, I spent fewer than 30 minutes with John and asked a lot of questions about the service and the physical environment. In particular, I asked who he worked with, who his supervisor was, and with whom he primarily interacted. I also asked practical questions about hours of operation, his hours of work, and his own schedule of volunteering. Any and all questions applied at this point because I didn't know what might prove to be important later during data analysis and write-up.

Following my grand tour observation of the addictions building, I decided for the next visit to spend some time with John in his personal workspace and gain an appreciation for this space relative to the larger environment. I spent the next few visits with John in the cramped library where he volunteered. For the purposes of this observational phase, I watched John perform his volunteer duties and asked only clarifying questions about what he was doing along the way. Although I was participating more at this point, I was still primarily interested in asking questions about what I saw, noticed, and observed in the setting. The interview would come later, and I could ask clarifying questions to alleviate any confusion I might be experiencing at that time.

The published results of this study are included in Part IV, Qualitative Research Studies of Occupation, Occupational Therapists, and Client Experiences, of this book.

A Research Process Example: The Women's Group

This exploratory study sought to understand the experience of occupational engagement from the perspectives of women with a mental illness who participated in a weekly, occupation-based mental health group. The original research design for this study planned to complement eight to ten in-depth interviews with audiotaping of the group in action. To this day, I am not sure what I was thinking when I thought of this strategy. I initially believed that audiotaping would be a respectful adjunct to the research process and that audiotaping would lend itself to greater honesty and sharing within the group. However, as the study began to unfold, two issues arose that required changes to the original design. First, the women would not consent to the group being audiotaped. Second, my recruitment of interview participants was becoming limited. Although I knew some of the participants in the group, many of the participants allegedly did not trust me due to my previous status as the director of rehabilitation. My suggestion of audiotaping the group seemed to heighten their distrust of the research process and of me.

This was my inaugural research project, and I was panicking. I had carefully planned the timing of data gathering for the spring and summer in order to spend the fall of that year in data analysis and write-up of my thesis. Without volunteers for the interviews, I would be short the required number of interviews for my thesis study. My academic preparation to conduct research did not prepare me for this, nor did it inform me as to what I should do if informants would not talk to me. From my reading, I learned that I needed to spend time in advance to ensure access and an informant pool; this, however, was of no use to me now. I decided to ask the few members of the group who had agreed to be interviewed about what I should do. They suggested that I should join the group for the summer. I had not considered participating in the group. I had intended to observe from a distance. I had not heard of participant observation at this point. My advisor had to put a name to it for my benefit.

Participant observation, although not

planned in the study design, proved to be my saving grace during this project. I suppose another reason why I had not considered being a participant in the group at the start of the research project was because I felt that in order to be a "real" researcher, I had to keep my distanced, observational stance apart from the group and take my requisite copious notes. It is worth emphasizing that this was my inaugural research project and with it came the pressures of it being my master's thesis. I wanted to not only pass this aspect of graduate school, but also to excel in it. My greenness is evident in how I originally designed the study. My naivete became even more profound as I immersed myself in the field and began to encounter problem after problem in the research process.

When I contacted my thesis advisor, she was thrilled that the members had suggested that I participate in the group. It was then that I learned there was actually a method called participant observation. She referred me to several texts, and I went about learning all that I could about this method prior to my anticipated start in the women's group. I did not know at that time how much I would learn on that personal research journey, nor how that experience would forever shape my future research endeavors and career path as an occupational therapist. Not only were the observations and comments from the group members instrumental to gaining a more indepth understanding of occupational engagement, but my own occupational engagement experiences also came to bear on the insights generated in the study.

Thus, participant observation, although not planned, was suggested and agreed on as an alternate data collection strategy. According to Jorgenson (1989), "the more information you have about something from multiple standpoints and sources, the less likely you are to misconstrue it" (p. 53). Participant observation occurred for a period of nine weeks from July 24, 1996, until September 25, 1996. Several of the members who were initially reluctant to participate in an interview subsequently agreed to be interviewed based on their exposure to my involvement in the group. This reaction is supported in the literature by Jorgenson (1989) who writes, "[P]erhaps the most important initial task of the overt participant in seeking to establish field relations is to overcome people's prejudices about you and the research" (p. 74). As one informant, Joan, stated, "[O]nce we knew you were a friend and not someone who was superior to us, that made all the difference in the world to me. Then I wanted to help you out." Jorgenson (1989) suggests that "the most effective general strategy for solidifying sympathetic field relations is to engage in joint activities" (p. 77). Participant observation occurred concurrently with the interviewing and data analysis processes, and although they were designed as distinct phases, they were overlapping and supportive of each other as the "insider's world of meaning" emerged.

Overall, I was involved with the women's group for a total of 25 weeks—16 weeks as a nonparticipant observer and 9 weeks as a participant. In those 9 weeks, I participated fully in many of the activities of the group. I made a trip to the White Rose crafts store to select something to do, which was difficult as I was not a craftsperson. I chose a cross-stitch bookmark, which I thought I could manage and also complete within a few weeks. I did not know on entering the participant observation phase of the research how long I would want to or need to participate in the group or how long the group would tolerate my presence. I went into the participant role feeling quite nervous but determined to learn something from the experience.

I had mixed feelings in the first few groups. First, I was not a craftsperson, and from what I had observed, the women's group did a lot of crafts. The women's group, although initially conceived to work on a large needlepoint quilt to be raffled for funds to keep the group going, had evolved into more "arts and crafts" where individual members worked on projects of their own choosing. I was definitely not a supporter of arts and crafts either in my personal or professional life. Actually, I hated the thought of doing any crafts and suffered tremendously over what in fact I might do in the group. Little did I know at the time that it did not really matter what I worked on because I would receive the needed assistance and support from the women to be successful. As a researcher, I would be learning regardless of the occupations on which I chose to work.

Second, I was unsure how to act, although to my advantage, I did know some of the women and decided that my pathetic level of skill in crafts was my edge with the group. Third, I was not intimately knowledgeable of participant observation as a research method, and I was always worried that I was not doing it correctly. I did not know at that time that just being myself and being respectful would be a good basis for being a participant observer. I spent the first few sessions focusing on my own project and just listening to the group discussions because I was so self-conscious. In particular, I tried to tune into the women whom I did not know and began to notice that things that had been described during the interviews were being confirmed for me by being a participant in the group. However, despite my good intentions of remaining somewhat removed from the group as an objective researcher, I gradually found myself feeling a part of the group and being treated like another group member, one that they obviously had great pity for due to my sad attempts at crafts.

Being a Participant Observer: The Researcher's Experience

The following passages are excerpts taken directly from my field notes and my written reflections on the women's group study. They will help the reader begin to understand my experiences, my mistakes, and how I learned from them. They will also allow the reader to identify when insights were learned and how I gradually merged into the culture and world of the women's group for a short but important period in my life.

Field Notes/Reflections: July 24, 1996

Today I began participant observation with the women's group. I was without a doubt anxious about starting, mainly because I was unsure about how each of the women felt about it. Specifically, I was certain that at least two of the women would boycott the group due to my presence. If that occurred, I would need to consider if ethically I had a place or a right to be there. I certainly did not want members missing group because I was there. Thankfully, the individual who has been most vocally opposed to this research project attended. I suspect that she showed up just to keep an eye on me. I felt very uncomfortable in the group today.

In trying to be a member, I do not know how successful I was at observing today. I did notice that everyone interacted fairly freely with each other. There did not appear to be any two people who dominated the group or any particular conversation. Those of us closest to each other tended to casually chat more often.

In general, the group interacted pretty much as I had remembered from my past experience with it. I guess time will tell how my presence influences what is said and done in the group. In particular, I want to be aware of nonverbals during the doing. Today, the doing was definitely the common focus

of the group with some casual chatting. Everyone's attention and energy were expended on learning the craft, doing the craft, and sharing materials and advice. How the doing contributes to the success of the group and what individuals get from this experience are still to be determined. Goffman's (1963) concept of "the own" rang true today, for there certainly was a level of comfort among the members. I think the comfort level contributed to the cooperation and interaction of the group. Time will tell, I suppose.

Field Notes/Reflections: July 31, 1996

Driving 500 km from our camp to attend the group, I arrived 10 minutes late. This was OK, since I did not want to appear too anxious or arrive early to each group. All members, except Jane, had arrived by this time, including Kay whom I met and chatted with casually about the blueberry season. Kay is the member who was reluctant to talk with me on the telephone, and I made the decision to wait it out with her instead of pressing for an interview. As it turns out, Kay went out for a cigarette, and I decided to go as well on the chance that I could chat with her. Another member, Jane, also went out for a cigarette but went in before Kay and I did. I apologized to Kay for calling her at home at what appeared to be a bad time, and she stated that she has not been doing well and had gone off her antidepressant. I told her that the interview was strictly voluntary, but that I would like to interview her about her experience in the women's group. She stated that it was best put on hold for now, and I stated that I would contact her in September. Kay went on to share some of her difficulties and how upsetting this has been for her. She also stated that she plans to resume her antidepressants. We left the discussion at that.

I do not remember how it came up, but Edith asked me if I had managed to get a nanny. I responded no and went on to share with the group the difficulties that I had in securing a reliable child care person this past year. Jane stated that she does not know how I have managed it all. In sharing the details of criminal activity of one of our baby-sitters, I felt a great deal of empathy and support from Julie, Edith, and Joan in particular. As I was driving home, I thought to myself that those women showed more empathy than a lot of therapists and physicians I have known. I understand a bit now how the support they feel in this group is important, even though I am not one of "the own." It truly felt nice to be able to share in the group, to take part, and to feel at this point that I am a part of the whole thing. Whether I in fact was, time will tell.

This week, I felt more a part of the group for a several reasons. One, I did not appear to be the focus of attention or such a novelty anymore. This occurred more quickly than I had thought it would. Second, I had the opportunity to give to others {the ribbon, assistance to Edith with her glueing, and the offer of the wedding dress to Julie) and also to take part and share a little of myself and my struggles with day care and juggling the master's program. I got the feeling that these revelations were important, especially for those who do not know me, to reveal that I am not perfect and have my own difficulties. We shared not so much as a researcher and women with chronic mental health problems but as women. It makes me wonder if the uniqueness that the women ascribe to this group has two domains of shared, common experiences—one of mental health problems and one of being women. It is something to think about.

It was a very comfortable experience today, despite my initial anxiety and reservations about participating. In my opinion, the group was not long enough and time passed far too quickly. I could easily have stayed another hour and continued either chatting

or working on my cross-stitch. The cross-stitch did not feel very rewarding to me. I liked it a lot better when I was able to finish a project and look at what I had done. I put the doll that I had made in the group (in a previous session) on the dash of my car, and as I looked at it, I felt somewhat pleased with myself.

I think it takes time to find out what makes you feel good, both short-term and long-term, and perhaps to discover what is personally meaningful for yourself. It makes me cringe to think about some comments from previous interviews and how clients felt when the OT gave them projects to increase their concentration, or whatever, and they were not at all interested in those projects. Maybe I feel the same way about this cross-stitch. I just want to finish it. I do not really feel a whole lot of joy doing it, but then again, I am half-attending to it and trying hard to be a good observer within the group at the same time. But seriously, this cross-stitch is boring me to death and killing me slowly!

Field Notes/Reflections: August 14, 1996

I arrived at group on time this week. On the way, I was worrying and thinking about my own family. I mused on all of this prior to group and, interestingly, did not think about it again until I was driving home after group. This confirms what others have said about no worries and the diversion from problems that the group seems to provide for its members. This is interesting.

I asked Anne if she has always done so many crafts, even when she worked full-time, and she said yes. I asked her why, and she said she has always done it. Margaret scooted over in her seat, and I thought this might be an opportunity to find something out from the two of them. I asked, "Can you guys tell me if accomplishing a project or a sense of accomplishment is related to the degree of challenge of the project?" Margaret said not for her. It was more a matter of completing it or finishing the project that contributed to her sense of accomplishing something. I asked, "Do you keep what you make?" Both answered no, they usually make things for other people. I asked why— and whether they had kept anything. Anne stated that she had kept one wall hanging because she had made it to match her home. I asked, "Did it feel any different making something for yourself versus making something for someone else?" She did not think so. I asked if making something that was a challenge versus something easy was a different experience. Both felt that the doing and accomplishing or completion was important to feeling accomplished, but they had not thought much about whether the challenge of the occupation was important. They would have to think about it. They both have always done things. I wanted to ask if it was more important since both were presently unemployed, but I did not because the conversation was feeling like an interrogation. I do not want to confuse my role here but probably already have.

Jane stated that she wanted to go for a smoke. It was 11:20. I said I would go with her and asked Joan if she wanted to come. She said yes. We went out and sat at the picnic table, and Joan immediately asked me how things were going with my research and whether I still had a job here. I stated that it was going slowly and I needed to finish the participant observation aspect of the research and three more interviews. She asked about what was involved in the interview, and I turned to Jane and said, "Ask Jane; she has been interviewed." Jane described how she perceived the interview as my tapping different perspectives about the group. I added that I was less interested in the group than in the occupational experience provided by the group. I told her what some of the informants stated, particularly about challenge and accomplishment. Joan

agreed that a challenge did seem important to the process of accomplishment. Joan asked if the interview would take a long time, and I said about two hours or so. She asked where this would occur, and I said wherever she wanted, at her home or at my office after the group. Joan stated that she would think about it. I said I would appreciate it as I wanted to know her perspective since she has been a long-standing group member. I stated that I could access past members but did not feel that they could provide as much insight about occupational engagement as the present members. Joan agreed. She added, "When this all started I was against it, you know. I don't know you very well, and I wouldn't talk openly with you. But since you've attended group, I trust you more and know you better, and I feel better about it. If you interviewed me before, I would have talked in general terms." I thanked her and acknowledged that I had made a few mistakes with the design and introduction of the research to the group. I explained that I would also do a member check in October to make sure that what I heard and understood from the interviews was correct in the group's opinion. Joan stated that she thought that was a good idea.

I felt joyous and absolutely pleased with myself. I was certain that Joan had enough information about the interview and trust in me that she would follow through and consent to be interviewed. Margaret asked Jane if she wanted some wool that was donated to the group by a friend of hers, and she dumped the contents of a bag on the table. Joan sorted through the wool and decided that she did not like any of it. Margaret explained that they have a relationship with this lady. If they give her stuff, she gives something back to donate to the hospital. If she gives them something, they give her something back in return—another aspect of the acts of reciprocity within the group of which I was unaware.

Field Notes/Reflections: August 21, 1996

This week the group was very busy making knickknack shelves, and I openly complained about how quickly the time went by and how it was not long enough for me to get done what I wanted to get done. I arrived early, and Margaret was already there. I had collected two bags of pine cones at the camp with my youngest son, and I put my offering on the table. I also offered some acorns that my eldest son had picked, as well as the small toys I collected from the bottom of our toy box in anticipation of the shelving units we were to make today. I thought to myself, only after the group, that the doing and planning for the doing gets all of us out of the house and doing other things to contribute to the various projects. The women do not just participate in the group but go to the malls, dollars stores, and various craft shops in addition to looking and searching at home for the various things that are needed or things that could be used by the group on projects.

It is interesting to see how I have become quite involved in the doing aspects of the group. The doing does not only occur in the group but before and after in anticipation of the doing. Occupation-as-means to other doing is somewhat like a spin-off of occupations. For myself, this week, I realized how I became involved in the doing outside of the group. I wanted to be able to give something to the group, to contribute. This was not something that was suggested to me or asked of me, but rather something that I just wanted to do. I am not sure if I wanted to do this to feel more like a member or to ensure fairness of the giving they have done for me—that is, reciprocity. I found myself thinking more of the group outside of the group and not with respect to the research, but more so about what we had planned to do the following week and about what I should bring or contribute.

I wonder how this planning and doing affects their sense of health or their sense of purpose. They say that without this group they would not likely get out of bed or do the other things in life that they are presently doing. For me at camp, it did give me something to do with Nicholas (picking the pine cones), and the picking was for a purpose (to contribute to the group). I did this so that my part in the group was equal and I was not just there taking from the members. It was a small token, but I felt better knowing that I also put something on the table.

As far as my involvement in the group, I was quite focused today. I did not anticipate the project to be hard, but perhaps the focus was because of the creativity involved in making my own unique shelf. I wanted it to be nice, and for this to happen, I had to put some thought into the design and colors and ornaments. The occupation required that of me. It also demanded that I pay attention to the samples that Margaret had made, search through the many ornaments placed on the table, and decide what to put on my shelf. I wonder how much this might challenge someone who was not feeling well. It certainly was a bit overstimulating for me. The activity and talking was quite high in the group today. As such, I needed to attend to my task in order to get done what I wanted to do in the group. So even though the project itself was not difficult, it was still a challenge for me to stay on task and progress through each of the steps. It is interesting how challenge for me does not necessarily mean difficult.

I am thinking about how this process and participation in the group are affecting me. I think I am more motivated to be a part of the group because of what I am learning from the members for my research. However, I am also motivated to be there to do something new and different from my daily routine. I definitely would not do these things on my own, but they are fun and a challenge. The people are nice, and I like the group. I am not sure exactly why I like it, but I do. This group gives me something to look forward to each week, something different to think about. Truly, during the group, I do not think about my thesis or family or any of the current worries I might be having. Time passes quickly for me during group, and I always leave thinking about what I will do next week. I think if I did not have anything to do in my life, this group could become very important to me as well. I think I am beginning to understand both the instrumental meaning and, somewhat, the emotional meaning that these ladies attach to the women's group.

Field Notes/Reflections: August 24, 1996

Really, I feel that I have very little to report today other than I announced that it was my last group. The members encouraged me to attend a few more so that I could make the Santa Claus with them. I will need to get busy and get my materials together so that I can be prepared. It was very easy for me to say OK and attend some more. I have the time, I like it, and I also seem to need a bit more time to work in those last interviews. Joan agreed to be interviewed today and asked that we not do it all in one shot, but for a one-half hour after each group until it is done. This might prove advantageous from a methods point of view in that I can try to member check with Joan each of the main ideas I think I have about the group doing to this point. I do not think that one-half hour will be realistic even then, but we will see.

Despite some talking, which is always present, the group again was totally focused on the various projects going on, sharing supplies and assistance. This appears to be the most accurate picture, as far as I can see, of what goes on in the women's group. It involves doing, and almost all of the activities are around or for the doing. I would think that it would be very boring if there were no activity and we sat there for two

hours and talked about our problems. I cannot imagine myself tolerating that for very long, and I wonder how long the group would last. It would also be very depressing to just talk about what is not right in their lives. With the activity, the members are automatically refocused on something they can control, do well, and accomplish. What a concept! Even if they are not directly participating, they are involved in the doing of others either by getting supplies for them, complimenting another's work, or offering technical or creative assistance. As I said before, the activity that occurs in this group is supported by various activities throughout the week and in between the groups. It is interesting. I know from my own experience that the activity was very important to my satisfaction from the group over time. It made time pass quickly and productively, and I had something to show for all of my efforts. I got recognition for my doing and the finished products. The tangible object made was proof of my efforts and confirmation of my capacity to do. The feedback from the members and from my daughter was the affirmation of the doing—that I was worthy and belonged and that my accomplishment meant something. I and it were of worth to someone!

I think that if one accomplishes something, the visible proof of one's efforts is important in confirming competence—"Gee, I can do it" or "I did it." Within the social context of a group of the own, not only is it safer to try and experiment with novel things, but also the very purpose of the group is doing and is in itself a reason to get out of the house and engage in various occupations. The initial feedback from the group provides one with the affirmation that encourages further doing or other attempts at doing that the occupation itself does not provide. This combined with positive affirmation from others perhaps secures that "feeling better" that keeps the occupational doing in motion or, rather, this idea of occupational spin-off.

Field Notes/Reflections: September 4, 1996

Although I did not know it at the time, this proved to be the last group that I attended as a participant observer. I made the decision after group that although I really liked being a group participant, I had learned a great deal at this point, and it was time to exit and allow the group to continue without me. But I could get used to this kind of support.

What I Learned from Participant Observation

There were many aspects of the group experience and, hence, occupational engagement that could not have been captured by interviews alone. Some of the issues raised in the interviews did not appear particularly relevant until these issues were considered within the context of the group experience, either through my own experience or by observing the group in action.

An important insight developed during participation as a group member was the importance of the social environment to the process of occupational engagement. The interrelatedness of reciprocity, of social feedback mechanisms in combination with feedback from the actual occupation, to the development of confidence and hope for the future became clear to me only as a result of my participation in the group. An understanding of how the social environment, "the own," and participation in occupations in this group contributed to "spin-off" (Rebeiro & Cook, 1999) developed through direct experience as a participant and by being accepted as a group member.

Finally, by being myself and sharing my own struggles (in group and in life), I became real to the participants and ultimately accepted. This acceptance resulted in the completion of the in-depth interviews and allowed me to understand the importance of

this group to the participants' mental health and well-being. Participant observation served as an important source of triangulation to the research project and confirmed, clarified, and expanded what I learned about the experience of occupational engagement from the interviewing process.

The results of this exploratory study generated three analytic themes and ten analytic categories that collectively reflect the experience of occupational engagement for members of the women's group. Some of the results were generated from nonparticipant observation and from participant observation. Some of the results were generated from the in-depth interviews with the members. However, most of the results were generated from both. That is, interview data were confirmed by or elaborated on by participant observation. Most certainly, I would not have gained an appreciation of how the participation in the group, which was not being articulated clearly in the interviews and was proving to be a great source of frustration to me in the research process, was related to the social environment. In the interviews, the women spoke eloquently and in great depth about the importance of the group members and how they cared about each other and supported one another through difficult times. These words only became real to me by experiencing this acceptance and support myself.

Occupational engagement was by no means an open process that could be described succinctly or directly. This perhaps explained the limited information gained in the initial interviews. This is not to say that important information was not obtained in those interviews, because it was. It is just that I did not understand the relationship between the doing and the social context of that particular group. I did not understand what the members meant when they kept telling me that it was the people who made the experience. After all, I was seeking to better understand the experience of doing. Nor did I understand how the doing extended far beyond the actual craft project in which the members participated. It was only by directly participating that I came to understand their experience and the meaning of being a member of the women's group. Participant observation is an awesome adventure and one that I fully intend to continue well into the future.

References

Bogdan, R. C., & Biklen, S. K. (1992). *Qualitative research for education: An introduction to theory and methods* (2nd ed.). Boston: Allyn & Bacon.

Goffman, E. (1963). *Stigma: Notes on the management of spoiled identity*. New York: Simon & Schuster Inc.

Jorgenson, D. L. (1989). *Participant observation: A methodology for human studies*. Newbury Park, CA: Sage.

Lincoln, Y., & Guba, E. (1985). *Naturalistic inquiry*. Beverly Hills, CA: Sage.

McCracken, G. (1988). *The long interview*. Newbury Park, CA: Sage.

Patton, M. Q. (1990). *Qualitative evaluation and research methods* (2nd ed.). Newbury Park, CA: Sage.

Rebeiro, K. L., & Allen, J. (1998). Voluntarism as occupation. *Canadian Journal of Occupational Therapy, 65*(5), 279–285.

Rebeiro, K. L., & Cook, J. V. (1999). Opportunity, not prescription: An exploratory study of the experience of occupational engagement. *Canadian Journal of Occupational Therapy, 66*(4), 176–187.

Spradley, J. P. (1979). *The ethnographic interview*. New York: Holt, Rineholt & Winston.

Spradley, J. P. (1980). *Participant observation*. New York: Holt, Rineholt & Winston.

Stringer, E. T. (1996). *Action research: A handbook for practitioners*. Thousand Oaks, CA: Sage.

Whyte, W. F. (Ed.). (1991). *Participatory action research*. Newbury Park, CA: Sage.

Yerxa, E. (1991). Seeking a relevant, ethical and realistic way of knowing for occupational therapy. *American Journal of Occupational Therapy, 45*, 295–299.

CHAPTER

Focus Group Research

Deborah Corring, M.Sc., OT(C)

> *To appreciate the potential of focus groups as a social and behavioural science research technique, one must first appreciate the value of qualitative methods in general.*
>
> —Asbury, 1995, p. 419

This chapter on the focus group method begins with a set of assumptions about the reader. I have assumed that you (the reader) would never have picked up this book if you were not at least intrigued by the idea of qualitative research. I have assumed that previous chapters in this book on other qualitative methods have kept you sufficiently intrigued to read this chapter. I have also assumed that if I do not do a good job of convincing you that focus groups have incredible potential as a research tool in the social sciences, you will not continue reading this text. Not wanting to be the one responsible for such a decision on your part, let us see if I can intrigue you further.

In the next few pages, I will endeavor to provide you with a brief history of focus groups, a definition, some of the basics you need to know before conducting focus groups, a rationale for their use, and examples of how they can and have been used in research. In addition, I will discuss their limitations, ethical concerns, fit and relevance of their use for occupational therapists, and some thoughts regarding the future. Finally, I will share some personal experience with this approach to data collection.

History and Definition

The development of the focus group technique began with Bogardus when he first published a description of group interviews in 1926. Robert Merton and his colleagues are credited with further development of the technique when they used focused interviews to examine the persuasiveness of propaganda efforts during World War II and the effectiveness of training materials in the early to mid 1940s (Carey & Smith, 1994). Although focus groups have been used in research since then, relatively few studies were published before the late 1970s, and most of these were in the field of marketing (Wilkinson, 1998). Social scientists appear to have rediscovered focus groups in the last ten to fifteen years. Morgan (1996), in a review of on-line databases, notes that research using focus groups was appearing in academic journals at the rate of more than 100 articles per year after 1986. In 1987, several books were published on focus groups by marketers; several of these are now in second editions (Greenbaum, 1998; Templeton, 1994). In 1988, social science followed with the first publication of David Morgan's work on focus groups as well as a subsequent book by Kreuger (1994). Other books and articles have been written since then, and focus groups have become an increasingly well-known method for collecting qualitative data (Morgan, 1997). In addition, focus groups have obtained increasing acceptability within academic institutions and now are considered acceptable for dissertations and as part of course work (Kreuger, 1995).

Definitions of a "focus group" range from Morgan's (1997) broad definition that describes "focus groups as a research technique that collects data through group interaction on a topic determined by the researcher" (p. 6) and Wilkinson's (1998) simplification that describes a focus group as "an informal discussion among selected individuals about specific topics" (p. 330) to more detailed definitions such as Carey and Smith's (1994), which states that the focus group technique "uses a semi-structured group session, held in an informal setting, for the purpose of collecting information about a designated topic" (p. 124). And with yet another twist, Asbury (1995) describes focus groups as "a data collection technique that capitalizes on the interaction within a group to elicit rich

experiential data" (p. 414). Whatever the definition, authors agree that the unique factor in this data collection strategy is the use of the group approach to data collection.

The Basics

There is no "one right way" to do focus groups.   —Morgan, 1997, p. 72.

The preceding statement by David Morgan (1997), a social scientist with considerable knowledge and experience in the focus group technique, might lead one to think that this approach has no particular rigor. But, taken in the context within which he makes this statement, the reader is challenged to think of focus groups as more than specific skills used to moderate a group discussion. Focus groups, Morgan stresses, must be thought of in terms of an overall research design requiring carefully formulated goals, areas of inquiry, recruitment issues and strategies, and analytical strategies, in addition to skillful moderation of the group.

There are many details to consider and work through prior to conducting a focus group. The following will highlight those noted by several authors in the field.

Rules of Thumb

Focus group researchers, as a rule, most often: use homogeneous strangers as participants; use a relatively structured interview with high moderator involvement; have six to ten people in a group; and complete a total of three to five groups as part of the overall research project (Morgan, 1997). Effectiveness of a focus group interview, as Merton et al. (1990) suggest, includes four broad criteria. These criteria are the covering of a maximum range of relevant topics; promoting group interaction to explore feelings in depth; providing data as specific as possible; and accounting for the effect of participants' personal context in their responses to the topic. Halloran and Grimes (1995) include the following as key principles in conducting focus group research: the selection of a homogeneous group of participants; flexibility in the number of participants in a group and total number of groups; selection of a comfortable nonthreatening environment; investigators serving as group moderators; and the direction of the analysis of results following study objectives.

Morgan (1997) notes that, in reality, it is "relatively rare for a project to achieve all of these criteria" (p. 34). Given the need for the project to attend to the specifics of the situation presenting itself, researchers make changes accordingly. Let us explore six areas further—namely, recruitment of participants, determining the level of structure introduced to the group experience, size of groups, total number of focus groups, analysis and reporting of focus group results, and practical issues such as room preferences and audiotaping—to see why such adjustments might be made.

Recruitment of Participants

Newcomers to qualitative research must often shed their ideas of necessary procedures for recruitment of participants promoted by advocates of quantitative research. As Morgan (1997) states, "[I]n selecting participants for a focus group project, it is often more useful to think in terms of minimizing sample bias rather than achieving generalizability . . . such bias is a problem only if it is ignored . . ." (p. 35). Morgan continues to argue that the shift away from generalization and random sampling to "theoretically motivated sampling" is necessary because of the

small number of participants involved in most focus group projects and the unlikely event that a randomly sampled group could be said to have a shared perspective on the research topic essential to generate meaningful discussion.

The need for homogeneity of participants or carefully controlled choosing of participants is known as segmentation. Segmentation allows for easier discussion between participants (Morgan, 1997), as well as enhancing analysis of results and the likelihood of saturation of data (Carey, 1995; Morgan, 1997). Saturation of data will be discussed further when discussing total number of groups in a research project.

The question of whether participants should be strangers or acquaintances speaks to issues regarding what people will discuss or not discuss in the presence of strangers or people with whom they may have already erected invisible boundaries and understandings around some topics. Although Morgan (1997) notes the use of strangers as one of the four common rules of thumb for focus groups, he also recognizes that this is often not possible due to practical concerns. He suggests careful attention be paid to group dynamics and their potential effect on research objectives.

Other practical issues in recruitment of participants include ensuring that enough participants actually arrive to participate in the group and deciding on the need and potential benefits/disadvantages of providing payment for group participation. Further discussion of these issues can be found in the description of my personal experiences with focus groups later in this chapter.

Determining Level of Structure

Choosing the level of structure you wish to achieve in a group will affect the development of your interview guide and the level of moderator involvement to be used (Asbury, 1995; Morgan, 1997; Templeton, 1994). Generally, more structured group approaches are useful when there is a strong, preexisting agenda for the research, and less structured approaches are useful for exploratory research (Morgan, 1997). Always flexible though, Morgan also suggests a third option, the "funnel approach," which allows the researcher to begin with an open, unstructured approach and end with a tighter, more controlled approach. Templeton (1994) argues that less structure is desirable and more conducive to the focus group strategy; she believes that direct questioning results in emotional disengagement from the topic, promotes a one-on-one discussion as opposed to a group discussion and therefore does not permit issues to emerge spontaneously, and may cause participants to respond without the same level of introspection.

Development of a semistructured interview guide with probes can help focus a discussion (Asbury, 1995). An effective interview guide can result in a discussion that manages itself and maintains a balance between the researcher's objectives and the group's spontaneous areas of discussion (Morgan, 1997). Interview guides must be able to channel discussion and keep topics on target, while avoiding a rigid ordering of topics and allowing the moderator to explore issues more deeply where necessary (Morgan, 1997). Interview guides should be constructed to accommodate a discussion of approximately 90 minutes. For an unstructured group, this might mean just two broadly stated topics or questions. For a more structured group, four or five specific questions with preplanned probes under each question should be considered the upper limit (Morgan, 1997).

Obviously, time spent on development of the interview guide prior to the focus group can be critical to its eventual success and accomplishment of research objectives.

Interview guides may also have to be adjusted and refined as the research process evolves (Corring, 1996). As Morgan (1997) points out, "[I]f a moderator has to work hard to force attention to a topic or keep attention from shifting to another topic, this should be a warning that there is something out of synch between the guide and the participants' perspectives on the topic" (p. 48). An example of an interview guide and the researcher's experience with using it can be found in the personal example of this writer's focus group research later in this chapter.

Several authors describe in detail the role of the group moderator (Bogardus, 1926; Morgan, 1997; Smith, 1995; Templeton, 1994; Then, 1996). They all speak to the crucial importance of the moderator in setting the tone of the discussion; encouraging participation of all members; maintaining a delicate balance of being both a leader and participant; facilitating interaction between group members; validating, acknowledging, and encouraging expansion of ideas and issues; keeping the discussion on track; and bringing appropriate closure to the discussion while remaining sensitive to group member needs. They all agree that careful consideration must be given to selection of the moderator. Although often the moderator is the researcher, Then (1996) cautions that "familiarity between the moderator and the participants may inhibit disclosure" (p. 29), and the moderator cannot be seen to have authority or control over the participants. Lindsey and Stajduhur (1998), for example, while conducting focus groups as part of a feasibility study for a respite care community home for people with HIV/AIDS, acknowledged the different levels of need and comfort with various participants by having the nurse researchers conduct focus groups with physicians and other specialists, while street workers conducted the focus groups with the street-associated people. As can be seen later in the description of this writer's focus group research experience, careful attention was also paid to this issue when conducting focus groups with individuals who consider themselves survivors of serious mental illness.

Size of Groups and Total Number of Groups

The size of a focus group is another important factor to consider. Generally, the range of participants varies from as small as four to as many as twelve participants (Dilorio et al., 1994). There are advantages and disadvantages to both small and large groups, and broadly stated, the ideal number depends on the research objectives. Small groups may not provide enough diversity of opinion, while large groups may make it difficult for all individuals to participate and share (Then, 1996). The number Morgan (1997) suggests for the desired size is between six to ten, but he cautions that overrecruiting by 20 percent to offset the possibility of no-shows is a prudent thing to consider.

The factor that affects the researcher's determination of when enough focus groups have been conducted for a particular research project is that of saturation (Asbury, 1995; Morgan, 1997). Saturation occurs when the researcher can anticipate what will be said next, which usually takes place after three to four groups (Asbury, 1995). Morgan (1997) agrees that "saturation," the point at which additional data collection no longer generates new understanding, usually occurs after three to five groups, but he further qualifies attaining saturation by considering three factors— variability of participants, degree of interview structure, and availability of participants. Generally, he argues that the more heterogeneous the participants, the less structured the interview and the greater the difficulty in

accessing participants, resulting in more groups being required to reach saturation.

Analysis and Reporting of Results

Analysis begins during the focus group session (Henderson, 1995; Then, 1996). It continues after the group through review of the process, analysis of audiotapes/transcripts, debriefing with any observers, and review of the purposes and objectives of the study (Carey & Smith, 1994; Henderson, 1995; Then, 1996).

Interpretation is the hardest, yet the most rewarding, part of the project (Templeton, 1994, p. 73). Interestingly, several authors note that one of the most common mistakes in the analysis and reporting of focus groups is the absence of comment regarding the impact of the group interaction and setting (Asbury, 1995; Carey & Smith, 1994; Wilkinson, 1998). Wilkinson (1998), for example, reviewed over 200 articles looking for the reporting of group effect in focus group studies and found that it was rare to find an analysis of group interactions, and even fewer articles included data illustrating participant interactions. Wilkinson noted surprise, as interaction between participants is such an important feature of the method. As Asbury (1995) notes, the whole purpose and value of focus groups rests on the group interaction. To not incorporate this dimension of the data is to suggest that a different methodology should have been used in the first place (pp. 418–419). Carey and Smith (1994) suggest that the researcher must examine the data on three levels—the group level, the individual level, and at the comparison level of individual with group data. Other skills needed for interpreting and reporting qualitative data include an ability to organize large amounts of data into categories, pull key themes out of the data, and report both negative and positive findings in a useful way (Henderson, 1995). Asbury (1995) stress-es that you must not "treat qualitative data as if it were quantitative" (p. 417). Comments are not to be tallied, counted, or taken out of context. Quotations are used to illustrate findings and give depth to reporting.

As to issues of credibility, usefulness, reli-ability, and validity, one must consult other authors for details (DePoy & Gitlin, 1994; Lincoln & Guba, 1985), but suffice it to say that when properly used, focus groups have proven themselves to be an effective data col-lection method (Carey, 1995; Kreuger, 1994; Morgan, 1997).

Practical Issues

The physical location for the group needs to be comfortable and accessible to participants. It needs to be a "safe" place to express views, and issues such as size, light, acoustics, tem-perature, and seating arrangements need to be considered (Asbury, 1995; Then, 1996).

Rationales for Using Focus Groups

Bogardus (1926), the first author to report on the benefits of group interviewing, con-cluded that "group discussion brings out points that otherwise would remain obscure . . . data is brought to the surface that a per-sonal interview would not likely touch at all . . . creative group discussion is a superior technique" (pp. 373, 380). Focus group inter-views work because they "tap into human tendencies . . . they are helpful when insights, perceptions and explanations are more important than actual numbers" (Kreuger, 1994, p. 31).

Wilkinson (1998) further explains that focus groups generate "interactive data that results in enhanced disclosure, access to the participants' own language and concepts . . .

they are an ideal method for exploring peo-ple's own meanings and understandings of health and illness" (p. 329). In addition, Wilkinson notes this method is particularly useful for accessing the views of those who have been poorly served by traditional research. This, then, makes such persons a good match for researchers employing par-ticipatory action research techniques dis-cussed in Chapter 2 of this book.

Focus groups can be used for many pur-poses. Straw and Marks (1995) note the important role these groups played in pro-gram development research for a community agency serving retired persons. Straw and Smith (1995) note their usefulness in con-ducting needs assessment, instrument devel-opment, implementation assessments, outcome assessments, meaning of results, policy development, and message testing.

An on-line search (Morgan, 1996) identi-fied three basic uses of focus groups in social science research. They are used as a stand-alone research method, as a secondary method to support or enhance the primary method, and as part of a multimethod study. Focus groups can systematically review mul-tiple viewpoints, identify areas of potential unintended effect, add meaning to results, and be helpful in understanding unexpected results (Straw & Smith, 1995).

Examples of the Use of Focus Groups

In a literature review, Morgan (1996) found hundreds of citations referring to studies that have used focus groups to collect qualitative data. I have selected three health care related examples to share with you in order to illus-trate how focus groups can be used. A detailed description of my own experience with focus group research follows these examples.

Quine and Cameron (1995) set out to exam-ine the feasibility of using focus groups as a research method with individuals who are physically disabled and elderly (75+ years). Participants were female, current inpatients in a geriatric rehabilitation ward, and had no cognitive difficulties. After the usual procedures for informed consent were completed and permission to audiotape the session was received, participants were asked to discuss their reaction to a new protective appliance (a specially designed undergarment), their willingness to wear it, perceived problems, and suggestions for improvement. An interview protocol was used, membership was restricted to six per group, group length was planned for 30 to 45 minutes, and five focus groups were completed. After review, coding, and analysis of transcripts, researchers reported that participants generally enjoyed the opportunity to contribute their views, issues regarding the use of the appliance were clarified, and new issues were identified that would have been missed in an individual interview or survey. The conclusion of the study confirmed the usefulness of the focus group technique.

Seals et al. (1995) used focus groups to describe the range of social service concerns that were experienced by woman infected with HIV. Eight focus groups were conducted over an eight-month period involving a total of 46 women. Each group met for two hours in a setting conducive to open discussion and was led by one of two moderators trained by the research team. Informed consent and permission to audiotape were obtained, and participants were paid an honorarium. A semistructured interview guide was used. The first four groups focused on family and daily living issues, and the second four groups focused on spirituality and alternative health care. Participants were also asked to comment on a Barriers to Use of Community Resources Scale being developed by the research staff. Following the analysis of results, researchers concluded that service concerns identified by women in

the study were consistent with other studies but added greater detail to the issues and, therefore, increased understanding of the issues these women faced.

Finally, Moore (1996) used a focus group method to examine the perceptions and experiences of women participating in a cardiac rehabilitation program. Ten women near the age of 72 years participated in focus groups of six and four members. A convenience sample was used, and a semistructured interview guide developed. Groups were held on separate days, scheduled for two hours, and were held in a small, comfortable room at a local outpatient clinic. An experienced focus group interviewer used the interview guide that was designed to promote discussion of the participants' reasons for agreeing to participate in the program, likes and dislikes, and suggested changes. Results indicated that prior to participation, the women had no idea what to expect. The features of the program they liked most were feeling "safe" during exercise, having a peer group during rehabilitation, and the pleasant, encouraging staff. They expressed a desire for more social interaction during cardiac rehabilitation exercise sessions, emotional support from staff throughout recovery, and exercise options other than cycle or treadmill. The author concluded that the focus group format provided unique data about attitudes and experiences that could serve as an adjunct to other forms of data collection.

A Personal Experience of Focus Group Research

I have used or been involved with the use of focus groups to survey the perspectives of individuals with serious mental illness on several occasions. As part of my thesis research, I talked to individuals with serious mental illness about a client definition of client-centred care (Corring, 1996; Corring &

Cook, 1999). As part of a client satisfaction exercise at the mental health facility where I am employed, I ran focus groups with individuals who were attending an outpatient geriatric psychiatry day program in order to discuss their satisfaction with the services offered. As part of my own business venture, I coordinated focus groups with consumers/ survivors of serious mental illness and their family members to explore quality of life issues (Corring, 1998). Finally, I supervised a graduate student in her use of focus groups with individuals with serious mental illness to explore their perceptions and experiences with employment (Willis, 2000).

Each experience had its unique features worth presenting, but in the interests of brevity, I will concentrate on the first project noted. I will explain why focus groups were chosen as the preferred data collection strategy, the recruitment strategies employed, the considerations that were involved in the development of the interview guide and the selection of the focus group moderators, and the experience of the observer (myself) in the groups.

Rationale for Using Focus Groups as a Strategy

The lack of knowledge concerning the client perspective of client-centred care was the critical factor influencing the choice of pre–data collection strategy. As Marshall and Rossman (1989) note, qualitative techniques should be used in the initial phase of an investigation that is largely exploratory. If the goal of the investigation is to understand how two groups (professionals and clients) communicate with each other, strategies such as focus groups are a good initial approach (Crabtree & Miller, 1992). This is particularly true if no preexisting expert consensus exists, you suspect a potential gap between professionals and the target audience, and you

want to control for a power differential between participants and decisionmakers (Morgan, 1993). Since an extensive literature review regarding client-centred care and related topics revealed that there were no examples of a client definition of client-centred care in the literature, it seemed wise to use the focus group approach.

Recruitment Strategies

Participants in this study were adults with a history of serious mental illness and experience with the mental health service delivery system. A total of 17 individuals participated in three focus groups. A self-selected "snowball" sample of convenience was utilized. Participants were drawn from the membership of two consumer/survivor agencies, and all groups were conducted on-site at the agencies. Recruitment was accomplished through the efforts of the executive directors of the agencies, informal meetings with the membership, advertisements in the agency newsletter, and posted flyers.

Interview Guide and Selection of Moderators

A semistructured focus group interview guide was developed to explore client opinion and perspective. Four broad topic questions were chosen to explore what client-centred care meant to the clients and how they would describe it; what services centered around their needs would look like; what services help or hinder clients to achieve their goals in life; and what would be their number one priority in service delivery. Specific probes were used where necessary to expand the discussion. All of the questions in the interview guide were posed during the focus group discussions, although the order of the questions varied in response to the groups' preferences for discussion. Due to the high degree of interest in the questions, the probes were often not needed except to clarify information discussed.

The selection of focus group moderators required special attention. Morgan (1993) suggests that when members of a focus group are part of a distinct culture, someone with the appropriate sensitivity and familiarity with the participants' point of view may be more effective than someone with professional credentials. Individuals involved with mental health consumer/survivor agencies can be said to be part of a distinct culture. In addition, the researcher was concerned about any effect she might have as a known service provider with the consumers involved as participants. Consequently, two individuals who were both self-identified mental health clients were used as group moderators. They both had experience in mental health self-help and advocacy services and possessed well-developed communication skills.

The Observer Experience

The researcher made a decision from the outset of this project to act as an observer rather than a moderator in the focus groups for the reasons noted previously. The role of observer allowed the researcher to experience the emotional atmosphere of the groups: warmth, tears, friendship, support, laughter, and deep sense of caring and commitment toward each other and to promoting change.

Initially, clients in the first focus group had considerable difficulty in focusing on the characteristics of client-centred care. Each one talked extensively of his or her past experience with mental illness, hospitalization, and professionals and his or her thoughts concerning the causes of his or her illness. Other group members listened patiently, providing support when necessary by holding a hand or putting an arm around a shoulder.

Individuals were often brought to tears as they remembered particularly painful incidents. One member remarked that she had never known until the day in the focus group that others also had a history of sexual and physical abuse. These people had known each other for some time, had spent hours together at the agency, but had not shared such personal detail. There was an accepting atmosphere in that group that day that somehow allowed them to share very personal stories. It was not an intended result but happened spontaneously. The moderators, with great sensitivity, allowed each person time to tell his or her story, and they too provided positive words of support. As they were able to, they pulled participants back to the topic at hand. They were responding to the message that was given by each of the participants that professionals never take the time to listen. The group took an hour and a half longer than scheduled, but no one seemed to mind. It seemed to be important to the moderators and group members not to repeat the same mistake as the unhearing professionals. The group ended on a positive note, and many expressed gratitude for the opportunity to talk. As the researcher, I was left with a feeling of shame that I had been part of such an uncaring health facility and had done so little to challenge the practices that participants had described. However, I was concerned that the specific criteria of client-centred care had not been discussed.

The second focus group brought new experiences. Participants did not have difficulty focusing on the topic at hand—client-centred care. As they discussed the existing problems with the service delivery system in the community, several participants became very energized and vehement concerning what was unacceptable and what had to change. Occasionally a participant would stop, apparently realizing that he or she had spoken very negatively about service providers, and wanting not to insult me, he or she would remark that I was different from the others. I was again left with a feeling of shame that, although I did not believe that I had personally behaved in the way participants had described, I had done very little to advocate for change.

The third group was again unique. The participants had all known each other for a considerable time and joked before the group began that they would have to support each other to get through this experience. The participants appeared somewhat anxious but eager to begin. They focused quickly on the topic. Participants took turns, each respectful of the others' opinions. When a participant spoke with a hint of anger in his or her voice when reciting a past experience with a professional, other participants demonstrated immediate support by acknowledging the anger with examples from their own past. When a participant was tearful while relating past experiences, other participants were quick to offer words of support. One member of the group was particularly articulate and insightful. He was adept at acknowledging others' contributions and adding depth to their comments with his own words. Other members responded warmly to his support and often voiced their admiration of his ability to express issues that were of importance to all of them. The sense of friendship and support was warming to me as an observer and left me with a sense that the determination for change expressed by the participants would most certainly produce results.

The three focus groups left lasting impressions on me. The participants' stories of their past experiences touched the heart and, as noted previously, left me with a sense of shame. The participants' sensitive support of their peers in time of need was full of warmth and sincere caring that perhaps only those who have known suffering could provide. The participants' sense of determination for

change left me with a deep respect and admiration for this group of people.

Limitations and Common Mistakes

All good things have limitations, and so one must consider not only the benefits but also the possible limitations of any strategy. As noted previously, there are numerous logistics problems that require attention. The physical environment must be one that promotes and encourages conversation, participants may be difficult to recruit, and homogeneity of the group may be difficult to ensure (Kreuger, 1994; Morgan, 1995; Then, 1996). A fundamental mistake might occur if one is attempting to use focus groups to meet objectives that are not possible in light of their capabilities and may scuttle a project from the start (Greenbaum, 1998).

Once one is sure that the logistics have been dealt with adequately and that it is the appropriate strategy to use, the researcher must then worry about asking the right questions, moderating the groups effectively, and ensuring accurate analysis (Greenbaum, 1998; Morgan, 1995). Such issues as maintaining sufficient "control" of the discussion, accounting for moderator influence, and the group's possible tendencies toward conformity and polarization need to be attended to in order to prepare for analysis of results (Morgan, 1997).

Lastly, one must be sure that one is clear on the distinction between focus groups and groups conducted to achieve clinical objectives. Focus groups require that moderators have an appreciation of group dynamics and how they might impact results. Individuals with clinical experience often have such skills but must be reminded that the objective of the exercise is data collection, not the creation of a therapeutic environment (Straw & Smith,

1995). Similarly, the objective is not to reach consensus, as focus groups are intended to pay attention to perceptions, feelings, and values as they pertain to the research question at hand (Kreuger, 1994).

Ethics

One cannot leave any discussion concerned with research of the human experience, especially with the possibility of involving those considered as vulnerable, without contemplating the potential ethical issues one might encounter. One of the more obvious potential trouble spots is the frequent use of "incentives" by researchers to encourage participants to engage in the group process (Then, 1996). Typically, these are not expensive items and include such things as the provision of refreshments or small gifts as tokens of appreciation. I have used honorariums of a small amount to recognize the value of the participants' input and offset any expenses they might incur by being part of the process. Clearly one must be sure that such incentives are used to facilitate and not to coerce.

The usual requirements of informed consent need to be attended to, but the issue of confidentiality has increased complexity because of the group environment. As Smith (1995) notes, the possibility of overdisclosure of personal information and, consequently, personal privacy must be recognized and appropriately managed. In addition, Smith underlines the need for the researcher to do some thinking about how he or she might respond to legally reportable incidents, such as child abuse, if they are discussed in the group. Techniques such as ensuring closure and debriefing participants at the end of the group are suggested for dealing with these types of concerns (Morgan, 1997; Smith, 1995; Then, 1996).

Fit and Relevance with Occupational Therapy

The fit and relevance of the focus group strategy with occupational therapy and occupational therapists almost seems too obvious to mention. Not wanting to be accused of either academic laziness or stating the obvious, I cite the following. In the "Joint Position Statement on Evidence-Based Occupational Therapy" by the Canadian Association of Occupational Therapists (CAOT), the Association of Canadian Occupational Therapy University Programs (ACOTUP), the Association of Canadian Occupational Therapy Regulatory Organizations (ACOTRO), and the Presidents' Advisory Committee (PAC) representing the provincial professional associations (see CAOT et al., 1999), it was clearly stated that "[T]he client provides expert knowledge crucial for determining occupational priorities. The client's perspective on medical, developmental, and social barriers to occupational performance is included as important information for understanding and taking action on issues. Also important are the client's subjective evaluation of present capacities, knowledge of personal and environmental resources and limitations, desired outcomes, acceptability of specific plans and criteria for success" (p. 267).

Clearly, this approach to information gathering for evidence-based practice fits with a research strategy such as the use of focus groups to examine the perspective, meaning, and values of those affected by the service. The education, professional training, and experience in conducting groups dealing with individuals with disabilities in client-centred care service delivery, and in a professional philosophy that promotes empowerment for individuals supports the conclusion that the fit between occupational therapists and focus groups as a research strategy is "natural."

The Future

Speculating on the future for focus groups was made easier for me by noting the comments of two noted authors regarding the use of focus group research in the social sciences, namely, David L. Morgan of Portland State University and Richard A. Kreuger of the University of Minnesota. Kreuger (1995) predicts more use of focus groups, more misuse of focus groups, increasing academic respectability for their use, increased collaboration between researchers and non-researchers in conducting focus groups, improved technologies to assist in analysis, and increased use of focus groups with individuals experiencing different cultures and life challenges. Morgan (1997) speaks to two challenges for the future—sharing the existing state of the art and advancing the state of the art. His first objective clearly requires information and experience sharing promoted to its maximum. His second, he states, will require increased attention to a systematic approach to research examining the effectiveness of the focus group method and advocating for a wider array of disciplines to become involved in conducting focus groups. I hope that occupational therapists will be active in that involvement.

References

Asbury, J. E. (1995). Overview of focus group research. *Qualitative Health Research, 5*(4), 414–419.

Bogardus, E. S. (1926). The group interview. *Journal of Applied Sociology, 10,* 372–382.

CAOT, ACOTUP, ACOTRO, & PAC. (1999). Joint position statement on evidence-based occupational therapy. *Canadian Journal of Occupational Therapy, 66*(5), 267–269.

Carey, M. A. (1995). Concerns in the analysis of focus group data. *Qualitative Health Research, 5*(4), 487–495.

Carey, M. A., & Smith, M. W. (1994). Capturing the group effect in focus groups: A special concern in analysis. *Qualitative Health Research, 4*(1), 123–127.

Corring, D. J. (1996). *Client-centred care means I am a valued human being.* Unpublished master's thesis, The University of Western Ontario, Canada.

Corring, D. J. (1998). *A report on quality of life issues.* London, Ontario: Client Perspectives.

Corring, D. J., & Cook, J. V. (1999). Client-centred care means I am a valued human being. *Canadian Journal of Occupational Therapy, 66*(2), 71–82.

Crabtree, B. F., & Miller, W. L. (Eds.). (1992). *Doing qualitative research.* Newbury Park, CA: Sage.

DePoy, E., & Gitlin, L. N. (1994). *Introduction to research: Multiple strategies for health and human services.* St. Louis, MO: Mosby.

Dilorio, C., Hockenberry-Eaton, M., Mailbeck, E., & Rivers, T. (1994). Focus groups: An interview method for nursing research. *Journal of Neuroscience Nursing, 26*(3), 175–180.

Greenbaum, T. L. (1998). *The handbook for focus group research* (2nd ed.). Thousand Oaks, CA: Sage.

Halloran, J. P., & Grimes, D. E. (1995). Application of the focus group methodology to educational program development. *Qualitative Health Research, 5*(4), 444–453.

Henderson, N. R. (1995). A practiced approach to analyzing and reporting focus group studies: Lessons from qualitative market research. *Qualitative Health Research, 5*(4), 463–477.

Kreuger, R. A. (1994). *Focus groups: A practical guide for applied research* (2nd ed.). Thousand Oaks, CA: Sage.

Kreuger, R. A. (1995). The future of focus groups. *Qualitative Health Research, 5*(4), 524–530.

Lincoln, Y. S., & Guba, E. G. (1985). *Naturalistic inquiry.* Newbury Park, CA: Sage.

Lindsey, E., & Stajduhar, K. (1998). From rhetoric to action: Establishing community participation in AIDS-related research. *Canadian Journal of Nursing Research, 30*(1), 137–152.

Marshall, C., & Rossman, G. B. (1989). *Designing qualitative research.* Newbury Park, CA: Sage.

Merton, R. K., Fiske, M., & Kendell, P. L. (1990). *The focused interview* (2nd ed.). New York: Free Press.

Moore, S. M. (1996). Women's views of cardiac rehabilitation programs. *Journal of Cardiopulmonary Rehabilitation, 16,* 123–129.

Morgan, D. L. (1988). *Focus groups as qualitative research.* Newbury Park, CA: Sage.

Morgan, D. L. (1993). *Successful focus groups: Advancing the state of the art.* Newbury Park, CA: Sage.

Morgan, D. L. (1995). Why things (sometimes) go wrong in focus groups. *Qualitative Health Research, 5*(4), 516–523.

Morgan, D. L. (1996). Focus groups. In J. Hagan & K. S. Cook (eds.), *Annual review of sociology* (Vol. 22, pp. 129–152). Palo Alto, CA: Annual Reviews.

Morgan, D. L. (1997). *Focus groups as qualitative research,* (2nd ed.). Newbury Park, CA: Sage.

Quine, S., & Cameron, I. (1995). The use of focus groups with the disabled elderly. *Qualitative Health Research, 5*(4), 454–462.

Seals, B. F., Sowell, R. L., Demi, A. S., Moneyham, L., Cohen, L., & Gillory, J. (1995). Falling through the cracks: Social service concerns of women infected with HIV. *Qualitative Health Research, 5*(4), 496–515.

Smith, M. W. (1995). Ethics in focus groups: A few concerns. *Qualitative Health Research, 5*(4), 478–486.

Straw, M. K., & Marks, K. (1995). Use of focus groups in program development. *Qualitative Health Research, 5*(4), 428–443.

Straw, R. B., & Smith, M. W. (1995). Potential uses of focus groups in federal policy and program evaluation studies. *Qualitative Health Research, 5*(4), 421–427.

Templeton, J. F. (1994). *The focus group: A strategic guide to organizing, conducting and analyzing the focus group interview.* Chicago: Probus Publishing.

Then, K. L. (1996). Focus group research. *Canadian Journal of Cardiovascular Nursing, 7*(4), 27–31.

Wilkinson, S. (1998). Focus groups in health research—Exploring the meanings of health and illness. *Journal of Health Psychology, 3*(3), 329–348.

Willis, A. (2000). *The role of work for people with chronic mental illness.* Unpublished master's of clinical science thesis, The University of Western Ontario, Canada.

PART

Personal Research Journeys

One of the limitations of published reports of research studies is that so much of the "truth" of the experience of conducting the research is omitted. This is usually due to the page length restrictions in journals, but it is also due to the reluctance of researchers to "tell all" for fear of appearing unscientific or indecisive in conducting their studies. Everyone who does research has "stories" to tell of the ups and downs of the process. Researchers who use qualitative methods more often discuss the trials and tribulations, joys and sorrows, and errors and brilliant decisions in their longer monographs, full-length books, and sometimes in their master's or doctoral theses. It is one of the valuable hallmarks of qualitative inquiries that the research study "evolves" and "develops" and insights "emerge" from the analysis of data collected. Usually in published reports, some brief description of the "development," "evolution," or "emergent" analysis is provided. Rarely, is one able to read about the subjective perspective of the experience by the author. Another limitation of journal articles is that, again due to limits on length, one seldom reads descriptions of how a single reported study fits with the researcher's overall research purpose and program of inquiries.

Part III includes several personal, subjective perspectives on the experiences of researchers. In keeping with qualitative tradition, they are written using the first person singular pronoun "I." They provide the reader with the kind of "tales of the field" (VanMaanen, 1988) that are often discussed with colleagues or in graduate methods seminars but are less often seen in print. The contributors to this text all agreed in discussions about the contents of this book that these types of stories are important.

Three of the personal journeys (MacGregor, Landry, and Nagle) are descriptions of certain aspects of the initial thesis research study undertaken as a graduate student. They illustrate the uncertainties, growing confidence, setbacks, personal pain, and ultimate satisfactions of pursuing qualitative research studies. The last two journeys (Segal and Rebeiro) describe how graduate study research evolved into an ongoing program of research. They provide a narrative of the way in which researching preliminary questions leads to more questions and motivates the researcher to use different strategies of inquiry and analysis.

All of the authors in this part discuss how they have been changed as professional clinicians, as researchers, and most of all as human beings due to their experiences of qualitatively exploring "occupation" with their research participants. We hope that students and novice researchers will identify with one or more of the accounts in this part of the text and realize that they are not alone in experiencing the "highs" and "lows" of what is, at certain times, a very solitary and lonely journey. All of the authors in this part describe how the journey is always worth the trip. We hope you, the reader, will agree and set out on your own journey.

References

VanMaanen, J. (1988). *"Tales of the field": On writing ethnography.* Chicago: University of Chicago Press.

CHAPTER

6

The Data Collection Journey: Variations on the "Tea Party" Theme

Laura MacGregor, M.Sc., OT(C)

> "Really, now you ask me," said Alice, very much confused, "I don't think— "Then you shouldn't talk, said the Hatter. . . . said Alice . . . It's the stupidest tea-party I ever was at in all my life!"
>
> — Lewis Carroll, *Alice's Adventures in Wonderland*

If someone had told me in 1989, when I finished my undergraduate degree, that I would be involved in research to the extent of contributing to a research textbook, I would have laughed. In my opinion, I was the last of my classmates who would ever pursue an additional degree or be involved in research. I was not even sure I liked the profession of occupational therapy. I had no sense of professional identity. I was frustrated by the lack of support for the activities I did on a daily basis. Working in psychiatry, given the extent of role blurring among the disciplines in this specialty, probably compounded the problem. I worked on life skills, but so did the social worker. I explored leisure issues but so did the recreation therapist. People thought all I did was crafts, which I hated. I was so frustrated with my career choice that for the first few years after completing my undergraduate degree I explored a variety of avenues that would get me out of the profession of occupational therapy. Then I discovered the M.Sc. program at The University of Western Ontario, which for me was a turning point.

Thus, I entered the program, disillusioned with occupational therapy. To further the problem, I believed that I was the sole cause of my angst. I believed that I was too stupid to understand occupational therapy and that within a few months my professors would realize this and politely ask me to leave the graduate program. It never crossed my mind that my issues with the profession may have stemmed from the state of the profession itself. Fortunately, I quickly learned that many of my issues with the profession related to the lack of empirical support for what we do.

The program was the ideal place for me. Rather than studying things that I was not very good at or interested in (for example, neurophysiology), I was encouraged to explore my issues with the profession. For the first time in my professional career, I discovered that it was okay to question the profession (in some cases, to "slam" the profession) and our activities. In fact, it was encouraged as long as it helped to define ways in which we could provide new research support for our profession. What an incredible feeling. Not only was I not the problem, but I could be part of the solution.

A requirement of the program, in addition to course work, was to complete an independent research project, otherwise known as a "thesis." I was one of the few students who had not come to the program with a burning research question or a clinical irritation that I wanted to explore. During a graduate level research issues course, I became fascinated with the idea of occupational deprivation—that is, with what happened to people who, because of illness or disability, could not participate in their chosen occupations. Obviously, this was a key issue in occupational therapy, but one that required exploration through research.

Prior to entering the graduate program, I had no real appreciation for qualitative research. In fact, as far as I was concerned, research involved a great deal of number crunching and entering data into a computer. The idea that I could explore individuals' stories was foreign to me until I arrived at The University of Western Ontario. On learning about the narrative, lived experience, and phenomenological approaches to research, I became genuinely excited about the idea that I could go and hear our clients' stories—that I could ask them to discuss occupation or the

lack of it and what that meant to their life. Thus, my research project quickly evolved.

Briefly, my research project explored the daily experiences of individuals, eight to be exact (as suggested by McCracken, 1988), who because of adult onset, chronic illness, or disability were unable to participate in the occupations of their choice. A snowball sample of convenience was used. The results of the study suggested that participation in occupations was important because it provided the individual with a source of identity and a sense of value, to both the individual and society.

Shortly after I decided on a research question, I approached Dr. Joanne Cook to supervise my project. I was thrilled to be working with her. She was a keen qualitative researcher who was known for her commitment to occupational therapy, qualitative methods, and her graduate students. She was the sort of professor, who in addition to supporting your research, would make sure you were eating, sleeping, and spending time with your family. Given that I had come to the graduate program with somewhat battered self-esteem and professional confidence, the very personal touch provided by Dr. Cook was truly appreciated (this is noteworthy, because at one point in my reflexive journal it is noted that I wanted to "kill this woman").

Professor Cook and I worked on developing a semistructured questionnaire. The chosen method of data collection was to be in the form of the long, in-depth interview. Dr. Cook had promised me that data collection was just plain fun. All of her other graduate students had apparently loved interviewing informants. According to Dr. Cook, the interviews often took the form of long, pleasant, informative chats over tea (hence this chapter's title). I could hardly wait. In my personal research journal at that time, I noted that I could hardly contain my excitement on getting the "go-ahead" from my research committee. For example, on September 9, 1994, prior to actually starting to interview, I wrote, "Hooray—yesterday I booked two more interviews. . . . Dr. Cook has made me promise to do no more than one per week. Oh well—that's already gone by the wayside." I would quickly learn that my experience would be very different from that of Professor Cook's previous students and that her advice should have been heeded.

This is NOT a Tea Party

When I reflect back on my interviewing experience, I honestly wonder where my head was. With the exception of one informant, I was interviewing people who had experienced an adult onset, long-term, and, in some cases, progressive physical or mental illness. What did I expect them to say? "Gee, yeah. I have this major condition, and I've experienced incredible losses. But you know, it's okay. . . . I love my life, and I love occupational therapists." Get real. Not unexpectedly, the interviews included incredibly painful stories centered on the experiences of change and loss. When you add that to the fact that qualitative research takes place in the realworld, not an ivory tower, and that as a researcher one may be experiencing real-world problems, my interviewing months ended up being one of the more stressful periods in my life.

The Informants' Experience: Pain, Bitterness, and Anger

Before talking about my experience with the interviews, it is important to give the reader some idea of the issues being discussed by my informants. As mentioned previously, my informants were adults, discussing their experiences with long-term, chronic illnesses

and how their illnesses interfered with their daily occupations. While I expected to hear stories about change and loss, the depth of my informants' pain, bitterness, and anger astounded me, and, to be honest, has profoundly changed me.

My informants were a hospitable group. They were brutally honest as they shared stories of immense pain with an individual who was a stranger. They cried. They swore. They talked about spouses and friends who had left them, either physically or emotionally. They talked about educational and professional opportunities lost because of failing abilities or discrimination. They talked about health care professionals (including, unfortunately, occupational therapists) who failed to listen. They talked about the pain of losing control. The list of losses was long. For example:

Informant 7: (Discussing the end of his marriage). Well, for one thing, it had a lot to do with the breakup of L. and I. I think it's just too much pressure on her after a while . . . all the seizures and everything just sort of built up, and she turned to drinking and stuff like that . . . so things just sorta . . . fell apart.

Informant 5: (Discussing the emotional distancing of her husband). There's a part of me that pines away. I want that intimacy back. I want that caring back. I want that life back (fighting tears) . . . Sexually I don't hold appeal anymore . . . and even as a companion, it can be strained.

Informant 5: (Discussing her disease). It's like . . . you sorta have this commitment or this belief that you can overcome anything, and it's like . . . you just don't let it happen to you . . . fight it, keep fighting it, that type of thing (crying). So to sort of see it happening, despite all your best efforts to rein in the devastation, really takes a shift in your mind.

Informant 6: (Discussing the effects of his progressive disease). For a long time when something would happen, I'd say to myself, How much can I take? What's my limit? . . . Throw at me whatever you want. I can take it, being the tough guy. But this last time, I was on the verge of becoming a quadri-plegic. I felt like this is it. This is all I can take. You can stop now. . . . It's scary. I'll probably adjust, but I don't want that to happen. I really don't.

Initially I was able to be empathetic during interviews, go home and transcribe the meetings, and not carry too much of the participants' pain with me. However, after completing several interviews and then reliving them while transcribing them, I found that their experiences began to take a toll. I think that is one thing about qualitative research for which you can never be prepared. To analyze your data, you immerse yourself in the data and live the experience. But in my case, the data and experiences were painful. What made the situation even harder was that the informants, in many cases, directed their anger toward health professionals and, perhaps because there was a captive occupational therapy audience, directly at occupational therapy itself.

> Informant 3: (Discussing OT). You are used to spending five and six hours reading texts, books, and studying (when you are a university student). All of a sudden, they have you hooking ice cream cone rugs, and they think you will be stimulated. Give it a rest . . . My experience with OT has not been great. It has all been crafts . . . Why don't you try a string art? Well, what the hell am I going to do with a string art?

> Informant 2: To be honest with [you], most of the workers with [Community Service], they're stuffed shirts. They come in all dressed up to the eyeballs pretending they know everything. They tell you what you need. They tell you what hours you're gonna get for homemaking . . . Literally, they tell you how to run your life.

> Informant 5: Bladder control is a major issue with people with [names condition] and she [the OT] just said, So . . . so like wear a diaper, big deal. And here she brings me these diapers where you wear, like babies, plastic pants . . . I mean her biggest drawback was

not putting herself in the client's shoes which I think you need to do. . . .

This anger directed at occupational therapy was simultaneously reaffirming and difficult. A part of me was relieved to hear that the client had issues with the profession similar to mine (that is, discomfort with a reliance on crafts). But it was difficult to hear stories about occupational therapists who did not listen or who were not empathetic. Initially, I would cope by telling myself that I was not one of those therapists. I was the good kind of therapist. I listened. I welcomed and valued clients' input. I saw them as people who were the sole experts on their life and condition. I never placed myself in a position of authority. However, as the research progressed and I immersed myself in the clients' responses and reflected on my clinical work, I began to realize that it probably was not true. There were times when I had not been the most empathetic or sensitive therapist I could have been. There were times that not only did I present myself as the expert, but I also wanted to be the expert, since being an expert helped deal with my insecurities about the profession.

Predictably, my angst about the profession grew. But now not only was I frustrated with the profession, I was also angry with occupational therapy. How could occupational therapists do this to our clients? How could we call ourselves helping professionals if these were the feelings we engendered in our clients? So rather than strengthening my commitment to the profession, this occupational therapy thesis was further eroding my commitment to occupational therapy. I became particularly angry about my undergraduate experience. I had been taught theories that not only failed to help the people with whom we were most concerned, but also perhaps heightened their feelings of pain and anger. So much for the idea that data collection was fun and exciting.

Give Me the Ivory Tower

By that time, data collection had become fairly stressful. Unfortunately that is when real life started to really rain on my tea party. When I started graduate school, I was recently married and happily living a newly-wed experience in a tiny apartment near the university. My husband had recently finished his year of articling (a requirement for lawyers that is similar to an apprenticeship or internship) and was completing the Bar Admission Course and the Bar Exams for Ontario, Canada. We were hopeful that he would find a job in the London, Ontario, area, so I could finish my M.Sc. However, four months into the program, he found a job with an excellent firm, one and one-half hours away in Cambridge, Ontario. While the distance was an issue, Bill really wanted to join this firm. They had a great reputation, he knew several people working with the firm, and the work he would be doing was appealing. He was incredibly excited, and I did not want to rain on *his* tea party. In addition, this was in the mid-1990s when a glut of young lawyers was hitting a recession-battered economy. Needless to say, such a solid offer was to be taken seriously.

Our first strategy was to maintain two apartments. Bill moved to Cambridge, and I moved in with a roommate in the student apartments. Although this worked, it was both financially and personally stressful. So after four months of this arrangement, we bought a second car, and I moved to Cambridge. This meant that I was commuting three hours, round-trip, on country roads during a Canadian winter. I knew no one in Cambridge, and all the fun was happening in London. To make matters seem worse, I had commuted a similar distance during my undergraduate years and had vowed I would never do it again. I quickly found that when you added the demands of research to the demands of the commute and my husband's

long hours, the situation became very stressful. In my field journal I noted, "I am feeling a little bit frazzled and tired today (and for that matter yesterday). I don't think it affected my interview skills though. However, after rushing home and doing the evening activities, I found I was not able to do my field notes and write in this journal. Both were completed today (the next day). I'm feeling a bit overwhelmed. I have to review informant 2's interview before tomorrow and then transcribe two more interviews."

Another exacerbating factor during the interview/research experience was that being a frugal graduate student, I had decided to transcribe all my interviews myself, rather than securing funding and paying someone. I also believed that by reliving the experience through transcription I would further immerse myself in the data. However, reviewing my field journal indicates that while I may have been more immersed, this also probably added to my stress level. I wrote, "Help—I am in Hell! My back is killing me, my neck is killing me, and my wrists ache. I HATE TRANSCRIBING (yes, it is in capital letters in my journal) . . . this transcribing crap is FROM HELL. I feel like I am falling way behind. I was relieved when my informant was not up to working on the interview. It gives me a bit of a chance to get my head above water—just in time to fall behind." In the end, I paid a typist to transcribe a few of my audiotapes.

As I have noted before, qualitative research works amid the bumps of daily life. Unfortunately, about this time when I really could have used Dr. Cook's famous personal touch, she experienced the terminal illness and death of her father and was required to leave town for several weeks. Although she tried to stay in touch and telephoned regularly, she had far too many demands to be worried about my graduate school experience. So later in my journal I noted, "I'm getting so bogged down. My thesis supervisor is incommunicado, which adds to the stress. Fortunately the fatigue is replaced by difficulty going to sleep . . . so at least I can get some more work done."

Dr. Cook's personal situation required me to get additional help. Another committee member, Dr. Helene Polatajko assumed the role of cosupervisor. As a graduate student, I had been thrilled to be in the same room with Dr. Polatajko. She had been (and still is) incredibly influential on the development of a rigorously researched knowledge base for occupational therapy. However, having cosupervisors, no matter how much I liked both of them, caused new and unexpected problems. For example, because Dr. Cook was away attending to family matters, I rarely met with both of them together. I would talk with Dr. Cook on the telephone and then later with Dr. Polatajko at the school. Unfortunately, what this often meant was that I got conflicting feedback about what to do, as indicated by one journal entry: "I have been crying on and off for the last half day. I had what I thought was a good chat with Dr. Polatajko yesterday. She suggested that I make changes to my data collection strategy. However, when Dr. Cook called last night, she said no. For someone who sings the praises about how flexible qualitative research is, she was pretty rigid." While I later noted in my reflexive journal that my frustration with Dr. Cook was irrational, it did not change the fact that I did not believe she could appreciate how overwhelmed I happened to be at that moment.

Another difficulty I discovered with cosupervisors was that while they were both genuinely excited about my research, it eventually seemed to me that it was becoming their research. In my understanding, this is a fairly common issue with novice qualitative researchers. I understood that I was doing the frontline work. In many ways, it

was their advanced research and conceptual skills that skillfully directed me along the research path. However, at times I became frustrated by the heated debates the two professors had about the interpretations emerging from data analysis. In my reflexive journal, I commented on conversations the "three" of us had that quickly became conversations between Dr. Cook and Dr. Polatajko. They would talk about Laura noted this and Laura discovered that, but they seemed to forget that Laura was still in the room. I think, common to many graduate students, that I wanted the ideas to be all mine; I wanted to have some sense of ownership of the data, and I was reluctant to share the experience.

Needless to say, when you add the previously noted supervisor issues, Dr. Cook's personal stresses, and my fatigue with commuting and transcribing to the pain and anger discussed during the interviews and in some instances directed at occupational therapy, I became quite distressed.

Reflections on My Tea Party: Lessons Learned

As I reflect on this experience five years after the fact, I must admit I am a little surprised by my reactions at the time. Realistically, I knew that my informants had experienced incredible losses, and the preliminary research I had completed included a detailed review of the sensory deprivation literature, which suggested that "not doing" was deleterious. I think in my excitement about actually doing real research, I was so consumed by my feelings that I may have briefly forgotten about my informants' feelings. While I do believe I was empathetic during the interviews, I had obviously not prepared myself for the extent of the emotional intensity my informants would express. In addition, I knew graduate school was a great deal of work and commuting long distances would not be fun. Yet, I committed to these activities during the first year of marriage. The fact that I was stressed was understandable. The fact that I was surprised by the level of stress I was experiencing, in my current view, shows some lack of forethought.

My first thought for someone embarking on their first experience with in-depth interviewing is to prepare yourself for the possibility that the experience may, indeed, be less than perfect and have some sense of how you will manage your stress level. Select your supervisor carefully, and if working with two or more individuals, be realistic about how the dynamics of this may unfold. I would not change my selection of supervisors. Dr. Cook was by far the ideal individual to supervise my research, and to this day, I am glad we formed the research and personal relationship that we did. I also am grateful that Dr. Polatajko became involved in my research at such a critical juncture. My only wish is that I had been better prepared for the complex dynamics of cosupervision. For example, I could have established a specific individual or group of individuals with whom to discuss my experiences, or perhaps I could have discussed the issue of cosupervision with students who had elected this option before me.

In the end, my experiences during this research project have had a profound effect on my current daily life, and I am grateful for the journey. I believe that I am a better clinician for the experience. I have a better understanding of the emotional and logistical struggles my clients experience on a daily basis. I have an appreciation for the depth of their losses and the meaning of their resulting victories. I think that, above all, I have a stronger commitment to the importance of occupation and the need for control over one's personal daily occupations. It was worth the personal and professional angst.

Epilogue—The Tea Party Continues

While I learned a great deal during my research journey, one thing that became abundantly clear to me was the notion of "there but for the grace of God go I." In all but one case, my informants had acquired their illness in later life and, in most cases, had no previous experience with issues of illness and disability. They had not planned for or expected illness or disability to touch their lives. No one does. These were things that happened to other people. While I, as an occupational therapist, academically understood that this, of course, was not true, emotionally I too expected my life to unfold accordingly. Illness and disability and their interrelationship with occupation were issues that I dealt with professionally, not personally.

However, on January 27, 1999, my view of this subject was altered forever. During the delivery of my second son, he experienced severe birth asphyxia. Initially, his very survival was called into question, and my husband and I were asked whether we wanted to discontinue life support. Suddenly, I was forced to collide head-on with my professional convictions about the meaning of life, illness, disability, and ability. It was time to put "my money where my mouth was." Six months later, Matthew was diagnosed with cerebral palsy, and my research journey, while very professionally meaningful, took on new meaning in my personal life. Life has a funny way of teaching us important lessons.

Reference

McCracken, G. (1988). *The long interview*. Newbury Park, CA: Sage.

CHAPTER

7

Nobody Told Me It Would Be Like This: The Trials and Triumphs of a Research Journey

Jennifer E. Landry, M.Sc., OT(C), O.T. Reg. (NS)

> *It is good to have an end to journey toward, but it is the journey that matters in the end.*
>
> —Ursula K. LeGuin

The Development of the Research Question

As it is often said, it all began simply enough. As a student occupational therapist, I had developed an interest in research and evidence-based practice that culminated in a fieldwork placement in research during my final undergraduate year. With my interest in research piqued, I knew at that time that I would be back for more. After working as an occupational therapist for a year, I returned to school to pursue a graduate degree in occupational therapy. I began graduate school with several ideas regarding areas of interest for research, but I had no clear topic area in mind. I decided that I would spend the time it took to complete the course work for my master of science degree exploring

many different avenues of potential interest for my thesis.

Early in graduate school, I discovered an article (Gage & Polatajko, 1994) about the construct of perceived self-efficacy and its relationship to occupational performance that sparked and held my interest. According to Gage and Polatajko, perceived self-efficacy relates to an individual's belief in his or her capabilities concerning a particular task. The mediating role of perceived self-efficacy on occupational performance for people without disabilities had been well established in the literature (Bandura, 1995; Maddux & Stanley, 1986). I wondered about the relationship between self-efficacy and occupational performance for people with disabilities. Would the relationship hold true for people with disabilities? Would it depend on the type of disability? If the relationship was different, what were the similarities and differences between people with disabilities and those without disabilities? I read all the literature I could find regarding perceived self-efficacy. My enthusiasm for the topic influenced my course work, and I tailored assignments toward discovering more about perceived self-efficacy and its relationship to occupational performance.

In reviewing the literature on perceived self-efficacy, I discovered several related constructs that are also said to influence performance, such as outcome expectancy, personal causation, attributions, and others. The more I read, the more uncomfortable I became with looking at perceived self-efficacy in isolation. I felt that self-efficacy and the other related constructs were possibly intertwined and that each was important. I felt that it would be difficult to meaningfully separate one construct from the others, but I was committed to the task. I had done so much reading and writing, and I had invested too much time, effort, and thinking to turn back now. Scholarship applications and course work deadlines were looming nearer, and both required a fairly well-developed description of my proposed thesis research, including a rationale or purpose, research design and methods, and the significance of the project.

I had to complete a research proposal as one of the requirements for a graduate level methods course in which I was enrolled. Presumably, the proposal prepared and presented for the course would serve as your thesis proposal. I designed a quantitative study to investigate the relationship between an individual's abilities or occupational performance components and perceived self-efficacy and that relationship's effect on occupational performance. The cross-sectional design was intended to determine if perceived self-efficacy was a mediator of occupational performance for a group of

young adults with nonprogressive, congenital disabilities and for a group of individuals with nonprogressive, acquired disabilities who were currently residing in the community. I had decided to study these groups for a number of reasons, including what I thought, at that point in time, was access to members of these groups of people through a local health care center. In addition, I chose nonprogressive disabilities to avoid having to consider all the issues surrounding dealing with an illness that has a downward trajectory in regard to occupational performance.

Developing the thesis proposal on the basis of the effect of perceived self-efficacy only heightened my sense that at the end of the day, I would not be satisfied with the results. There were so many factors, in addition to perceived self-efficacy, that influence occupational performance, and I was uneasy with focusing on just one of those factors. My commitment was already wavering. My confidence in the project was already shaken. I had been told (as I am sure many embarking on their thesis had) that I would come to hate even the most beloved research project at some point during the process, so I had better make sure the project was something that inspired me. I was not inspired by my research project in its current form.

Without stating my uncertainty regarding the project, I had conversations with a number of fairly established researchers. I distinctly remember one conversation with an epidemiologist, who had a fairly good knowledge of occupational therapy. This faculty member had assisted me in determining an appropriate design for my research and had read the final draft of my proposal. He told me that it was a "nice little project," and I would get my master's degree and possibly a few publications from it. However, he had to ask me if I really thought the project held meaning for me. Given my original interest and questions, would the depth of understanding I was looking for be possible with such a proposal? Initially, I was taken aback and somewhat defensive. I had spent so much time on the proposal, and I had received positive feedback regarding the project. Besides, this was a master's project, and it would be only a small piece in a much larger puzzle. How meaningful can you expect one small piece to be?

With my nose still somewhat out of joint, I soon came to recognize that the faculty member's comments really echoed some of my own misgivings regarding the proposed research project. Consequently, I returned to the original questions that led me toward perceived self-efficacy. These questions arose from observations I had made during clinical practice and other interactions with people with disabilities. What are those internal factors unique to the individual that determine one's capacity or potential to engage in daily living? Why do some individuals, despite challenges, appear to actively engage in daily life, while others appear more limited by their disability? In my interactions with people with disabilities, I had noted that some individuals appeared to live their lives as "disabled people," while others gave me the sense that they were "people with disabilities," independent of the degree of disability or, rather, my perception of the person's "functional status."

Following this discussing, rethinking, and soul searching, I gave up on my original research proposal and started over. As I write about it, I can clearly remember how difficult the decision was for me to make. To me, it was a decision that meant a great deal of time and effort had been wasted and it was a decision that would put me behind schedule.

During this period, I was in the process of completing a graduate course in qualitative methods. I had very little exposure to qualitative methods prior to graduate school. As an undergraduate student, scientific inquiry was presented almost exclusively within the quantitative paradigm. Given my background knowledge, there was only one view of science, and "ways of knowing" were restricted to the traditional positivistic perspective. Legitimate, systematic investigation or research was predicated on hypothesis testing and quantification. The qualitative methods course presented me with new ways of approaching research.

From my reading, course work, and discussions with established researchers, I knew that a number of aspects must be considered when selecting an appropriate research approach. These factors included the research question(s), rationale for conducting the study, and level of knowledge development in the area to be investigated. The researcher's views regarding the nature of reality, preferred ways of knowing and thinking about phenomena, and what is considered to be valuable knowledge are also important considerations when determining the approach. I had heard or read many references to "preferred ways of knowing." At this point, I do not think that I had what could be referred to as a "preferred way," but I felt much more comfortable with "in-depth exploration from the participant's perspective" than I did with "quantification." Although quantitative approaches were more familiar to me, when I answered all the preceding questions, I realized that this familiarity did not equate with a "goodness of fit" for me and my research issue.

Having defined an initial area of research interest, completed a review of the literature, increased my knowledge of quantitative and qualitative research approaches, and reflected on my newly discovered "preferred way of knowing," it became apparent to me that a qualitative research approach would best suit the research question, my views regarding what constitutes meaningful knowledge, and the state of knowledge in the research area of interest. I concluded that the issues of personal resources and occupational engagement are highly complex, individualized, and subjective, and that a qualitative approach would provide the opportunity for open, in-depth exploration of the meaning of these phenomena from the viewpoint of the participant.

Soon after completing the qualitative methods course, I began broadening my reading beyond qualitative methods and examples of the qualitative approach in action to include the disability literature. On reviewing the literature, I noted a paucity of information regarding occupational engagement, particularly for women with physical disabilities, and even more notably for women with congenital disabilities. With some notable exceptions, such as Frank's (1984, 1986, 1988) work with Diane DeVries, much of the research dealing with individuals with congenital physical disabilities appeared to be from the professional's or caregiver's perspective. I was interested in hearing the participants' experiences from their perspective. Given the paucity of information, combined with the fact that a member of my committee might be able to assist me in gaining entrance to a site that could be helpful in linking me with potential participants, I decided to explore the link between personal resources and occupational engagement for a group of women with nonprogressive, congenital disabilities.

My fieldwork journal has enabled me to recreate the research journey and has reminded me of what I was experiencing at the time: all of my challenges and triumphs, successes and failures, and impressions of the research process.

The Pilot Interviews

The research project had three phases. The first phase involved the development and pilot testing of the interview guide, which was then revised based on the pilot test. Phase two involved recruitment of participants, and data collection and analysis. Phase three consisted of member-checking and writing the thesis.

The initial interview guide was developed with guidance from the original members of my thesis committee. The interview guide was meant to organize, lend structure and continuity to each of the interviews, and outline areas to be explored within the interview sessions. Development of the initial interview guide was directed by my research questions and the literature. I decided to use semistructured interviews to gain an understanding from the participants' perspective. My questions were geared toward gaining insight into the nature of the experience of engagement, with particular emphasis on personal resources that enable or disable occupation. Probes or prompts were used to further explore relevant concepts or ideas and to encourage the participant to elaborate on or clarify information.

In truth, my first pilot interviews were disastrous, and I felt like I was a complete washout. The initial interview guide was far too structured and set up a survey-type atmosphere for the research context, rather than being more open and conversational in nature. Preliminary analysis of the data from the pilot interviews indicated that detailed responses from the participants were not forthcoming. The participants responded to questions very briefly and often appeared to be waiting for the next question on the list. The data derived from these interviews did not adequately capture the women's experiences and perceptions of living with a disability. I felt as though I was back at the beginning again.

Revision of the Question and Strategies

Following the rather unsuccessful pilot interviews, I returned to the literature once again and found a dearth of research regarding the experience of living with a disability. As a result of my continued examination of the literature regarding women with disabilities, and consistent with the emergent or continually developing nature of qualitative inquiry, the research questions changed and developed throughout the initial stage of my project. I revised my research question and the interview guide to better reflect the research area I was interested in pursuing. In the end, the exploratory study used a qualitative approach to gain insight into the lived experience of women with nonprogressive, congenital disabilities.

My research questions were:

1. What is it like to go through daily life as a woman with a disability?
2. What does it take to get through daily life as a woman with a disability?

During the interviews, each of the participants were asked those two questions. Again, in contrast to much of the current literature but consistent with client-centered practice, I was dedicated to describing the experience of living with a disability from the perspectives of the women involved in the research project. Without downplaying the agony of having to go back to the beginning more than once, I must admit that with every revision to the research project I felt closer to capturing what I was really interested in studying.

Searching for Participants

Searching for participants for my research was a fairly long and difficult process. It took me almost 15 months to interview eight women. Despite what I had expected and for reasons far beyond my control, I was unable to access participants through local agencies and health care centers. Very disappointed but still undaunted, I contacted a number of agencies in other areas who were involved with individuals with physical disabilities

and approached colleagues, faculty members, and the participants to assist me in identifying individuals who met the inclusion criteria of being women, between the ages of 21 and 65, with a nonprogressive, congenital disability. Mine was a "snowball" sample of convenience. This approach is somewhat akin to the saying, "I told two friends, then they told two friends, and so on." In particular, I am indebted to the participants, a few faculty members, and one agency that really rallied behind me and helped me with recruitment. The participants really enjoyed being involved in the research and were definitely the best advertisements for involvement in the project.

While McCracken (1988) indicated that participants should be strangers to the researcher to encourage candor, only six of the eight participants were strangers. Due to difficulty in accessing potential participants, two women with whom I had prior contact were also involved in the study. While the effect of a prior relationship cannot be determined, both participants with whom I had previous relationships appeared to speak quite openly and candidly with me regarding their experiences as women living with disabilities.

The Real Thing—Interviews

My revised interview guide was far more flexible and much less directive than the original version. I purposely avoided looking at the interview guide during the interviews, except near the end of the interview to confirm that we had covered everything. Topic areas were addressed as they "emerged," that is, as the participants brought them up, and additional questions were used as indicated.

I started with my grand tour question: "I am interested in your life as a woman with a disability. Tell me what it is like and what it takes to go through daily life with a disability.

Introduce me to your life, past and present, and you can start wherever you like." Probes were used as needed, and the questions were rephrased when participants indicated they were unclear. The actual probes that I used, of course, varied depending on the course each of the interviews took. Examples of some of the areas raised are: impact of disability on life, if any; successes and failures; facing challenges; new situations; doing; time use; occupations engaged in; independence; and resources and barriers. More significant than the actual revised interview guide, however, was my revised approach to the interviews. During the interviews, I tried to foster an atmosphere that was conversational in nature.

The Interview Struggle

Prior to my undergraduate degree in occupational therapy, I had obtained a degree in physical education and had worked as a fitness counselor and as a kinesiologist. These jobs involved initial interviews and assessments, so I was somewhat familiar with the process of gathering information from people, at least in regard to their health status. As a student occupational therapist, I felt fairly comfortable with interviewing, both in the classroom "mock" interviews and on fieldwork placements. I was confident with my social, interpersonal, and communication skills prior to the formal interview training I received as an undergraduate in occupational therapy. My ability to interview was considered by me, my preceptors, and supervisors to be one of my strengths.

From my experience, the "typical" occupational therapy interview involved information gathering through interview and assessment. I usually completely directed the interview and had a fairly standardized list of questions and assessments to carry out as quickly as I could. I had to cover as many

occupational therapy related issues as I could in the shortest time possible. Often, this included addressing issues related to the person (cognitive, affective, and physical), their environments, and occupations during a one-hour appointment.

As a student occupational therapist and as a practitioner, I was encouraged to take on the role of the "professional" with my clients. My interviews were typically structured more to meet my needs for documentation and treatment planning than to meet the needs of the client. Based on their other health care experiences, clients typically knew what I was there to do during the initial interview and adopted the role of "patient" by answering the questions asked but not elaborating too much.

The sessions were typically brief question and answer periods, combined with "hands-on" assessment and observation. There was a fairly standard set of questions that occupational therapy was to cover. While at times the clients spoke about issues or things that were on their minds (immediate worries, concerns, and so forth), I was trained to briefly acknowledge those issues, indicate (if appropriate) that those were things we could address as we worked together, and then redirect the client back to the question I asked. In this manner, I was able to, in most cases, proceed fairly routinely through the initial interview/assessment. Although the occupational performance issues varied, one interview seemed very much like the next.

This type of interview typically required very little "thinking on one's feet" regarding my responses to the clients' concerns. Indeed, once mastered, I had some pretty stock comments that I was able to adapt slightly to suit each client's issues and get me quickly "back on track" with the interview.

I believe my communication reflected a genuine concern for the people with whom I worked, but "getting the information" and "carrying out the interview properly" were concerns of equal importance. I often found myself half-listening to the client, while the other half was problem-solving. What are the issues I can address here? What is most important in terms of my role as an occupational therapist? What can I do about intervention with this person? In fact, by the end of the hour-long interaction, I often had my problem list, goals, and at least part of the treatment plan created. While I always asked my clients what was important for them to be able to do in their daily lives, I often played the expert in the interview situation. I was in control, I directed its course, and if it got "off course," it was my responsibility to bring it back on course as quickly as possible. Techniques like "paraphrasing, summarizing, and reflecting back" to the client were so ingrained that my personal communication style outside the clinical situation also reflected these techniques.

My first introduction to qualitative research interviewing was in the qualitative methods course I took during graduate school. As indicated earlier in this chapter, prior to that course, I had absolutely no knowledge of qualitative research methods in general or of the "semistructured interview" format. Although I was intrigued, the mention of words like *semistructured, open, emergent,* and *exploratory* in class and in the literature made me anxious just thinking about that type of interview.

The flexibility and relatively unstructured nature of the qualitative research interview was difficult and provoked anxiety for me. This interview method did not come as easily to me as the occupational therapy practice interviews. I felt much more comfortable with the thought of memorizing a list of questions and asking each one in succession. Again, I was familiar with a survey interview format where I would ask a question, the client would answer, and when the client was finished answering that question, I would ask the next one on my list.

I knew I would have to be less directive and more flexible in a research interview, but old habits are hard to break and definitely die hard. Following the participant's lead, thinking on my feet, truly focusing on what the informant was saying (versus thinking about my next question), and enabling smooth transitions to tie the threads of the discussion together proved to be very difficult for me. The insecurity of being less directive in the interview came from anxiety related to getting "anything good" (that is, rich data) from the interview, anxiety regarding getting "the information that I wanted from the participants," and also letting the interview flow.

Again, with the first few pilot interviews for my thesis, I took in a big list of questions and early on set the tone of a question and answer or survey-style interview. After my first few less than successful pilot interviews, it was suggested that I do a few more pilot interviews before I try to pursue the "real" thing. It was a blow to my confidence. Communication had typically come easily to me. I was often told it was one of my strengths, yet this new type of qualitative interview interaction felt awkward and foreign.

A few verbal communication habits that I had fallen into were pointed out as interfering with the qualitative research interview process. I stifled discussion at times by saying things like "right," which may have indicated to the participant that she had said enough, that I had "gotten" what she was saying and it was time to move onto something else, instead of encouraging her to "tell me more." Additionally, I often assumed understanding without asking the participant to explain further. For example, my understanding of the concept of "motherhood" may be very different from the participant's perspective on motherhood. I had to learn to make sure I explored "meaning" with each participant from her perspective and not to assume shared understanding.

In contrast to clinical interviews, I felt more pressure "to do it right" because this was for my research project. I believed that I did not have the luxury of going back to the participant if I did not get what I needed the first time. Clinically, I would typically see my clients every day for at least one week, usually much longer. Anything that I missed, I could ask later. With the research interviews, while I knew that I could and would go back to clarify and ask further questions, I really felt that I had only one chance to conduct a good interview. After all, these were busy women with full lives.

During clinical interviews, I assumed that I had a right to ask potentially sensitive questions because I was the professional there to help and the client was seeking occupational therapy services. That was my role. I was able to ask the questions in a direct manner under the guise of my profession, just as a physician asks and expects his or her patients to answer very personal questions in a forthcoming manner. In general, the relevancy of the information to be gathered was determined by what the facility had judged to be important to have on the client's medical chart.

I was less comfortable asking questions during my research interviews. There was pressure in the research interviews to establish rapport as soon as possible because I knew I was asking the women to discuss some fairly personal information with me. I did not have the luxury of developing rapport over a more extended period of time. It was difficult asking participants personal questions about themselves, as most of the women were unknown to me except for a telephone call or E-mail to set the interview time. There was also a sense of not really having the right to be asking the women to share their lives with me. These were people with whom I was unfamiliar, and they owed me nothing. Generously, they were willing to share their time and life with me. Yet, I somehow felt unworthy.

During the research interviews, there was an awkwardness about me that was not typical of my personality. I had always considered myself as quite socially adept, but my sense of my abilities in the research situation was tenuous, unlike my confidence in carrying out clinical interviews. My transition between topics felt awkward and jumpy at times. My perceived self-efficacy regarding my ability to conduct a solid qualitative research interview was quite low

I was also very concerned about being respectful and even felt hesitant about directly addressing their disabilities. Calling them "women with disabilities" and asking them to tell me about their lives as women with disabilities indicated that I was assuming life with a disability was different from living without a disability and that the difference was such that I would be able to study it. What would these individuals think about my questions? Would I unintentionally offend them? With a group of women without disabilities, would I be so bold as to assume such similarity in experience?

I was hesitant to give up my list of questions and my control over the situation. However, when speaking to the women, I often found that I lost myself in the conversation. The women spoke in very compelling ways about things that were important to them. They offered information that they felt would answer my main question of "tell me about your life as a woman with a disability." The conversational atmosphere of the qualitative research interviews completely drew me in. Unlike occupational therapy practice situations where I left interviews knowing what was addressed and what was not addressed and needed to be, several times I left the research interviews not really knowing whether the interview had covered the areas that I had set out to address.

However, I was always amazed at what would come out of each of the research interviews, including the things the women would share with me about their lives and the important information that could be gleaned from the interviews. Sometimes, the feeling of déjà vu was very strong because the women would describe experiences that were surprisingly similar.

The flexible nature of the interview allowed me to follow up on things the women spoke of that I had not previously considered. My preconceptions were altered after the first few interviews, and I was able to enter into the subsequent interviews with a more open mind and less of an agenda. My agenda became to really hear the women as they spoke.

Most significantly, the women did not want to speak to me about intrinsic factors or personal resources. The women indicated that, as a group, they were no more similar to or different from a group of women without disabilities. What was different for these women were the challenges they faced. The women indicated overwhelmingly that it was the sociocultural environment that facilitated or hindered engagement in daily living. It was the messages they received, including the attitudes and expectations of others, and the effect those messages had on women that significantly influenced their occupational engagement. Each spoke of how supportive or unsupportive sociocultural environments significantly influenced their ability to actively engage in meaningful occupation, be it in the context of the family, work, school, or with friends.

I have no permanent record of exactly what I said and did in my occupational therapy practice interviews, whereas with the audiotaped qualitative research interviews, I do have a permanent record, so I can be more critical of my performance. However, I honestly do not remember struggling as much with clinical interviews, and usually I felt reasonably satisfied with my performance on the whole. Again, feedback from my clients and supervisors highlighted empathy and

communication skills as my strengths. I can honestly say that I was not completely satisfied with any of the research interviews I had conducted up to this point. However, I was able to see improvement with each interview. With each participant, I found myself more completely engaged during the interview, fully attending not only to what was being said, but also to how it was being said.

The Researcher as the Main Research Tool: Assumptions

In qualitative inquiries, the researcher is the main research tool. However, I do not think I truly understood what this meant until I was completely "immersed" or, to be more reflective of how I felt at the time, "submersed" in analysis. I knew that "objectivity" was impossible and in fact undesirable, but that it was very important to be aware of the impact that the researcher had on the process. I brought to the research journey a broad range of experiences. My professional and personal experiences, graduate course work, as well as preliminary review of the literature led to the development of an area of interest and subsequent research questions. However, these background experiences also led to certain biases and assumptions (Strauss & Corbin, 1990).

From my professional background, I brought a belief that engagement in daily living is essential to health and that active engagement in life is something desirable. I embraced the Canadian Model of Occupational Performance (Canadian Association of Occupational Therapists, 1997), which describes occupational performance as resulting from an interaction between the person, the environment, and the occupation. Consistent with the philosophy of occupational therapy practice in Canada, I valued holism and believed that the experience of living with a disability or engaging in daily life with a disability cannot be meaningfully reduced to specific, clearly defined variables. Regarding human behavior and experience, I believed that the whole is much more than the sum of its parts.

Prior to engaging in data gathering, I speculated that I would find that intrinsic factors within the individual (such as perceived self-efficacy, self-esteem, and personal agency) enabled or conversely disabled engagement in daily life. While recognizing the significance of the environment or context, I was initially more captured by the internal factors that influence engagement. Although I understood and respected the role of the environment in engaging in occupation, my interest was in the person and those internal things or personal resources that an individual brings to and that influence occupational engagement. I asked each participant the following question. What are those things about you personally that have helped you in engaging in everyday life?

However, with each subsequent interview and in analyzing my data, I began to see that for this group of women at least, I was off the mark in focusing on intrinsic factors. From the women's perspective, it was not their personal resources that made their lived experiences different, but rather the sociocultural environment that enabled or disabled engagement in daily life.

The Analysis Challenge

I may not have gone where I intended to go, but I think I have ended up where I intended to be. —Douglas Adams

The management of data, analysis, and interpretation require judgment and creativity because there are only procedural guidelines and suggestions when taking a qualitative approach (Patton, 1990). Indeed, Lincoln (1995) asserts that "the entire field of interpretive or qualitative inquiry is itself still emerging and being defined" (p. 275). So not surprisingly, the analysis of qualitative data is challenging. It is like setting out on a journey without a map and little in the way of orientation. Instead, the map is created along the way. The creativity involved in analysis provided both the beauty and, at times, the frustration of a qualitative research project.

My research project was conducted over a two-year period, which allowed initial analysis to be conducted concurrent with data collection and enabled me to sufficiently immerse myself in the research area. As expected, given the evolving, emergent nature of qualitative research and the fact that I was intent on letting the data speak for itself, immersion was accompanied by challenges from the data to some of the assumptions I had made before I began collecting data.

Each of the eight interviews I conducted were audiotaped and transcribed verbatim. Some of the interviews I transcribed myself, and others I paid someone else to transcribe. Doing your own transcription as opposed to having someone else transcribe the interviews for you is the subject of some controversy and is a personal decision. Although having someone else transcribe my interviews saved some time, I ended up spending a fair amount of time listening to the audiotapes and "correcting" the transcriptions to truly reflect the conversation. More than half of the women interviewed had mild to moderate dysarthria, which at times made it difficult for the transcriber to understand what was being said. I also found that I had better knowledge of the content of the interviews I transcribed myself. As I was transcribing, I found myself transported back to the interview context. I thought about the setting, the person, and all the nonverbal information that was available in my face-to-face interactions with the women.

I was one of those people who amaze Morse (1997) and "try to do qualitative research by reading manuals" (p. 181). While I had committee members working with me who had expertise and had engaged in qualitative research, all were unfamiliar with the narrative approaches that I was interested in using to analyze my data. So I relied on the literature regarding narrative approaches and read extensively (Coffey & Atkinson, 1996; Cortazzi, 1993; Mischler, 1986, 1995; Polkinghorne, 1988; Reissman, 1993). I was intrigued by the "storied" nature of human discourse, and based on my reading, narrative analysis sounded fairly straightforward.

In analyzing narratives, we look at how experiences or events have been constructed and interpreted by the storyteller to make the narrative meaningful. Human beings are said to organize their experiences and make sense of their lives through stories (Coffey & Atkinson, 1996; Polkinghorne, 1988). Within the narrative approach, there are a number of different analytic strategies. The strategies typically consider both the structure and function of the stories told (Reissman, 1993). My focus was on the function or the point of the narrative, such as what the stories told me about the individual and how the individual framed and made sense of a particular experience or set of experiences. The goal for narrative research is to move beyond specific stories to more general stories that provide unity to an individual's story and perhaps to the group of participants involved in the research (Cortazzi, 1993; Reissman, 1993).

As with most qualitative research projects, analysis began by listening and relistening to the audiotapes and poring over the transcribed interviews. I had hoped to be able to use a narrative approach for analyzing my data. In order to identify the narrative, I began by looking at structure, including identifying the abstract, the orientation, the complication, and so forth. This type of analysis definitely helped me get started. However, my primary focus or interest was function or the meaning of the narratives, and I looked for key events, turning points, influences, and figures.

However, following the initial stage of analysis that involved identifying sections of text as narrative and examining structure, I got stuck. I could not seem to get beyond the initial stage of narrative analysis. I could not figure out how to proceed, how to reduce the data to make it more manageable yet maintain and be true to the participants' narratives. In addition, some of the study's participants frequently spoke in narratives, while others did not. Some of the interview data appeared to be forms of discourse other than narratives, and I felt that a lot of important data were not captured when I focused on the narrative discourse in the interview text. I guess that being a novice researcher contributed to the failure to elicit narratives from the participants or, perhaps, to identify narratives in the data.

This description of my experience with narrative analysis will undoubtedly fail to capture the struggle in which I was engaged. True to character, I read extensively and continued to pore over my data, trying to make narrative analysis work for me. I kept going in circles, hoping for that "aha experience" where everything clicks and analysis begins to come together or "emerge," as is often described in the literature on qualitative research. I have pages and pages of notes documenting my initial attempts at analysis. Far from making the data more manageable, I was creating another stack of papers equal in magnitude and no more refined than the original, transcribed interviews.

Once again, I realized I was back to the beginning. I had come to a standstill using narrative analysis. I needed more guidance than any of the literature I had read could give me. The narrative approach fascinated me, but because I had support from my committee members who had expertise in grounded theory and I had a small amount of background experience from the qualitative methods course, I decided to use grounded theory's constant comparative approach. However, throughout the analysis and interpretation of my data, I was still conscious of unfolding plots or storylines, and the initial analysis I did using a narrative approach, where I looked for the meaning of the stories the women told me, was very helpful. I went back to it when I felt fragmented, as though I had lost sight of the whole and lost sight of the participants' experiences.

Consistent with the constant comparative approach, the transcripts were reviewed to identify key concepts and relationships. Following the initial review, I focused on those units of text that appeared to be relevant to an understanding of the disability experience. As each interview was completed, I reflected on the data collected. To facilitate analysis, I asked questions of the data and of myself. What is she really saying? What is she trying to tell me? What is the point?

My initial impressions of the data appeared to correspond with the person-environment-occupation (PEO) model (Law, et al., 1996). The model was used as a framework for organizing my analysis of the data. Analysis proceeded in reference to the PEO model, while recognizing the need for continued vigilance to ensure that the analysis emerged from and reflected the data. However, grouping the data along the lines of person, environment, and occupation failed to bring coherence to the data or provide any meaningful insight. The categories remained too large and unwieldy and failed to capture the women's experiences of living with a disability. In addition, I recognized that using the model imposed a structure on the data, rather than allowing the analysis to emerge from the data. It became clear that an organization consistent with the PEO model did not reflect the data, but rather my theoretical orientation.

Consequently, use of the PEO model as a framework was abandoned, and over the next several months, I had very little contact with the data. I needed a break. I felt as though I was spinning my wheels. This was a fairly dark period for me. I felt as though I had made every mistake possible, starting with my quantitative research proposal and the disastrous pilot interviews, to having to let go of narrative analysis, and finally having to abandon my second attempt at formal analysis. I began to think that maybe qualitative research was not for me. I decided to take some time away from my data, and I returned to clinical work. I knew that I would persist and finish the project I started. I owed it to myself, my advisors, and most importantly to the women who shared their lives with me. I also knew that I needed to distance myself for a period of time. It was one of the smartest decisions that I made during my journey.

By taking a break from the research project, I was able to return to the data "fresh," and with the assistance of one member of my thesis committee in particular, I finally allowed the women's discourse to focus and shape the analysis. My thesis, therefore, reflects my third venture into the analysis of the qualitative interview data I collected from eight women with congenital disabilities. To prevent me from going back to the data in the same manner that had caused me trouble before, one of my advisors strongly suggested that, without looking at the transcripts (which I had not reviewed in over four months), I write down in one page or less what I thought each of the participants was telling me. It was through this process in collaboration with my advisor that I finally achieved that "aha experience," where things just seemed to click and fall into place like the pieces in a puzzle. My analysis made sense to me and my committee and seemed to take shape in a way that was congruent with the women's stories. I was energized and excited about making sure my interpretations or "answers" to these questions accurately reflected what the participants had told me. I took my results back to the study's participants for feedback to find out if my interpretations accurately reflected their experiences.

The Triumph of Member Checking

Analyzing the data and writing the thesis were fairly solitary activities that were quite different from my experience as a clinician, where I was constantly interacting with other people. The process was frustrating at times. For every hour that I spent with the participants, I spent countless hours alone in front of my computer. However, on a few occasions in particular, I found others who appeared to be truly interested in my research. Both member checking and the oral examination of my thesis provided me with treasured opportunities for discussing my research.

I was rejuvenated by the discussions I had with each of the participants during member checking. Each participant offered her comments and criticisms, letting me know where she felt I had really captured her experience and the spots where she felt I was somewhat "off the mark." These women were my toughest audience. I knew I was on the right track when, following some revision, three of the women told me that they felt as though I was "telling their stories." Despite the fact that the results were presented in an collectivized way, the results reflected the participants' individual experiences. Another participant indicated that it was a great relief for her to know that other women with disabilities had experiences similar to her own. She stated that while she had never met any of the other women involved with my project, she felt a connection to them and a

lot less alone in her struggles with the sociocultural environment.

My conversations with the women during both the interviews and the member checking are aspects of the research process that I truly cherish. It was my interactions with these women that inspired me. They spoke very frankly and poignantly about their experiences and had important messages to relate regarding the experience of living with a disability. While I understood that my project was a small piece of a very large puzzle, I felt that others needed to hear from these women, and so I persisted through analysis, wrote my thesis, successfully defended it, and continued to work with the data in hopes of further widening the audience through the submission of manuscripts to journals.

Six of the women indicated that they would like to continue being part of the process in a number of different capacities, including reviewing any manuscripts based on the research that I planned to submit to journals. I was then and continue to be excited by the collaborative research relationship I have with some of the women.

Epilogue

One's destination is never a place, but rather a new way of looking at things.
—Henry Miller

During the oral examination of my thesis, I felt energized by the group of examiners who knew my work and, for the most part, appeared eager to discuss the research project and the related literature. Rather than a student-examiner relationship, I felt as though the examination involved a group of colleagues (including myself) discussing my research and its implications. This is not to say that the examiners did not ask me challenging questions. Thankfully, they did. I had put so much effort into the thesis that I truly would have felt "ripped off" had I been let off easily. Rather than making me feel "defensive," or "under the gun", the atmosphere that was created made me feel challenged, yet respected for my work. For me, this was scholarship. In terms of my project, the examiners came with highly relevant expertise, and each of them offered insights and feedback that strengthened the final version.

I still struggle with a variety of issues, such as imposing myself on the data rather than letting the data speak for itself. I am often unclear about the data and question myself. I question the interpretation of my results, that is, I sometimes think "everybody already knows that" or, "that is just common sense." I struggle with the inability to generalize, struggle with analysis, and struggle with the whole process.

So, no one told me it would be like this—no person or book. The process was a difficult, frustrating, and painstaking endeavor. However, nothing prepared me for the joys the process would bring either. In particular, there were the interviews with the women and the sense of connection and purpose that those intimate conversations brought. There was also the excitement of those "aha" moments when the data first began to speak to me in a language that is shared, when the participants indicated that my findings and interpretations did indeed capture their experiences, and the complete satisfaction that came with the knowledge that, despite the challenges, through thick and thin, I persevered and found a way of knowing that truly resonated.

References

Bandura, A. (Ed.). (1995). *Self-efficacy in changing societies.* New York: Cambridge University Press.

Canadian Association of Occupational Therapists. (1997). *Enabling occupation: A Canadian occupational therapy perspective.* Ottawa, Canada: Author.

Coffey, A., & Atkinson, P. (1996). *Making sense of qualitative data: Complementary research strategies.* Thousand Oaks, CA: Sage.

Cortazzi, M. (1993). *Narrative analysis.* London: Falmer.

Fearing, V. G., & Clark, J. (2000). *Individuals in context: A practical guide to client-centered practice.* Thorofare, NJ: SLACK.

Frank, G. (1984). Life history model of adaptation to disability: The case of a "congenital amputee." *Social Science Medicine, 19,* 639–645.

Frank, G. (1986). On embodiment: A case study of congenital limb deficiency in American culture. *Culture, Medicine and Psychiatry, 10,* 189–219.

Frank, G. (1988). Beyond stigma: Visibility and self-empowerment of persons with congenital limb deficiencies. *Journal of Social Issues, 44,* 95–115.

Gage, M., & Polatajko, H. J. (1994). Enhancing occupational performance through an understanding of perceived self-efficacy. *American Journal of Occupational Therapy, 48,* 452–461.

Law, M., Cooper, B. A., Strong, S., Stewart, D., Rigby, P., & Letts, L. (1996). The person-environment-occupation model: A transactional approach to occupational performance. *Canadian Journal of Occupational Therapy, 63,* 9–23.

Lincoln, Y. S. (1995). Emerging criteria for quality in qualitative and interpretive research. *Qualitative Inquiry, 1,* 275–289.

Maddux, J. E., & Stanley, M. A. (1986). Self-efficacy theory in contemporary psychology: An overview. *Journal of Social and Clinical Psychology, 4,* 249–255.

McCracken, G. (1988). *The long interview.* Newbury Park, CA: Sage.

Mischler, E. G. (1986). *Research interviewing: Context and narrative.* Cambridge, MA: Harvard University Press.

Mischler, E. G. (1995). Models of narrative analysis: A typology. *Journal of Narrative and Life History, 5,* 87–123.

Morse, J. M. (1997). Learning to drive from a manual? *Qualitative Health Research, 7*(2), 181–183.

Patton, M. Q. (1990). *Qualitative evaluation and research methods* (2nd ed.). Newbury Park, CA: Sage.

Polkinghorne, D. E. (1988). *Narrative knowing and the human sciences.* Albany, NY: State University of New York Press.

Reissman, C. (1993). *Narrative analysis.* Thousand Oaks, CA: Sage.

Strauss, A., & Corbin, J. (1990). *Basics of qualitative research: Grounded theory, procedures and techniques.* Newbury Park, CA: Sage.

CHAPTER

The Right Way,
The Wrong Way, My Way

Susan Nagle, M.Sc. OT(C)

> *The investigator who has received the agreement of the respondent groups on the credibility of his or her work has established a strong beachhead toward convincing readers of the authenticity of her work.*
>
> —Lincoln & Guba, 1985, p. 315

Introduction

As a practicing occupational therapist and master's student, my research journey began, progressed slowly, and continues to this day because of my quest to do things the right way. While my genuine desire to do things well is a motivator, it also serves as a stumbling block. Time and time again, my longing to do things perfectly encouraged me to continue pursuing my qualitative research project, but it also sometimes stopped me in my tracks. The researcher is the key instrument in all stages of qualitative inquiry (Bogdan & Biklin, 1992; Patton, 1987). As a novice researcher, I found this to be exciting but often overwhelming. My struggles are well documented in the volumes of field notes that I kept throughout the research process. I turned to these notes to reconstruct and reflect on my research journey. My story demonstrates the "emergent" nature of qualitative studies, as well as the pitfalls novice researchers can fall into as they learn to trust in the power of qualitative methods.

The Clinical Irritation

My research questions stemmed from my clinical practice as an occupational therapist and case manager in a hospital-based, psychosocial rehabilitation program serving persons with severe and persistent mental illness. Many of the clients I saw stated that they wanted to obtain employment. Despite great efforts and time invested by both the clients and me, clients were unsuccessful in obtaining and keeping jobs. As an occupational therapist, I was viewed by both clients and other members of the treatment team as an "expert" in vocational rehabilitation. Thus, my inability to help clients meet this personally important goal frustrated and challenged me. I felt angry that clients who wanted to be productive, contributing members of society were shut out from the working world. This clinical irritation prompted me to explore and research the area of work with persons with mental illness.

School Days

After several unsuccessful attempts at research, I realized that my undergraduate degree in occupational therapy did not equip me with the skills to pursue meaningful research in a timely and cost-effective way. To alleviate my lack of skills, I enrolled in a master of science degree program in occupational therapy. I assumed that once I learned how to conduct and complete research in a rigorous way, I could discover ways to improve the effectiveness of my clinical practice.

Returning to formal education after a substantial time away presented me with many joys and challenges. While I was thrilled to return to the role of full-time student, it meant temporarily leaving my role as a paid clinician. This meant a change in city, financial status, social network, and daily routine. While I had to dust off previously learned essay writing and statistical skills, obtaining other needed skills was a real challenge. The advent of computers meant new ways of learning, researching, and writing. I will never forget losing a painstakingly entered reference list with one hit of a wrong key and a due date hours past! After completing the course work, I returned to full-time clinical work and attempted to complete the thesis requirements of my degree on a part-time basis. This presented me with a host of new

challenges. Balancing school, work, and family roles left me feeling guilty and panicky most of the time.

Hitting the Books

With the course work complete, my next step was to delve into the vast literature on work and persons with mental illness. I accumulated boxes and boxes of references that reiterated, again and again, the importance of work in our society. Work is valued not only for the resultant products and services (Parker, 1983; Schleuning, 1990), but also for the opportunities work provides for individuals to meet instrumental, psychological, and social needs (Warr, 1987). Despite the importance of nonremunerative work, in everyday use people understand the word *work* to mean a paid job (Warr, 1987). Getting and holding a job is an important measure of success and source of social approval (Stauffer, 1986). Entering or reentering the workforce is a profoundly meaningful, yet daunting, goal for persons with severe mental illness (Jeong, 1996). Like everyone else, persons with mental illness want real jobs (Pape, 1997). Nevertheless, very few persons with mental illness have success in finding and keeping jobs (Anthony, Cohen, & Farkas, 1990).

My confidence in the importance of my chosen research area was bolstered by my discovery that the published research echoed my clinical experience but did not illuminate for me how I could improve vocational outcomes. I was left with the gnawing feeling that I just had to keep reading. With all the volumes dedicated to the topic, I felt the answers to my questions had to be there. Again, my quest to do everything thoroughly was a motivator as well as a barrier to my research path. I did not want to pursue a project that had already been done and did not need to be replicated. I wanted to do something that mattered. I wanted to learn something that would improve my clinical practice. I did not know when to stop reading. I did not know when to stop collecting boxes and boxes of photocopied references. In retrospect, I probably spent too much time in the literature. Instead of uncovering answers to my questions, all the reading I did clouded the clarity of my original clinical questions.

Determining the Question

At the outset of my literature review, I wanted to know why the clients I saw were not successful in obtaining and keeping jobs. I had been frustrated by clients who appeared ready to take active steps toward employment but were unable to carry through with agreed-on steps. My mind raced with research questions. None were clearly defined. I knew I could not answer all of them, but it was hard to isolate and feel content with one area of inquiry. The broad scope of my questions concerned reviewers of my proposals. One reviewer's comments were: "The lack of focus for the research gives me some concerns. I would like to see this reduced, sharpened, and resubmitted." I continued to read, trying to clearly define my questions. One year and eighteen research proposals later, I had yet to settle on my research project. (Hint: Remember to number drafts! I didn't and spent hours trying to chronologically order my work.)

Despite all my reading and reflecting on my clinical practice, I was unable to isolate or define categories to hypothesize relationships to be studied quantitatively (McCracken, 1988). I was still left with questions and major concepts that could be explored. When it appeared that a qualitative research design was indicated, people would repeatedly needle me with "what do you want to know?" until I would blurt out something specific that could be answered quantitatively. They would then exclaim, "You can

use a standardized measure to study that." I would plead, "But that really isn't my question." I would leave these encounters feeling demoralized. Peer debriefing can provide an external check to ensure truth value (Lincoln & Guba, 1985) and an opportunity for catharsis, but in my pursuit to do everything perfectly, I sought the opinions and approval of too many people. Though well-meaning, these people eroded my confidence and detracted me from my true research questions.

I felt like I was going around and around on a gerbil wheel as I struggled to find a doable research question that was meaningful to me. I started to question the validity of all research. I began to doubt the value of pooled research findings, when each individual is different. I asked myself, "Why not just ask individuals in therapy what they think?" At times, I wanted to completely abandon my topic and find something new. Despite all my self doubts, I always returned to the same spot. The literature had supported my understanding of the importance of work and validated my experiences in working with people with mental illness, but it left many questions unanswered. I finally came to terms with the fact that I could not answer all my questions. Personally and professionally, I was genuinely interested in learning about clients' perspectives on work. To do this, it was necessary to look at informants' subjective perceptions through qualitative methods. I decided that I was going to use in-depth, long interviewing using an interview guide as my research technique. I narrowed my focus to persons with severe and persistent mental illness who were unemployed.

In my reading I had discovered a model that struck a chord with my experiences. The Vitamin Model (Warr, 1987) outlined opportunities important to well-being that work and nonwork environments could provide. My initial interview guide was based on this model. I set out to explore the occupational experience of unemployed, persistently and severely, psychiatrically, disabled adults in perceiving and utilizing opportunities in their environments to meet the needs often associated with competitive work. Still plagued with nagging doubts about my competence and readiness, I was bolstered by getting ethical approval from two universities, as well as securing research funding after several unsuccessful attempts. With renewed confidence, I set out to pilot the study interview guide.

I was encouraged after my initial pilot interview. A field note reads, "I can't wait to do more." Still, the piloting demonstrated that, once again, I had gone down a wrong path. Armed with pages of questions, I discovered that by asking the first "grand tour" (Spradley, 1979) question, my informants gave me a wealth of enlightening information. Given my time and attention, they were eager to share their worldviews with me. They did not need a long, structured interview guide or standardized measure to do so. Since the intent was not to test the Vitamin Model (Warr, 1987) but to understand the informants' occupational experiences from their point of view, the study questions were revised to be more exploratory. It was important to provide an opportunity for informants to elaborate on their occupational lives rather than superimpose Warr's model on their experiences. Finally, I recognized that it was important to strive to understand the meaning that persons with mental illness give to their everyday occupational experiences. I realized I was hampering the interview process and constraining it by using the Warr model to guide it.

Again, my project evolved. My revised project sought to understand what persons with severe and persistent mental illness do in the absence of competitive work. In keeping with qualitative research, the interview guide was revised to explore what informants did on a typical weekday; what other things they did, for instance, on the weekend, a special day, a good day, or a bad day; and what things they were not doing presently but would like to do. From the boxes of photocopied journal articles, stacks of earmarked books, and folders of proposals slashed with red pen emerged a one-page, four-question interview guide. I had learned to trust in the power of the qualitative research process. More important, I learned to trust my informants.

As with other research styles, demographic information had to be collected. A brief questionnaire was used to obtain descriptive information about the informants using closed or short answer questions to screen potential informants, describe the informants, and analyze the data (McCracken, 1988). A letter of information was handed out and consent forms were signed. In later interviews, the Descriptive Information Questionnaire was administered after the long interview. It became apparent to me that starting the interview with the questions that required only short answers could set a tone for the interview in which the participant was not actively involved and discouraged long descriptive answers (Patton, 1990). Filling out the Descriptive Information Questionnaire after the interview took very little time because often almost all the information needed had already arisen naturally in the interview.

The Joy of Interviewing

Now the fun began. Obtaining the eight informants I required was a "breeze." Several factors helped me connect quickly with informants and possibly precluded the need for longer engagement with them. I was aware of some aspects of the context because I had worked at the site of research for seven years. My clinical experience gave me the skills to build rapport quickly with the informants, who may have trusted me because they knew of me as an occupational therapist/case manager at their treatment setting. I was still relatively uninvolved personally because the informants were not my clients. My experience as a clinician helped me to recognize when informants needed assistance from their support network. The research funding enabled me to pay my informants for their time. Being paid to participate in a research project demonstrates that the informants' experience in the mental health system is valued (Reville, 1991).

Finally things were going smoothly. Not even the burden of transcribing lengthy interviews could dampen my glee. With each interview, I got more excited about what I was discovering. This made it difficult to stop. If eight interviews were so enlightening, would not sixteen teach me even more? My thesis advisor reminded me about McCracken's (1988) recommendation that eight informants are sufficient in a study using long interviews. I questioned whether that was right. I enjoyed this part of the research process so much. Finally, I agreed it was not necessary to expand the final number of informants because the eight interviews provided an adequate amount of variation of information. Preliminary data analysis showed that informational redundancy was experienced during the last interviews. With some reluctance, I stopped interviewing.

Drowning in the Data

Thank goodness I did stop interviewing informants. The three pilot interviews and eight long interviews produced binders full of transcribed information. During the analysis stage of qualitative research, researchers are often said to drown in the volume of data collected as they struggle to discover the important themes that inductively should emerge in their studies. I was overwhelmed while trying to bring order to this rich data. I read everything available about data analysis. Again, my confidence as a researcher was challenged. Data handling, analysis, and interpretation require judgment and creativity because there are no rules, only guidelines and procedural suggestions (Patton, 1990). Again, I was back to spending hours alone figuring out how to approach the task ahead. This was in stark contrast to the energizing time spent interviewing informants. The sheer volume of time spent in introspection was a challenge to my usual social nature.

I devised contact summary sheets for each of my interviews, coded all the interview transcripts with descriptive, interpretive, and pattern codes, and cut and pasted quotations. Four copies were made: one for safekeeping, one from which to photocopy, one to write on, and one to cut and paste. Despite doing this, most cutting and pasting was done on the computer. The result was a large code book of codes and paper everywhere. A field note from this time reads, "I'm going to code notes today. Is this a waste of time? It sometimes feels that way." I felt uncomfortable with the process. I was drawn to qualitative research because data is collected in words or pictures rather than numbers (Bogdan & Biklin, 1992). In coding the transcripts, I felt as though I was reducing what the informants said to small bits and losing the big picture.

I took a step back and reflected on all that I had learned. I wrote a case narrative to present a discrete, holistic portrayal of each informant. I found it helpful to display data visually in order to represent and reflect on the themes uncovered with each informant, to begin theorizing about the social phenomenon under study, and to get an overall understanding of patterns without being lost in the details. As recommended by Miles and Huberman (1994), I drew many of diagrams with lines showing the relationships between concepts that presented themselves in each case and cross-case. I checked the informants' transcript to ensure that the informants' words supported the conceptual model that was emerging.

Paralyzed in Fear

Despite following data handling, analysis, and interpretation guidelines found in the literature, I was fearful that the emerging themes did not accurately reflect the experience of the people I interviewed (Cobb & Hagemaster, 1987; Glesne & Peshkin, 1992; Krefting, 1991; Lincoln & Guba, 1985; Lofland & Lofland, 1984; Marshall & Rossman, 1989; McCracken, 1988; Miles & Huberman, 1994; Patton, 1990; Strauss & Corbin, 1990). I spent months staring at the computer, going over my transcripts again and again, making lists and lists and lists. My walls still bear the marks of tape and pushpins from hanging up lists on every bare space. Binders of field notes are testimony to my turmoil. Finally, my thesis supervisor insisted I stop. I did so, but reluctantly, as I was still questioning my work. I wanted to be true to the people I interviewed. I was afraid that I was seeing in their words only what I wanted to hear.

Member Checking

Though qualitative research does not use the same statistical tests that quantitative research relies on, there are criteria by which to judge the trustworthiness of qualitative research (Lincoln & Guba, 1985). The four criteria to evaluate qualitative research for trustworthiness are truth value, applicability, consistency, and neutrality. To meet the criterion of truth value, researchers must establish credibility in their research. After analysis, the researcher can demonstrate the credibility of the findings and interpretations by having them verified by the people being studied, through member checking (Lincoln & Guba, 1985). I had included a formal member checking group in my research design to ensure trustworthiness, and the group proved to be beneficial on several other levels.

Once all the interviews were completed and I had decided on the themes that emerged through data analysis, all the informants were invited to attend a member checking group. Since it is difficult to take notes and facilitate a group, the two-hour long member checking group was audiotaped. The informants were provided with a pizza lunch and paid for their time. During the meeting, informants chose pseudonyms for themselves and approved brief biographical sketches to be used in the thesis manuscript and future reports, publications, or presentations resulting from the study. At the member checking group, a summary of the research was presented. Simple diagrams were used to visually depict the research themes. As I explained my interpretations, the informants interjected with their insights on the themes described. I asked them to reflect on their occupational life course since their initial interview and apply the themes to their experience. Possible implications of knowledge gained in this study for health professionals were also discussed.

I approached the member checking group with some trepidation. What if they told me I was all wrong? Although I knew the researcher does not have to accept all the criticisms, only hear and account for them, I still hoped that I was on the right track. The member checking group proved to be an enjoyable, confirming experience for both me and the informants. New information was collected that added to the research findings and confirmed what had already been discovered. The group bolstered my confidence in the qualitative research process, as well as my own research skills. When I shared my results, the group enthusiastically clapped, taking me by surprise. When I asked them if what the analysis showed rang true for them, one informant said, "Sure it does." Another informant said, "It makes sense because I may have brought it to you." The informants also challenged me to think of the themes in a new way. The three integral themes, "doing," "social connections," and "health," were illustrated using a triangle. I had not determined that one of the themes was more important than the other. For no particular reason, health appeared on the top of the tri-angle. During the group, a debate ensued among the informants about whether social connections or doing should replace health at the top position. They helped me see that each of the three concepts could be at the top of the triangle depending on individual circumstances.

Member checking provided an opportunity for me to give back to the informants who were interested in hearing the research results. At the end of the group, I shared the working title of my thesis, which was "'I'm Doing as Much as I Can': Pathways to Occupational Choice." In response, the group clapped again. Another member emphatically exclaimed, "I agree with it. I agree very much. . . . Can I write it down? . . . I'm going to a family event after, and they wanted to know all about this." At the end of the group, this member looked like she wanted to say something, but when she was invited to do so, she said, "Oh nothing. I was just smiling." After discussing the findings over the telephone with an infor-mant who could not attend the member checking group, he ended our call by saying the "conversation was a pleasure." The informants felt they had been heard. I had put the informants' thoughts and feelings into words. It felt good to have them vali-date my analysis and interpretation.

Writing It Up

The member checking group convinced me that I had collected and synthesized valuable information. I was reassured that I had accu-rately heard what the informants had to say. Now I felt the responsibility to take the mountain of quotations I had collected from my interviews and put it together in a read-able, reasonable length thesis that still hon-ored the individual and collective messages. I wanted to include "in-depth, thick descrip-tions" of the context of the study to allow readers to decide if the findings were applic-able or transferable to their settings (Denzin & Lincoln, 1994). I organized and reorga-nized the outline. Every day I was going to write the thesis a different way. Again, I was on that familiar gerbil wheel. A looming uni-versity deadline to complete my degree forced me to take a leave from my full-time clinical job to immerse myself once more in the research work on a full-time basis at the university. I went through mountains of paper and gallons of black coffee as I strove to complete the thesis. Security guards would visit me to warn me that I was the only per-son in the large, university building where I toiled late into the night. On the white board in my office where I had penned my last attempt at an outline a colleague had written across it "Just do it!."

The Thesis Defense

With the clock ticking I finished. Many drafts and 270 finalized pages later, I had com-pleted my work. The result was exhilaration and exhaustion rolled into one. But the best was yet to come. While colleagues had dreaded their defense date, I looked toward mine with anticipation. It proved to be one of the best days of my life. Three professors were going to read my work and take time to talk to me about it. The day started with my public lecture. I was as high as a kite. I was thrilled to share the words of my informants and buoyed by the genuine interest of those in my audience. Although the examiners asked some very thought-provoking and challenging questions, for the most part they provided an arena in which to share the views of my informants with a small group of informed and committed individuals. It was over all too quickly.

Since Then

The joy continued as I presented at local, national, and international conferences. It continues now when I share my findings with individual clients and groups in my clinical practice. Again and again, people tell me my findings ring true. The findings continue to inform my practice. They have helped me to make sense of the stories that clients tell me. They have helped me to understand when to encourage clients to do more and when to support them in their continuation of their current daily occupations.

Writing this has given me an opportunity to reflect on my research experience as a graduate student. I was nervous when I dusted off the old field notes, but the experience of reviewing them was actually cleansing. My field notes bore titles such as " Going to Get This If It Kills Me (or My Friends)." They speak of the joys on the days when I was experiencing "flow" (Csikszentmihalyi, 1993), and of other days when I wrote comments such as,"I feel like crying, but I won't." (I did). I remember the months and years of trying to determine my question. In looking back, I realize it was all part of the emergent nature of my completed work. The years spent reading and clarifying my question

were indeed the beginning of my analysis. The length of time I was involved in the study, as well as my involvement in clinical work, gave me time to carefully identify and reflect on reappearing patterns. By default, it was a way to ensure truth value and credibility (Lincoln & Guba, 1985) in the study.

In the end, the qualitative research process is very powerful. It holds power in providing a way to tap into unanswered questions and requires researchers to be humbled in front of those they study. It fits well into my understanding of what occupational therapy is and my vision of myself as an occupational therapist. My experience was sometimes frustrating and embarrassing, but for the most part, it was empowering. The student/researcher role was one I embraced and found hard to let go. I am left with trying to find out how to manage the clinician/researcher role in light of my many other roles. But my quest for perfection continues to haunt me. Is my work good enough? Can I write in a manner that is truthful to my informants? Although the qualitative research process does not give researchers and authors the confidence of statistics to stand behind, it gives us so much more. No research method is foolproof in unearthing the truth, but qualitative research methods give us a way to be open to the messages our informants want us to hear. They give us a window to informants' perceptions, feelings, and thoughts (Lord, Schnarr, & Hutchinson, 1987). The spoken words of my informants and the importance of their stories help me to continue to strive to convey their messages. I hope that you do the same.

References

Anthony, W. A., Cohen, M., & Farkas, M. (1990). *Psychiatric rehabilitation.* Boston: Center for Psychiatric Rehabilitation.

Bogdan, R., & Biklen, S. K. (1992).

Qualitative research for education: An introduction to theory and methods (2nd ed.). Boston: Allyn & Bacon.

Cobb, A. K., & Hagemaster, J. N. (1987). Ten criteria for evaluating qualitative research proposals. *Journal of Nursing Education, 26*(4), 138–143.

Csikszentmihalyi, M. (1993). Activity and happiness: Towards a science of occupation. *Occupational Science: Australia, 1*(1), 38–42.

Denzin, N. K., & Lincoln, Y. S. (Eds.). (1994). *Handbook of qualitative research.* Thousand Oaks, CA: Sage.

Glesne, C., & Peshkin, A. (1992). *Becoming qualitative researchers: An introduction.* White Plains, NY: Longman.

Jeong, G. (1996, September). Enabling people with cognitive disabilities to join the workforce. *OT Practice*, 40–45.

Krefting, L. (1991). Rigor in qualitative research: The assessment of trustworthiness. *The American Journal of Occupational Therapy, 45*, 214–222.

Lincoln, Y. S., & Guba, E. G. (1985). *Naturalistic inquiry.* Newbury Park, CA: Sage.

Lofland, J., & Lofland, L. H. (1984). *Analyzing social settings: A guide to qualitative observation and analysis* (2nd ed.). Belmont, CA: Wadsworth.

Lord, J., Schnarr, A., & Hutchinson, P. (1987). The voice of the people: Qualitative research and the needs of consumers. *Canadian Journal of Community Mental Health, 6*(2), 25–36.

Marshall, C., & Rossman, G. R. (1989). *Designing qualitative research.* London: Sage.

McCracken, G. (1988). *The long interview.* Newbury Park, CA: Sage.

Miles, M. B., & Huberman, A. M. (1994). *Qualitative data analysis: An expanded source book* (2nd ed.). Thousand Oaks, CA: Sage.

Pape, B. (1997). Editor's notes. *Forum: A National Mental Health Policy Report from the Mental Health Services Work Group, 9*, 1–3.

Parker, S. (1983). *Leisure and work.* London: George Allen & Unwin.

Patton, M. Q. (1987). *How to use qualitative methods in evaluation.* Newbury Park, CA: Sage.

Patton, M. Q. (1990). *Qualitative evaluation and research methods* (2nd ed.). Newbury Park, CA: Sage.

Reville, D. (1991). *What about work and other questions?* Toronto, Canada: Queen Street Mental Health Centre, Users Designing Future Project.

Schleuning, N. (1990). *Idle hands and empty hearts.* New York: Bergin & Garvey.

Spradley, J. P. (1979). *The ethnographic interview.* New York: Holt, Rinehart & Winston.

Stauffer, D. L. (1986). Predicting successful employment in the community for people with a history of chronic mental illness. *Occupational Therapy in Mental Health, 6*(2), 31–49.

Strauss, A., & Corbin, J. (1990). *Basics of qualitative research: Grounded theory and procedures and techniques.* Newbury Park, CA: Sage.

Warr, P. (1987). *Work, unemployment and*

CHAPTER

9

From a Personal Interest to a Research Program

Ruth Segal, Ph.D.

> *We have followed Tocqueville and other classical theorists in focusing on the mores—"the habits of the heart"—that include consciousness, culture and the daily practices of life.*
>
> —Bellah et al., 1985, p. 275

Introduction

My purpose is to demonstrate how a personal interest area evolved into a research program. The research journey is a story, a section of my life story. A narrative becomes a story when it has "a human interest," when others find that narrative interesting (Toolan, 1988). Similarly, an interest area has to be interesting to others to become a research program. Additionally, a good story has to have a beginning, middle, and end. The middle, or the muddle, should consist of complications, resolutions, and unexpected turns of events. Those features of a story are the features of how my area of interest evolved into a research program.

A Beginning: Becoming a Parent

When my first child was born, I found myself in awe of the extent of changes in routine that occurred in my life and my spouse's life. I was intrigued with issues such as how did we make those changes? How did we adapt to having a child? We stopped doing a number of things but never thought of it as a sacrifice. Why not? When these life changes occurred, I certainly did not think of these issues as a research topic. They were conversation items when people asked me about parenting.

At this time, I already had my advanced master's degree in occupational therapy from the University of Southern California.

In the course of pursuing that degree, I had taken the seminar on adaptation, given by Dr. Gelya Frank, as an elective. It turned out to be one of the most transforming educational experiences I had. This was the first time I read ethnographies of life experiences of the people with whom we work. I cannot recall being introduced to these subjective aspects of patients and clients in any other class. This also was the first time I experienced an educational method in which the instructor encouraged the course syllabus to evolve based on the students' interests, needs, and requests. I liked that style, and I decided to ask Gelya to be my master's thesis supervisor.

At the time, I saw myself as a practitioner in the mental health field, and my chosen thesis topic at the master's level was about the meaning of "grave disability" as a criterion for nonvoluntary hospitalization of people with mental illness. I collected the data through observations of writ hearings in court. I also interviewed the judge, district attorneys, and public defenders. My thesis committee included Dr. Florence Clark and Professor Martin Levine, who held a joint chair in law, gerontology, and psychiatry. This ethnographic study of the legal system in action was very gratifying. I enjoyed the research process, and I enjoyed working with Gelya. Professor Levine tried to recruit me to go to graduate school in law. I wanted to do more research.

When I came back to the University of Southern California for my doctoral studies, I knew I wanted to work again with Gelya Frank, and I was committed to qualitative research methods. Both of these commitments were directly related to my experience completing my master's degree under the guidance of Gelya. I also decided that my specialty area should be qualitative methods. I believe that a sound grounding in methods

and methodological issues is essential for good research.

The Middle

The Doctoral Studies and Dissertation

Coming back to the University of Southern California was fun and exciting. I took my courses in the first year, made new friends, developed relationships with colleagues, and met with old friends. I did not think too much about a dissertation topic. I am sure, though I cannot recall the specific details, that I talked about the lifestyle changes we went through when my child was born. By the beginning of the second year, I knew I was interested in studying families. I did not know what I wanted to study in that broad field. So, I decided to read about families in the context of each course and seminar I took.

The first opportunity came in the seminar on temporal adaptation taught by Dr. Ruth Zemke. One of the seminar assignments was to fill a time log twice per week. In one of our meetings, I told Dr. Zemke that I did not really fill out the time log as instructed, as soon as the activity was finished, but rather, I filled out the time log in retrospect. I added that it seemed to me that qualitative interviews about time use would be even better because they would allow the researcher to engage in in-depth investigation of time use. Dr. Zemke's response was, "Well, I think you may have the topic for the seminar project." It turned out that both my doctoral dissertation and the seminar research project were launched at that moment.

For the seminar project, I decided to interview four families about their daily schedules, routines, and occupations. I consulted with a colleague, a pediatric occupational therapist, about parents who might find daily schedules and routine a challenge. She suggested parents of children with attention deficit hyperactivity disorder (ADHD). She and her colleagues in the clinic helped me to recruit four families (four mothers and one father) who agreed to be interviewed. They also put me in contact with another mother who did not become a participant but later became an important gatekeeper for my dissertation.

For the seminar project, each parent was interviewed one or two times about their daily routines. In the first interview, they were asked to describe a typical day from the first person who gets up to the last person who goes to sleep. In the second interview, they were asked to describe the previous day, evaluate whether it was typical, and explain what made it typical or atypical. Additionally, they were asked to identify and explain the best, worst, and most routinized parts of the day.

During that term, I also took the final seminar on qualitative methods in the sociology department. In that course, we were expected to develop the methodological aspects of a project of our interest. I chose to work on the project for the seminar on temporal adaptation. When I decided to use the same project in the two seminars, I was not aware of the great advantage that would be. The methods seminar was designed so that we moved along with our project as we read and discussed the relevant material, basically a step-by-step process of a research project from the beginning to its end (the writing of a paper). In this seminar, my interview guide was developed and critiqued on the basis of its methodological aspects (the how), while in the temporal adaptation seminar that same interview guide was critiqued on the basis of the content it aimed to elicit (the what). This same process continued throughout until the project was completed.

Throughout that term, I considered the project a class project, and based on class discussion that class projects do not need to go through the human subject ethics review board, I did not apply for approval. Since the colleague who had helped me review participants was a classmate, I assumed that she was aware of this situation. As it turned out, she was not, and she and her colleagues in the clinic discovered this situation and were very concerned about the lack of ethics approval. Consequently, the interview data from this class project were never used in my doctoral dissertation, conference presentations, or publications. This was a great loss. Not only could I not use the data that I had already collected and analyzed in my dissertation, but I also could not continue to work with that clinic and had to search for other places to get participants. The move to other sources, especially to support groups, necessitated a change in the children's ages from 4 to 5-year-olds to 7 to 12-year-olds because of patterns of parental participation in these support groups. Children's ages are reflected in the type of adaptive strategies that parents can use.

In the process of data collection and analysis for the seminar project, I developed four memos that I showed Gelya, asking her whether there was anything in them that could be used in my dissertation. I remember that her eyes lit up. Without saying much, she referred me to the paper (1996) she presented in one of the occupational science's symposiums and to the paper that Mary Catherine Bateson (1996) delivered in the same symposium. These papers helped me to conceptualize the memos into the concepts of "unfolding occupations" and the "construction of daily routines and occupations" as powerful means for socializing children into their culture. These memos were not well developed, but they were the initial ideas that were later developed in my dissertation. These original memos were a real discovery for me. At the time, I was not aware of any literature discussing the use of time or the construction of occupations as an adaptive strategy. Now that I have read widely in this topic, I know there is no literature about time use as an adaptive strategy other than Gelya's work. Gelya conceptualizes and demonstrates adaptation as the organization of occupations or activities for the purposes of enhancing quality of life and increasing life opportunities (Frank, 1996, 2000).

As the term progressed, my project went very well in terms of my occupational science classes, and it also went well in terms of gatekeepers and entering the field. I met a mother who was described as "very active and involved" by my friend at the clinic. I will call her Eileen. The relationship that developed never permitted taking out the tape recorder and audiotaping a formal interview with her. But we talked a lot and met quite often, and in a way we became friends and colleagues. She was involved with a regional center as a parent who was trying to develop a family support group for families of children with special needs. The attempt had been going on for quite a while and had not gone anywhere. Thus, the center hired someone to work at developing this group, and Eileen suggested that I come and get involved. I came in, and slowly my role evolved into helping with minor organizational issues such as heading the group when it was geared for men only (at which time the speaker, as well as the fathers, did not appear except for one father). This involvement began before I was formally collecting data and continued until I left Los Angeles. I did not consider it part of my dissertation, and I did not keep a field journal or notes of any type. However, in participating in the groups, I learned in the process of introductions that parents of children with special needs always looked to see whether I had a wedding band on my finger. Then they would ask if I had any children and whether

they had any special needs. Later, in the course of interviewing for my dissertation, I always made a point of revealing at least this marital and parental aspect of my personal life.

Eileen told me one day that she saw a newspaper advertisement for a meeting of a parent support group called CHADD, geared toward parents of children with ADHD. The meetings were in the evening and quite far away. Eileen suggested that we drive together. She would do the driving, since she was familiar with the area. I drove to her house where I met her husband and two young children. Her young children were diagnosed as having ADHD, and when we left them, the father was trying to convince them to stop swinging on the curtain rods.

We drove together to several meetings, and then Eileen could not attend any meetings for some time because she and her family moved to a new house. However, this support group turned out to be a gold mine for recruiting my research participants. Gelya and I built my advisory committee with two people from the sociology department who were experts in the study of families and minorities, and two people from occupational science, Dr. Florence Clark and Dr. Diane Parham (who eventually withdrew). I prepared my proposal and passed the qualifying examination. In the qualifying examination (which is the proposal defense), one of my committee members, a sociologist who studies family organization, suggested that I read Edward T. Hall's (1983) *Dance of Life* for the concepts of monochronic and polychronic time and the latter's similarity to Bateson's (1996) "enfolded occupation." Although I read this book as part of the readings for the seminar on temporal adaptation, I had somehow missed this point. So, I reread the book and also read Zerubavel's (1981) *Hidden Rhythms*. These books were essential to my later analysis of my data.

After passing the hurdles of the proposal and the qualifying examination, I had to pass the hurdle of the human subject review committee. My first request for approval was rejected because I did not have a substantial description of the "statistical analysis" of the data. I was devastated. I went to Gelya, and within 45 minutes, she wrote a letter to the committee explaining some of the basics of qualitative research. She also instructed me how to write the letter of response in which I would politely refuse, without offending the committee numbers, to add a statistical analysis based on the premises of qualitative methods. She also told me that one committee member who was knowledgeable about qualitative research and occupational therapy called her on his own and apologized about this response, explaining that he had been unable to attend that particular meeting. We attached our letters to a request for approval, and this time I was successful.

In the meantime, I checked on the CHADD support group. I took some information flyers to the meetings, and I talked with the organizers. I learned that it was a national support group with at least three chapters in the Los Angeles area. I got the telephone numbers of the organizers and contacted them about the possibility of recruiting participants for my research. All three told me that each meeting begins with announcements and I could ask to make one. They also suggested that I prepare flyers to hand out at the meetings, as well as for them, the organizers, because there would be a table with flyers at each meeting.

I printed my flyers on bright lime-green paper that was bold and would stand out from the other flyers. Armed with the flyers, I went to the first meeting, and I tried to recruit participants. I attended four meetings to get enough participants for my dissertation (21 participants). In three of the meetings, I made an announcement and handed out flyers. To another chapter of CHADD, I just mailed the flyers, and some potential participants contacted me. The meetings

occurred on a monthly basis, so I had time in between to interview each family at least once. The data collection was finished within three months from the time it began. It was fun and exhilarating. Data analysis was something else.

I remember sitting with my first interview transcript trying to analyze it over and over again. I tried to reconstruct the family schedule and who was doing what at what time. I created tables, but they were not interesting (that is, insightful). I tried to break the transcript down based on occupational classification (work, leisure, self-care) and got nowhere. I was certain at the time that since my seminar project could not be used, I had to ignore the previous conceptual memos as well. I also wanted to approach the analysis by suspending all preconceived ideas and theories, as indicated by grounded theory. So, I was stuck.

All this was occurring while I kept collecting data, and the transcripts and documents were piling up. I could not stop collecting data because my spouse and I would soon be moving to Canada for his employment. I tried harder. I made a point of listening to the interviews in the car on my way home from every interview. In this way, at least I could have some follow-up questions for the interviewees.

I managed to see some patterns in the family stories, in particular, how mothers worked with their children on homework. They talked about how difficult it was either to get a diagnosis or to get a diagnosis with which they agreed. The participating parents in my dissertation study identified their children as being "high need" babies in the past and having problems the parents believed required a diagnosis and intervention. I also looked at how much energy and time the parents invested in finding appropriate interventions for their children. These interventions often did not follow only the mainstream type of intervention; many other avenues were used as well. I never formally analyzed the family stories, but I read them in order to understand the families. I learned to care for these people and to respect them. I respected the hard work of raising children.

Eventually, after I interviewed the fifth family, I had the breakthrough, or perhaps it was a breakdown. I decided to look at the memos from the seminar project. I had thought about the memos for awhile, but I was determined not to use them. I considered them data rather than grounded concepts that came from the interaction between the seminar data and me. I decided to retrace my steps, and I read again Frank's (1996) and Bateson's (1996) works and eventually came to work with some of their concepts—organization of occupations and enfolding, respectively. Looking closely at my data with these concepts in mind, I found that the mothers in my study adapted routines by reorganization of occupations, particularly by removing occupations from one part of the day to another or by temporal relocation. Additionally, mothers commonly stated that enfolding occupations did not work well with their children with ADHD, and they adapted their schedules by, what I called, unfolding of their previously enfolded occupations (Segal, in press). These concepts were not identical to the memos from the seminar project, but I think the differences in children's ages can explain this discrepancy. It was important to me that they were different. In this way, I felt I did not use this data, but rather it influenced my thinking.

Once I began working with these concepts, the analysis flew. I went through the process of grounded theory and developed a model to identify the time use related processes by which families attempt to enhance their quality of life and increase their children's life opportunities. This model was never published. It took a long time to learn how to divide the dissertation into publishable sections. Attempts at publication did not go well.

However, I began presenting my findings at the conferences of the American Occupational Therapy Association (AOTA), Canadian Association of Occupational Therapists (CAOT), and World Federation of Occupational Therapists (WFOT). The presentations always attracted a good audience. The most memorable presentation was my first AOTA conference where, at the end, a person approached me and gave words of encouragement about the good work I was doing. I do not know who she was because she did not wear her identification. However, she seemed to be somebody embedded in the field of occupational therapy, and somehow her comments were very important for me.

Once the data collection was done, I moved back to Canada to the University of Western Ontario. I defended my dissertation in December. I had to do some corrections, but I did not have to go through another defense. The main correction was to add a "plot" to my literature review because the defense committee thought it was too boring. I completed the corrections and formally graduated in May 1995.

A Faculty Position and Continuing Research

The publication ordeal began, but I was encouraged because of the positive and enthusiastic responses I received at conferences and in meetings with friends from school. My first publication began in 1998 (that is, submission in 1997), three years after finishing my dissertation and after five rejected manuscripts.

The move to the university meant not only publishing, but also continuing with further research and data collection and analysis. My dissertation findings came from interviews with families of children with ADHD. Were these findings, therefore, only applicable to such families? What about families with children with different special needs? These were my continuing research questions.

When I came to The University of Western Ontario, I was assigned to teach the qualitative methods class for graduate students. I took this course over from Joanne Cook who gave me her previous course outline with the clear and strict instruction to change and adapt it in any way I liked. I made some changes and read the books she had on her reading list. This was the first time I read Spradley (1979) and McCracken (1988), and I was impressed with their books, particularly Spradley's, which greatly influenced how I wanted to conduct my next project.

Teaching is an interesting phenomenon. Although my cognate or specialty in my doctoral studies was in qualitative research methods, I felt quite insecure about teaching this course. But the process of reading for teaching, as well as working with the material for and with the students and reading their work, greatly increased my knowledge and understanding of research methods. Additionally, my interactions with Joanne not only enhanced my understanding, but also developed it into a real area of interest. I kept reading methods books as though they were fiction novels.

I applied for research funding and eventually obtained it. I designed the project to be similar to my dissertation but focused on families with children who had physical disabilities. Instead of two interviews with the homemaker and one interview with the other parent, I planned on conducting three interviews with the homemaker and two interviews with the other parent. Originally, I wanted to meet approximately four times with each participant in order to really explore his or her world in the way that Spradley (1979) suggests. However, the research review committee at the agency through which I wanted to recruit participants felt it would be too much of a burden

on the families and asked me to reduce the number of interviews with each participant.

This project unfolded somewhat differently from what I anticipated. First, I obtained only eight families out of a proposed twenty because of personnel changes in the facility. The previous program director had agreed to my request, but the new director decided that her population did not fit my criteria.

Second, the stories people told me affected me very strongly, and my focus shifted away from the construction of routine, at least for the present. This change of focus occurred because the daily routines of these families were not the primary issue for them. Yes, the routines presented challenges, but these were challenges they could overcome with resources (money, hard work, getting organized, and other support). However, they faced other challenges they could not overcome. In particular, the families with children with Duchenne's muscular dystrophy (DMD) worked hard, but the thing they want most could not be achieved, that is, for their children to have a long life.

I am still intrigued by the fact that the family stories from my dissertation were not particularly interesting to me at that time. They were good stories, but they were peripheral at the time to my interest in the construction of daily routines and occupations. They described many issues pertaining to daily routines and occupational performance as they related to the children's development and growth; however, in the family stories of the families with children with physical disabilities, the life stories, experiences, and meanings were not about the issue of routines and occupations. They were much more about emotional issues related to raising children with disabilities and nonemotional issues related to dealing with the education system and various agencies in the health system. My doctoral participants had also described difficulties with systems, but these agency system issues looked much more difficult when the children had DMD and the agencies were viewed by the participants as a lacking in understanding of DMD and in care and sensitivity, which was much more painful.

Now I was ready to move away from the more structured, prescriptive grounded theory or, as Gelya referred to my dissertation, the "scientist" perspective. The element of personal development cannot be discounted, but perhaps it was not just development. It was the data. I used the constant comparative (grounded theory) approach to my data analysis. I had a hard time with it because it did not fit the data. It took away from the power of the story. As I was playing with the analysis and pondering, I focused on one interview with a caregiver who was a natural storyteller. It was the first time that I really saw "the story" in the interview. It was presented with dramatic turns of events. It had a clear beginning, middle, and end. That interview was a complete story and needed to be dealt with in that way.

Some Turning Points

These realizations, of course, were not clear in the beginning. I worked with the data—using the constant comparative method to develop concepts and categories. I took it far enough to develop a presentation for a WFOT conference. However, I could not deny the feeling that I was not getting to "it," whatever "it" may be. As I kept reading the interviews, and talking with Joanne, I slowly began to see that at least one of the interviews began like a story. The participant began his narration with an idyllic background of marriage, birth of children, and purchasing the first and second houses before he presented the catastrophic event in which both his sons were diagnosed with Duchenne's muscular dystrophy.

I began a search in the literature and read a number of books as I looked for an approach that would fit better. I was wondering and thinking seriously about how to treat this story, do it justice, and present its power.

I worked with my data using Cortazzi's (1993) guidelines from each field of study and eventually settled on literary, structural analysis. In order to feel confident in what I was doing, I read relevant resources that Cortazzi (1993) used for his chapter on literary narrative analysis. I began with Toolan (1988), Rimmon-Kenan (1983), and Bal (1997). Finally, I read the French structuralists, Bremond (1970) and Greimas (1983). Since I could read only the work that was written in English or translated into English, I used Rimmon-Kenan's work to supplement my reading and help my understanding of their approach to analysis. Using Bremond's work, I looked at the development and nature of the events of the story. Using Greimas's work, I looked at the nature of the characters and their actions in the story. I think using this approach maintained the integrity of the story and highlighted the tragic unfolding of events. It was in many ways like a Greek tragedy.

In the course of data collection, a mother remarked that her son's response when he heard I was interviewing her as a mother of a child with DMD was to ask, "Why isn't she talking with me?" Additionally, coordinating a course on psychiatric diagnoses, I became friendly with a child psychiatrist, and we discovered a mutual interest in children with DMD and their families. We met, talked, and formed a group of people interested in the topic. The discussions went on for a long time. By the time we were almost on the verge of writing a research proposal in which I would interview children with disabilities, I moved to New York and was unable to continue the collaboration.

During the same period, in the course of discussions with a colleague, it was mentioned that I should do some work with parents of children with developmental coordination disorder. Eventually, this project materialized. My colleague, who is a pediatric therapist, collected data with the children themselves, while I interviewed the parents. In my next proposed project, interviewing the children will be an integral part of the proposal.

To summarize this story, it all started with an observation about my own life changes related to having a child in the family, and it evolved into a research program with families of children with special needs with a look at daily routines, occupations, time use, adaptation, experiences, and life stories.

There Is No Ending

In this story, I have no ending yet. I have not finished with any of my work. I feel that my dissertation data could be analyzed further, especially the family stories. Much of my other data is not fully analyzed as well. There are many grounded ideas that appear as work in progress that have not materialized yet. There are numerous books, papers, conferences, and other sources on methods, methodology, philosophy, and content specifics with which that I need to become familiar. It is only the beginning of the rest of the story.

Discussion

In this section, I will synthesize some of the threads that enabled and shaped the development of my research program. As individuals, we are part of our social and cultural environments. The interactions with the environment allow us to influence, as well as be influenced. My observation about the changes in my personal life occurred at the right time and the right place. It was not long after my first child was born that I began the doctoral studies that gave me the opportunity to explore issues not related to my practice in mental health. I chose to pursue my doctoral work at the University of Southern California where doctoral students were encouraged to embark in new fields that were not necessarily directly related to the practice of occupational therapy. These were the initial conditions that allowed for this research journey to evolve.

The same thing is true for the evolution of methods used. My familiarity with and understanding of qualitative research methods were greatly influenced by my teaching and my friendship with Joanne Cook. This is a friendship embedded in common interests and mutual respect for each other. The differences that we have encourage our development and deepen our friendship. This environment allowed me to grow and enhance my research program.

Chance meetings and interactions also shaped the evolution of the research program. When I challenged the use of a time log, Dr. Zemke's response actually redirected me to the observation on the changes in my daily life as a result of having a child. The decision to interview parents of children with ADHD for the seminar project was based on convenience—one semester is a very short time for collecting data, analyzing data, and writing a paper. So, I asked for markers that would define a relatively large group. As it turned out, daily routines and schedules are a major issue for families of children with ADHD. As my later data collection shows, this is not a major issue for other families. This is another important environmental aspect—the participants and their life experiences also shape the research program, from including the children to changing the methods of analysis. I will undoubtedly continue to adapt, alter, and develop both my interests and research strategies as I continue this program of research. It is not just the journey itself that is satisfying, but as in any trip, the planning and anticipation are also rewarding. I look forward to "packing my bags."

References

Bal, M. (1997). *Narratology: Introduction to the theory of narrative* (2nd ed.). Buffalo, NY: University of Toronto Press.

Bateson, M. C. (1996). Enfolded activity and the concept of occupation. In R. Zemke & F. Clark (Eds.), *Occupational science: The evolving discipline* (pp. 5–12). Philadelphia, PA: Davis.

Bellah, R., Madsen, R., Sullivan, W. Swidler, A., & Tipton, S. (1985). *Habits of the heart.* Berkeley, CA: University of California Press.

Bremond, C. (1970). Morphology of the French folktale. *Semiotica, 2,* 247–276.

Cortazzi, M. (1993). *Narrative analysis.* Washington, DC: The Falmer Press.

Frank, G. (1996). The concept of adaptation as a foundation for occupational science research. In R. Zemke & F. Clark (Eds.), *Occupational science: The evolving discipline* (pp. 47–55). Philadelphia, PA: Davis.

Frank, G. (2000). *Venus on wheels: Two decades of dialogue on disability, biography and being female in America.* Los Angeles, CA: University of California Press.

Greimas, A. J. (1983). *Structural semantics: An attempt at a method* (D. McDowell, R. Schleifer, & A. Velie, Trans.). Lincoln, NE: University of Nebraska Press. (Original work published 1966).

Hall, E. T. (1983). *The dance of life: The other dimension of time.* New York: Anchor Books.

McCracken, G. (1988). *The long interview.* Newbury Park, CA: Sage.

Rimmon-Kenan, S. (1983). *Narrative fiction: Contemporary poetics.* New York: Routledge.

Segal, R. (1995). *Family adaptation to a child with attention deficit hyperactivity disorder.* Unpublished doctoral dissertation, University of Southern California, Los Angeles.

Segal, R. (in press). Adaptive strategies of mothers with children with attention deficit hyperactivity disorder: Enfolding and unfolding occupations. *American Journal of Occupational Therapy.*

Spradley, J. (1979). *The ethnographic interview.* New York: Holt, Rinehart & Winston.

Toolan, M. J. (1988). *Narrative: A critical linguistic introduction.* New York: Routledge.

Zerubavel, E. (1981). *Hidden rhythms: Schedules and calendars in social life.* Los Angeles, CA: University of California Press.

CHAPTER

In Order to Make a Difference:
A Research Journey

Karen L. Rebeiro M.Sc., OT(C)

> *Our role consists in giving opportunities rather than prescriptions.*
> *There must be opportunities to do and to plan and create, and to*
> *learn to use material.*
>
> —Adolph Meyer, 1922

Introduction

What began as a research project intended to meet the requirements of a master's degree in occupational therapy evolved into a personal research journey that, to date, has yet to end. What was initiated through clinical irritation about occupational therapy mental health practice being poorly understood evolved into a better understanding of the complexities of what we, as occupational therapists, attempt to do in practice, as well as a clearer clinical vision of what should be done in mental health practice.

This journey yielded insights but also generated many more questions than answers. To say that I was naive when I started this research journey would be an understatement. If I believed that one study would

answer my clinical questions and bring me to a comfort level with my practice, I was wrong. What research did for me was to open a Pandora's box of unknowns that further complicated what I already knew and ultimately compelled me to pursue a series of research projects in order to gain a better understanding of the issues on which to base my clinical practice. I make no claims to hold any expert knowledge of research methods or the practice of occupational therapy in mental health. I merely share my own struggles with clinical practice and attempt to detail my own research journey. I share my mistakes and confusion in the hope that the reader will not be afraid to attempt research and make mistakes. I share this journey to offer some of the incredible insights into practice that I have gained by working collaboratively with my clients and research participants. These understandings have forever changed the way I practice.

I began this research journey in graduate school with a thorough review of the occupational therapy research in mental health. Specifically, I was looking for research conducted on the use of occupation-as-means to mental health. What I discovered was very discouraging. A great deal of what we as occupational therapists claim to do has very little support in research (Rebeiro, 1998). Further, occupational therapy theory regarding the use of occupation as the primary means of therapy rarely gets fulfilled in community practice. This is not to say that occupational therapists do not act with good intention, for I believe we do. It is just that the systems within which occupational therapists are traditionally employed are not structured to support the work that occupational therapists aspire toward—enabling occupation. E. Townsend's (1998) book, *Good Intentions Overruled: An Institutional Ethnography of Occupational Therapy Practices*, provides insight into the ways in which occupational therapists' good intentions are not supported by the systems and institutions within which they work. This book has been a valuable resource to my own understanding of why I have, for years, banged my head against the proverbial brick wall. I recently realized that there was a back door through which I could travel and by which I could ultimately enact my good intentions and make a difference. This back door was only opened to me by traveling the road with clients and extensive listening and paying attention to everything I did not learn in school. The most useful insights were discovered during research and given generously by the "real experts"—persons who live daily with a mental illness.

The deeper I went into the research process, the more clarity I achieved in thinking about my own role and purpose as an occupational therapist. The more I learned, the more I recognized that enabling occupation was a complicated undertaking. I became intimately aware of the issues facing persons with a mental illness and angry at the system on more than one occasion. The system's continual focus on the person being the problem, and all resources, both human and fiscal, being dedicated to fixing the person, allows service providers to pay less attention to the multitude of social issues faced by persons with a mental illness (Rebeiro, 1999). Further, the tremendous focus on the biochemical nature of mental illness often leaves the person with mental illness in a position of dependency and without much hope. If it is the person's genetic makeup or flawed chemistry, then it must be "of the person," and if medication does not work, then the person must not be trying very hard.

I also became angry with the profession for its sole reliance on the medical model of intervention and treatment of mental illness. I became discouraged because of the stories I heard regarding clients' occupational therapy experiences. What I read in the occupational therapy literature about our client-centered practice and our enabling or empowering approach to therapy certainly was not being supported by my field research. What I learned was that many occupational therapists remain stuck in their practice and attempt to fit their ideas of occupational therapy to the system. Unfortunately, this does not work. The prescriptive use of activities may help occupational therapists to explain their use of activities to others (for example, that working with mosaic tile may help clients with frustration tolerance or planning). However, there is no evidence in the literature to support a theory that completing a mosaic tile will assist the client to resume volunteer work or maintain activities of daily living once discharged from the hospital. If we are about enabling occupation and fostering the occupational performance of our clients, then this needs to happen in a real way in the clinic or community. There must be evidence that our enabling strategies within the clinic have real value in the real world, or else, what is the point?

There have been many calls for occupational therapists to research and provide evidence of what we do. I understand that we are all busy and find it difficult to find the time to meet our clients' needs, let alone conduct research and publish the results. However, if we aspire to have recognition from our clients and from other professions, we must provide evidence that what we do with clients makes a difference. I have suggested elsewhere (Rebeiro & Allen, 1998) that single-case studies can provide a means by which occupational therapists can collectively develop a knowledge base that supports the use of occupation-as-means to mental health. Qualitative research methods are a natural research strategy for occupational therapists and are methods well-suited to conducting single-case studies within busy practices. One case at a time, the professional can substantiate a practice so that it can withstand jurisdictional challenges (Abbott, 1988) from other professions.

Collaboratively, clients and researchers are gaining an understanding of the complexities of illness and its impact on daily function. For me, this journey was never walked alone. I always walked with someone who had been there. I always checked any understanding or insight with the authority, the client. I always positioned myself as an empty vessel, learning more, receptive to challenges to any growing insights, and always assuming a humble stance in my role. I felt very grateful for the stories and experiences that were shared with me during the past three and one-half years and for my own personal development, both in knowledge and spiritually. The process of reflecting on the past three years for the purposes of writing this chapter was a difficult undertaking for me, and many of my experiences were hard to articulate. I learned so much in a short period of time and have so dramatically altered the ways in which I view the issues of mental health and illness that it becomes for me a chicken and egg equation. Which came first? It probably does not matter.

This research journey was not an easy one for me. I spent a great deal of the time confused, bewildered, angry, frustrated, and unsure of what to do next. Just when I thought I could "see the light," I would speak to someone else who would complicate the issues further, and thus complicate or nullify the great insights I had. Little did I know at the time that my research would be a continual journey. I now know that it will most likely never end. The more I learned, the more I realized I needed to learn more and know more to truly make a difference. I have not felt anything more than transient comfort or confidence with my knowledge in the four years since entering and leaving graduate school. This is a good position for a researcher because it compels you to keep going and wanting to study and learn more. However, this is an extremely frustrating position for a clinician. At some point, I would like to think that I am ready to "just practice," but I am certain that will not happen for me in the near future. For certain, all of my research is being put into practice, and this is detailed in the description of the Northern Initiative for Social Action (NISA) study included later in this chapter. I do not think I would be interested in research that did not have an impact on clinical practice. However, I am infected with this "I don't know enough yet" syndrome that compels me to research further and continue this research journey.

This narrative of one research journey is about people, real people, who live with the daily reality of a serious mental illness. This journey is about them, their lives, their struggles, and about how I began to make these struggles my own. This description of my research journey up to the present ends where it began, in Building Two of a mental health facility in northern Ontario, where my first research project about a women's group took place.

The Beginning of the Journey: The Women's Group Study

When I was first approached to write about my own personal research journey, I was slightly hesitant to write about it because my journey was a bumpy one with many peaks and valleys. The Women's Group study was my first research study, and I did not realize how this would open up my world and direct my career on a path that was very different from the one I was on prior to graduate school. I made a lot of mistakes. As a long-distance graduate student, I learned qualitative research methods primarily from textbooks and designed my research study based on known, described methods. This design required many adjustments and changes throughout the study.

The original research design was to audio-tape the group meetings (thinking that this would be less intrusive and more client-friendly). However, this was seen as extremely intrusive and rejected by the group from the beginning. I initially believed that my knowledge of the group to be studied would be an asset to the research. As it turned out, my status as the director of the rehabilitation department at the facility where the research took place was seen as a deterrent to the group members, and my intentions were questioned openly. The women perceived my position as one of power. In reality, I felt extremely vulnerable as a novice researcher. Initially, I thought I would have little difficulty accessing the group and obtaining interview participants/ informants, but in reality, I struggled to obtain the minimum requisite complement of

informants. I thought that I would obtain all the information and insights I needed through the in-depth interviewing process. Instead, I learned little of the experience of occupational engagement through this method and actually learned more about the group by being a full participant in the process. Where I believed the methods I had learned in graduate school would help me conduct quality research, I realized that the tools and clinical skills I brought with me as an occupational therapist, having worked in psychiatry for ten years, were invaluable assets to me during my journey. I realized that by being myself, having a good healthy sense of humor, and being honest about my intentions and my mistakes, the participants could relate to a well-intentioned, but imperfect, me, and this eventually made for excellent field relations.

The Women's Group study was an important project for me personally for several reasons. First, I learned the basic rudimentary skills for conducting research. Second, I made several mistakes in the learning, and I ended up learning a great deal more because of those mistakes. Third, I refined the art of listening and paying attention, which opened up many learning opportunities for me. Fourth, I began to appreciate what I could do for the clients and what changes I might make within the system. Fifth, I realized I needed to do more research.

Historical Description of the Women's Group

The Women's Group is an outpatient, women's mental health group that was developed in 1990 by the Department of Occupational Therapy at a northeastern Ontario mental health facility. The group was developed in response to the significant number of women who were readmitted to the hospital on a regular basis, were frequently at risk for suicide, and/or did not appear to benefit from the more traditional, verbal-based therapies available to them within the community clinics system.

The original objective of the Women's Group was to provide a place where the women could meet on a weekly basis for support and resolution of issues, and cooperatively participate in an occupation-based project. A quilt was prescribed as the occupation of choice for the group because it offered a long-term project in which each of the women could participate and was conducive to both cooperative and parallel work.

The Women's Group was somewhat unique at the research site in that it was the only known occupation-based mental health group in the region. In general, all other mental health programs in the region were largely psychoeducational and used verbal-based therapies. The absence of occupation-based groups in the community provided the original rationale for developing the group. The Women's Group started in January 1991 and has continued since then on a weekly basis. Fifty-four women have participated in the group, and new members have joined on a regular basis. Of the original four members who began in January 1991, two have continued to attend the group.

In late 1994, the incumbent therapist began to discuss the possibility of the Women's Group being self-run with the assistance of a volunteer. This decision was driven primarily by a shortage of occupational therapists at the facility and the need to maximize a consultative role in the face of budget cuts to the department. Initially, there was a great deal of concern voiced by the members with respect to their capacity to handle a crisis without professional involvement. It was agreed that an occupational therapist would remain "on call" for the group for as long as they deemed it necessary. At the time of this writing, the Women's Group considers itself a self-help

group. A description of the research design, analysis, and results of this study (Rebeiro & Cook, 1999) is reprinted in Chapter 15 of this book.

The Women's Group: What I Learned

The Women's Group study opened up an appreciation of the things that I would need to do differently within the mental health system if I truly wanted to make a difference as an occupational therapist. This section highlights some of these discoveries and the suggestions for clinical practice that evolved from the knowledge gained in this study.

The original intention of this research was to better understand how participating in an occupation-based, weekly, mental health group affected the members. Although I went into the project strongly suspecting that the members were doing well and staying out of the hospital because of their involvement in occupation, I learned that this was only part of the picture. Clearly, their involvement in meaningful occupation was beneficial from their perspective. However, what they stressed as most important to the success of the group and their individual successes was the social environment that was fostered within the Women's Group. Insights into the social environment of the group were only realized by my direct participation in the group.

In this study, the experience of occupational engagement was explained in the form of a conceptual model, namely, occupational spin-off. I learned from participant observation that the provision of an opportunity to gather and belong in a social environment with individuals who were considered to be in the same situation contributed to the women feeling safe and comfortable. Further, the women did not have to expend excessive mental, emotional, or physical energy to control for illness identity or manage stigma. The women did not fear that they would be judged because they had a mental illness. They were able to share freely within the group.

In this study, I also learned about the importance of unconditional acceptance and affirmation of the individual and how important this was to the women's desire and confidence to participate in occupations. This story of the personal experience of occupational engagement for the members of the Women's Group is unique in its conceptualization of how occupation as therapeutic means may contribute to one's sense of mental health.

Implications for Clinical Practice

Members of the group spoke loud and clear about how being in the group, and being with "the own," contributed to their capacity to engage in occupations. I have borrowed Goffman's (1963) term *the own* to conceptually describe what the members of the Women's Group said about the other members and how this affected the social environment. According to Goffman (1963), "the own" are

> sympathetic others . . . who share his [sic] stigma. Knowing from their own experience what it is like to have this particular stigma, some of them can provide the individual with instructions in the tricks of the trade and with a circle of lament to which he can withdraw for moral support and the comfort of feeling at home, at ease, accepted as a person who really is like any other normal person. (pp. 20–21)

An integral aspect of being with "the own" was the absence of a perceived hierarchy in their group relationships and how this contributed to their ability to talk and listen to each other. If our clients perceive that their opinions are both desired and valued, they may feel more confident to participate in therapy. If therapists acknowledge that the client comes to the therapeutic relationship with a personal history of strengths and a knowledge of what is meaningful and helpful to them, therapists may be more inclined to plan interventions based on client-expressed needs, as opposed to fixing the assessed deficits that contribute to the individual's disability. Listening and acting on client-expressed needs appears to be essential for the client's voice to "carry authority" in any therapeutic relationship.

This study suggested that the provision of occupational opportunities in an environment that supports an individual's strengths is more desirable than the provision of assessments that focus on what the individual cannot do or on the limitations imposed by the individual's disability. It suggested that occupational therapists focus on creating a therapeutic environment that is conducive to affirming the humanness of clients through active listening, instead of focusing on fixing the person.

A second clinical implication of this study concerned the creation of a supportive social environment. The informants suggested that there were several elements of their group environment that contributed to the group being relaxing, safe, and comfortable. In general, the social milieu was largely a result of the provision of opportunity and choice with "the own." This included the right to choose whether the members attended, when they exited the group, and the occupation on which they worked. Members suggested that if choice was not provided regarding the occupation, they would likely become bored with working on it and abandon it. In addition, members suggested that the provision of choice stimulated both interest in and anticipation of future group projects. This study implies that the provision of choice is likely to stimulate greater interest in what the client works on, facilitate engagement in the occupation until completion, and ultimately encourage participation beyond the therapeutic environment.

A third clinical implication of this study concerned the composition of the group and its impact on the social environment of the doing. In this study, gathering with "the own" was essential to the social environment. Traditionally, therapists have based group composition on pragmatic considerations such as the physical location of the client (for example, inpatient versus outpatient; ward versus unit), the purpose of the group (stress management versus community living skills), or by referral (doctor's order versus team recommendation). The informants in this study stated that gathering with individuals who are the same (diagnostically and in terms of gender) created a social environment that was safe and accepting and was conducive to their engaging in occupations.

This study suggested to me that the creation of a supportive social environment and the provision of occupation based on client-expressed needs will have an impact on the person's confidence to engage in therapy and the person's desire to maintain occupational engagement into the future. A focus on client strengths and not on assessed deficits or limitations imposed by disability is essential. Acknowledgment of the importance of a supportive social environment to engaging in occupations will encourage therapists to identify and address those aspects of the hospital and community environments that pose a social handicap to the person and limit, as opposed to enable, occupational engagement. The provision of opportunity will enable therapists to better address individual human needs and create individual road maps that can guide the therapeutic process. Opportunity, not prescription, will give the client "authority" in occupational therapy practice.

The Middle of the Research Journey: The Labyrinth of Community Mental Health

After completing the Women's Group study, I discovered that too many questions remained in my mind regarding the opportunity for meaningful occupation within the community and, more important perhaps, how I might be helpful as an occupational therapist in a community-based setting. For instance, despite the encouraging findings from the Women's Group study, the participants had clearly told me that they remained at a hospital-based location because they did not perceive that there were the same opportunities for them in the larger community. In general, they did not perceive the community to be safe.

I decided that I wanted and needed to learn more about the provision of occupational opportunities in the community for persons who were described as seriously and persistently mentally ill. This was the target population for mental health reform (Ministry of Health 1988, 1993) and also the client group with whom I was likely to be working. I knew from working and living in this community that there were few occupation-based programs. I also knew that occupation was rarely, if ever, discussed as a discharge goal for clients. Medication, housing, and income support usually dominated any discharge or planning process in which I had been previously involved. It was largely assumed that if these three issues were dealt with, then the client would be fine. When I worked on what was referred to as the "chronic team," the case managers encouraged clients to be involved, but there were few programs clients were interested in attending, or the hours of operation were deemed to be "better suited to the needs of the staff than the clients," according to one participant. I knew that the outpatient program at the local general hospital consisted mainly of psychoeducational groups. The "clubhouse" downtown was not a place where any of the Women's Group members wanted to go. I had heard it was scary and "not safe" from members of the Women's Group, although I had not been there for awhile. I knew little at this point about Ontario Psychiatric Survivors Alliance (OPSA), now known as Sudbury Mental Health Survivors Inc. (SMHS).

I also had mixed feelings about conducting more research. I felt mentally tired after graduate school. I was unsure as to whether I wanted to delve into another study so soon after my thesis. However, I still did not feel that I had all the answers, or any of them for that matter. I still did not feel confident. I suppose I knew a little more about the importance of the social environment to enabling occupation and the benefits of engaging in occupation for a small group of participants. But I did not feel confident to begin work in the community setting, which was much larger than the environment of the Women's Group. I felt that I needed to have a better grasp of what was missing and what was needed in the community. It seemed the more I learned, the less I felt I knew about what was needed. Thus, came my decision to conduct more research.

The Research Question

The research question that guided this next stage of the research journey was: What are the opportunities for participation in meaningful occupation within the city of Sudbury for persons with serious and persistent mental illness (SMI)? Although this was a fairly broad question, I felt that a better knowledge of the existing opportunities would lead me in the right direction. Once I knew a bit more about the available opportunities for participation, I would have a better appreciation of

the clinical programs and interventions that would be required.

The Research Design

A qualitative design was chosen for reasons similar to those for the Women's Group study. The phenomenon under investigation was one that was not extensively reported. People who were diagnosed as having SMI and resided in the community were chosen as the study group. The study was designed to capture both objective data and the subjective, personal experiences of daily living in the community.

Phase One: Survey Questionnaire

A survey questionnaire was used to identify those programs, services, and resources (fiscal and human) that were dedicated to the provision of opportunity for participation in meaningful occupation. The survey was sent to the eight known services and agencies within the city of Sudbury that were mandated to provide services for persons with SMI. The results of this survey confirmed my experiential knowledge, based on working in the system for twelve years, that few human, fiscal, or program services were dedicated to providing opportunities for participation in meaningful occupation. The survey results were utilized as a basis for the in-depth interviews with participants to examine the service sector responses and also to ascertain participants' reasons as to why or why not they attended certain programs.

Phase Two: In-depth Interviews

In the second phase of the research, four in-depth interviews were conducted with volunteer participants. Participants were recruited by enclosing a poster with the surveys that were sent to the service sectors.

Participating agencies were requested to hang the poster with the request for participants in an area that would likely be seen by most clients. Participants contacted the researcher directly by telephone.

The in-depth interview began with the following grand tour question: "Tell me a little bit about how you spend your time on a daily basis." Prompt questions that were used to further explore responses included: "Can you tell me why you go to X or why not?"; "Can you tell me more about what you do and why you choose to do this?"; and "Are you satisfied with how you are spending your time?" The information gathered from these interviews was used as the basis of phase three, participant observation. A daily personal journal of my thoughts, ideas, insights, and feelings was kept throughout the study period.

Phase Three: Participant Observation Phase And What Was Learned

Phase three was a lengthy phase lasting from June 1997 until August 1998. During the participant observation phase, I "hung out" at community drop-in centers, participated in a review of the local consumer-survivor development initiative (CSDI), had coffee with consumers, and, in general, did a great deal of listening and observing rather than talking. I was fortunate in that I had filled out a membership form for the local CSDI and was, therefore, invited as a nonvoting member (because I was not a consumer) to all meetings dealing with the review, including the involvement of Ministry of Health officials, membership meetings, and annual general meetings. These opportunities were extremely helpful, if not crucial, to my understanding of some of the current struggles within consumer-directed programs.

I was also fortunate to have the opportunity to participate in two well-established community programs. The first was the local CSDI project, which consumers told me was started as a true alternative to current programming available within the system. The second was the local psychosocial clubhouse, run by the Canadian Mental Health Association (CMHA) and founded on psychosocial rehabilitation philosophy and principles.

This opportunity to participate intimately with the agencies enabled me to observe, listen, learn, and compare/contrast information that I had already learned from the surveys and the first four in-depth interviews. I also had knowledge from the Women's Group and was always looking for affirming and supportive social environments. It was an incredible learning opportunity for me. I was directly involved, and I could observe and document what I learned from the perspective of being both a participant insider and an outside observer. I also had the opportunity to give something back during the research rather than just taking from the consumers for my own purposes or those of research alone. McCracken (1988) states clearly that the best possible situation for participant observation research is participating in joint activities. I learned from the Women's Group study that participating with them reduced barriers (perceived or real) between the researcher and participants, increased trust of the researcher, and increased the group's support of the research. This was also true of this research study. Consumers stated that they had participated in many research studies conducted by outside agencies (that is, the local university). Once the surveys or questionnaires were completed, they did not see the researcher again, let alone have the opportunity to review the results. Consumers stated that they felt used by the researchers. In contrast, by being active participants in this research, they shared ownership of the study and were motivated to participate and ensure that I had it right.

This study took me to a level of understanding about the issues that face persons with a mental illness that I would not have realized had I remained in the clinic or conducted research in an office or controlled environment. I now realize how limited any one of my research projects would have been had I not participated actively and had I not spent time with participants in the field.

The prominent issues that were identified in the labyrinth study had more do with the struggles inherent in navigating a convoluted system of services and programs, which ideally was developed and funded to help people but in reality was often confusing, contradictory, and essentially nonhelpful. These issues had to do with money, food, shelter, transportation, access to leisure activities, and struggles with the pervasive, extensive stigma that exists within the larger community and also within the mental health system. I learned that many, if not most, of the twenty-five people who participated in the study not only struggled with a serious mental illness, but also struggled with extreme poverty. Thus, individually and collectively, they struggled not only with the stigma of mental illness, but also with the stigma associated with poverty, unemployment, and being recipients of a disability pension (at the subsistence level of funding) each month. The bureaucratic complexity and inconsistency that I observed firsthand was identified as the single most limiting barrier to successful participation in personally chosen occupations within the community. Thus, I began to use the metaphor of a labyrinth as the guiding theme of the study findings.

The labyrinth metaphor did not emerge in the in-depth interviews. In those, I learned only what people were and were not doing on a daily basis. Nor did I learn about the labyrinth presented by the various social services agencies by shadowing any one participant in the community. The labyrinth metaphor emerged from all the different sources of data. That is, in isolation, any one of the sources of data (survey, eight in-depth interviews, participant observation, or questionnaire) would not likely have yielded the major findings of this study. The system intended to help people with a serious mental illness was exhausting their physical, emotional, spiritual, and financial resources, so much so that any hopes of seeking, finding, obtaining, and maintaining meaningful occupation became difficult, if not impossible, for many people.

I learned that the issues in the community for persons with serious mental illness had more to do with social issues than issues of the illness or issues of personal problems. This was also a significant insight for me in the Women's Group study and caused me to ask myself why I had spent so much time in school learning about illness. That is not to say that people with a serious mental illness do not experience personal, illness-related problems, because they do. However, when the system continuously places the onus for recovery on the individual and invests all of its resources into fixing the person, it becomes somewhat problematic for the system when the person does not fix. This labyrinth lends itself to hopelessness and a cycle of despair. Instead of the system reevaluating its own level and effectiveness of care, the recipients of the ineffective care are labeled noncompliant, uncooperative, or nonresponsive when they do not get better. They are shuffled from one service agency to another, oftentimes receiving contradictory information. The system figuratively scratches its head, and health care professionals act perplexed as to why their interventions have not worked and why the clients are not doing better.

The participants spoke of their struggles in managing a serious mental illness. However, once people gained some pharmacological control of the illness, the issues spoken about were almost exclusively of a social nature. People spoke about the need for acceptance, a friend, a safe place within which to recover, and a place to build the trust that had been eroded over the years. Participants spoke extensively about the stigma of living with a mental illness and how stigma impacts an individual's self and social identity, which in turn affects one's confidence to participate fully within the community. Sadly, the participants spoke extensively about a system that was perceived to be one that addressed the professional's schedules and needs, more so than the needs of the people for whom it was intended.

In addition, people spoke about the lack of opportunity to participate in something challenging and meaningful and more than a "make work" project. People identified that the "next step" or opportunity beyond what was currently being offered was a missing link in the system. They also spoke of the risks involved in taking that next step, especially the risk of losing their disability benefits as a result of attempting to become involved in volunteer or paid occupation. The perceived risk of being denied their income derived from government benefits was a major barrier to becoming more involved in the community.

The labyrinth study was a turning point for me with respect to my clinical perspectives and theoretical orientation. I now knew that I could no longer practice within the safe confines of a clinic and so-called "professional boundaries" if I wanted to make a difference for persons with a mental illness. I could no longer pretend that what I saw in the clinic was also happening in the community, that is, if the clients can do it here, they must be able to do it at home and in the community. I could no longer regard my clients with a limited eye to the signs and symptoms of mental illness and their impact on "function," nor could I base any clinical information or decision-making within such a limited perspective. I knew that poverty was real and must be factored into any equation

that sought to improve the quality of life of persons with mental illness. I realized that advocacy in many forms must become an integral part of my practice because the system was confusing to everyone, including me. I knew that I had to figure out the labyrinth and a way to simplify it in order to be helpful.

I also became consciously aware of the many learning curves to be climbed. These would involve increasing my familiarity with and understanding of three levels of government and a variety of social and health policies. I realized that I would need to learn a great deal more about enabling occupation within a multileveled community system and that this process would be extremely complicated from a clinical point of view. Finally, in learning about these participants, these people who had become my friends, I developed a deep, personal need to help them in any way that I could. I suppose I professionally crossed that sacred boundary that we as professionals are advised to maintain. I began to care deeply about their lives and about them as people. They were people who deserved better from the system, from society in general, and I suppose, most importantly, from me.

Phase Four: In-depth Interviews Again

By the time I was ready to resume the latter part of the project and conduct the final four in-depth interviews, I had a fairly good appreciation of the opportunities that were available in the community. The final four interviews served to largely confirm and expand what I had learned in the participant observation phase of the research. Whereas in the first set of interviews I was most interested in understanding and learning about what people did on a daily basis, I now wanted to know how they did what they did. I wanted to learn about their individual strategies for navigating the labyrinth. I wanted to understand how people had over-come environmental or systemic constraints to their pursuit of occupation, if they in fact had overcome them, and I wanted to learn what the system and professionals within the system needed to do to better enable their pursuit of and participation in occupation.

Phase Five: The Member Check

In the fifth and final phase of the study, after approximately one and one-half years of data gathering and analysis, I mapped out the labyrinth as I understood it and the various personal and social constraints that existed as barriers to clients' pursuit of and participa-tion in meaningful occupation within the community. The number of participants had expanded to twenty-five at this point and also included participants in the Northern Initiative for Social Action (NISA) program, which evolved logically out of the labyrinth study. I prepared a slide show for ease of pre-sentation during the member check. I had taped 5″ by 7″ index cards to the wall of my office in an attempt to organize and visually map out the labyrinth. I asked every con-sumer who came into my office to give me feedback on this conceptualization and to suggest any changes that he or she would deem necessary, including placement of the cards. I also made a point to have all mem-bers read and edit my synopsis of the research that I had prepared for a presenta-tion at the World Congress of Occupational Therapists in June 1998 in Montreal, Canada.

I received a warm and unanimous confir-mation of the portrayal of the labyrinth and also of the systemic and professional strate-gies that would be needed to eradicate the labyrinth and successfully enable occupation. The participants were all attentive and car-ing. Each of them had participated in the study, and they were major stakeholders in the results to be presented and published. In the end, in the acknowledgment section of

the presentation, I thanked them all for what they had shared with me, for what they had taught me, and for being my friends and col-leagues during the study. This is when I cried. I was so glad to be finished, or so I thought.

The Ongoing Journey: Putting Research into Practice

The NISA project, although described here as the last leg of my research journey, was in fact in its infancy or conceptual development prior to the completion of the labyrinth study. Many of the initial members of the NISA project were also participants in the labyrinth study and participated in the mem-ber checking group. In addition, these same participants were involved in, corrected, or amended the study findings for publication and enthusiastically agreed to be involved as participant observers on the research team in the development of a consumer-run initiative and any proposed evaluation study of NISA. Thus, many of the people who initially enlightened me as to what was problematic within community mental health were now collaborators in a program aimed at correct-ing the problem(s) and a research project to study its effectiveness. I begin this section with a brief description of the NISA program, its objectives and program initiatives, and then describe the evaluation study of its effectiveness over an 18-month period.

Northern Initiative for Social Action (NISA)

The Northern Initiative for Social Action (NISA), established in 1997, is a nonprofit, charitable organization developed by and for consumers/survivors of the mental health system. The organization's objectives were clearly derived from the Women's Group and labyrinth studies and are as follows: to provide a safe and supportive work environment within which to gain confidence and skills; to provide opportunities for participation in personally meaningful and socially valued occupations; and to support and empower consumers to become contributing members of society. An accepting social environment in which all persons are considered equal and capable is a cornerstone of NISA.

The aim of NISA is to promote the capabilities of consumers through its variety of program initiatives and by enabling consumers to actively participate in and contribute to the social fabric of the community. The following programs are being offered at NISA at the time of this writing: The Writer's Circle, *Open Minds Quarterly*, ParNorth Research Unit, Warm Hearts/Warm Bodies, The Artist's Loft, Northern Computer Recycling Depot, and The Community Kitchen.

At the time of this writing, NISA has 38 participants, with an international outreach to more than 300 consumers/survivors through the Internet, The Artist's Loft, and *Open Minds Quarterly*. Forty-two percent of NISA participants have a diagnosis of schizophrenia; 16% have a diagnosis of bipolar affective disorder; 23% have a diagnosis of chronic depression, and 19% have other diagnoses. Eighty-four percent of people who attend NISA are currently seeing a psychiatrist; 81% take some form of medication; and 90% are on supported income. In the two years after attending NISA, participants collectively accrued a total of three hospitalization days.

The NISA Study

The Northern Initiative for Social Action (NISA) program was driven by a hospital and provincial government mandate to develop a consumer initiatives program. When I returned to work after graduate school, my employer gave me two empty folders. The first was labeled *research,* and the second was labeled *consumer initiatives.* I really did not have a clue as to what consumer initiatives were or what they were supposed to look like. A recent document outlining mental health reform, *Making It Happen: Implementation Plan for Mental Health Reform* (Ministry of Health, 1999), briefly highlighted the importance of involving consumers/survivors in the design, planning, and implementation of a reformed mental health system; however, it was severely lacking in any direction or structure for the development of consumer initiatives.

At the time of my return to work, I was fortunate in being quite involved with consumers/survivors within the community due to the labyrinth study. This gave me ample opportunity to chat with them about what a consumer/survivor initiative might be and what they would like to see developed. The NISA initiative was based on my research and the ideals of the dedicated group of consumers with which I was working. Several things that we knew from the research and experience would become integral to the developing consumer initiative known as NISA. For example, we knew that there was a lack of opportunity for participation in meaningful occupation for consumers/survivors of the mental health system within the community. We also knew that any new program must address the extensive social issues that were identified in the labyrinth study. We knew that any consumer/survivor program must provide a supportive social environment and be based on the provision of opportunity rather than the prescription of occupation. Although we began NISA with little direction, and with no promised resources or funding other than a building and an occupational therapist, we did know that what we would create would be very different from any program that currently existed within the system. This program initiative would be directed by those most affected by system change and who had an intimate knowledge of the needs of persons with a serious mental illness. We hoped that the program we developed would rectify many of the problems and social issues now known to be disincentives or barriers to participation within our community.

The labyrinth study was instrumental in identifying some of the barriers to participation within the larger system. We knew that we would need to pay attention to the economic barriers to participation, one of which was access to transportation. I initially had NISA participants sign on as Network North (my employer) volunteers because I had heard that they would then be covered by the hospital's insurance and I could access transportation funds to subsidize participants' bus costs. However, three months into the project, the volunteer coordinator informed me that too many people were coming and there was no more money to cover bus costs.

We also learned that access to programs and the hours of operation of other programs were problematic. Thus, we eliminated the need for a referral to the program, and I informed consumers who came by with a "doctor's order" that they did not have to come to NISA. We initially made the program as flexible as possible, and consumers set their own hours and frequency of participation.

I realized early on in the development of NISA that we would need more than a building and a clinician to develop a program well-suited to meeting consumers' needs. I realized at this point that I would need to lobby the administration for operational funds for the NISA program, as well as the space and office supplies needed to create a suitable working environment. I did not know at this point what we would be doing, who would come, what the outcomes would be, or how often people would participate.

Thankfully, my employer had faith in the basic premises that were being applied to the NISA program and granted us $15,000 per year to apply to operational costs. It was a huge relief that we did not have to worry about finding money to cover transportation costs or secure the basic supplies we would need.

We also knew that NISA would have to address other issues related to poverty, including food and nutrition needs. Many of the participants in the research who were coming to NISA did not eat on a regular basis, and when they did eat, they did not eat well from a nutritional standpoint. I knew that the operational budget we had been given was insufficient to meet the nutritional needs of the NISA members, and I began to lobby the hospital to help meet these needs. We were very fortunate to be able to negotiate a deal with the dietary department to receive any foods that were offered for sale in the staff cafeteria and that were deemed edible but nonsalable the next day. Refrigerator number 4 became the NISA refrigerator, and each day NISA members transported any food items from the hospital to the NISA building. I believe that our capacity to meet nutritional needs was a drawing card for some members. We also instituted "pot lucks" early in NISA's history as a means to bring people together and nourish our members. Interestingly, this gathering for food and nourishment was perceived to be a spiritual experience for many of our members.

We also realized early in the development of NISA that we would need to provide evidence of effectiveness in order to receive any funding for the program into the future and be in a position to fully develop the initiative based on what members most wanted to do. The original two members of NISA were interested in conducting research with me on the social and self-identity impact of being a person with schizophrenia. However, our research proposal and design were turned down by my employer, who cited confidentiality and questioned the ownership of the data/results as the reasons for denial. After this disappointment we decided to complete an ethics application and submit our design to an outside ethics board for approval. We were successful in this attempt, with assistance from a colleague at The University of Western Ontario. I believe that our acceptance by a higher authority ethics board gained some respect and recognition for NISA and our capacity to design and conduct research. Most certainly, when we applied to the local ethics review board to approve the later NISA formative evaluation study, we received approval quickly.

Since the NISA project aimed to develop a program designed by the people who participated, that is, to be a truly client-driven initiative, it was important from the beginning to evaluate whether the program was in fact meeting the members' needs. We also realized that if we were to develop program initiatives based on what participants wanted to do, we would need money to do this. We spent a great deal of time in the first year writing funding and research proposals, including a research proposal to the Canadian Occupational Therapy Foundation (COTF), to fund our research. In July 1998, we learned that we had been successful in our application to COTF and would receive the necessary funds to conduct the NISA study.

The NISA Formative Evaluation Study

The NISA study was designed from its inception to be a formative evaluation study, that is, to identify early in program development what worked and, most importantly, to identify what did not work so that it could be corrected. Essentially, all of the helpful strategies identified in the Women's Group and

labyrinth studies were incorporated into the NISA program. In addition, an attempt was made to eliminate or reduce all known barriers or constraints to one's fullest participation in meaningful occupation. For example, referral processes that limited, delayed, or denied access to services were eliminated; limited hours of operation and/or limited time frames for recovery (that is, six- to twelve-week programs) were lifted; and any signs or symbols of professional dominance, authority, or socioeconomic status (that is, dress, office decorum, and physical setup of the offices that symbolized hierarchies in the workplace) were removed. I no longer had to wait for "dress-down day" for the United Way to wear jeans to the office.

We decided to create an environment that provided choice and did not limit consumers' participation by having a professional decide what was meaningful for the consumers. We tried very hard to implement real work versus make-work opportunities. Wherever possible, all NISA projects were intimately connected to the larger social community and were valued by the community. The NISA program also aimed to learn from both the Women's Group and labyrinth studies in providing a safe, supportive, and affirming social environment. The opportunity for economic self-sufficiency was an issue raised early in the development of the NISA program.

The research team identified the dependent variables that were most important and that they hoped NISA would address as the following: quality of life, including improved socioeconomic status; self-esteem; self-identity; decreased stigma; and improved participation in the social fabric of the community. It was decided that a quality of life measure would be administered to NISA participants at the start of the research project (T1), at six months (T2), at twelve months (T3), and at eighteen months (T4). A consumer member survey would also be concurrently administered at each time interval to look at empowerment and mastery variables in addition to subjective quality of life.

In addition to the more formal program evaluation, the following variables were tracked throughout the NISA research study because of their importance to the Ministry of Health and other significant funding agencies: diagnoses, last hospitalization admission dates, total days hospitalized, and NISA attendance. Later we also began documentation of NISA participants who successfully graduated to the competitive workforce. These statistics were deemed to be important to the Ministry of Health, which we hoped might fund the program in the future. Evidence of cost savings via reduced hospitalization days was important to this funding agency. Unfortunately, NISA was being developed based on local research and not what the funding agencies deemed to be "best practices," which had largely evolved out of and were based on programs in southern Ontario. Further, Sudbury, like most areas in the province, was undergoing a process of hospital restructuring, and very few programs were being granted money at that time.

The independent variables in the study would be participation in one or more of the NISA programs that were occupation-based and self-chosen, as well as the degree and extent of participation. Participants could work within any NISA program, switch programs if they preferred, or initiate or develop a program of interest. Participation could occur during any hours the building was open from 8:00 A.M. until approximately 5:00 P.M. In general, there were only two rules governing the NISA program. The first was a courtesy agreement regarding behavior that new members were asked to read and verbally consent to; the second was a decision to work with consumers/survivors who resided in the community, that is, not with inpatients. Although I worked closely with

the occupational therapist on the inpatient unit, we decided that the extensive use of sharp instruments at NISA with the Warm Hearts/Warm Bodies program warranted excluding inpatients for the safety of NISA participants, inpatients, and myself. I was the only clinician working at the NISA program, and some days up to 20 people participated. No individual member can keep track of the sharp instruments at NISA all the time. Inpatients who were interested in participating would be oriented to the program by the inpatient occupational therapist. Once the individual identified a program of interest, the inpatient therapist arranged with the person to attend NISA after discharge from the hospital.

The Research Design

Although the NISA study was designed to incorporate several different measures to track effectiveness, it was primarily designed as successive focus groups over a period of one year. We utilized Morgan's (1997) rule of thumb of six to eight participants for the focus groups. The first two focus groups had eight participants, the third focus group had ten participants, and the final member checking focus group invited all registered NISA members.

Focus Group One: October 1998

The research questions that guided the first focus group were: "Why did you initially come to NISA?" and "Why do you keep coming to NISA?" All focus group sessions were audiotaped and later transcribed verbatim. I led all focus groups while the research team members participated as NISA members during all focus groups. Members were offered the opportunity to lead the focus groups but chose not to do so. Rules of order were applied to the focus groups for the clarity of transcription and also as a sign of respect for each person's contributions. I asked people to speak in turn and to go around the table. This method worked well for the group. Following the focus group, the audiotapes were transcribed and given to the four members of the research team. The team then met twice per week for analysis of the transcripts.

Data Analysis

The research data from the focus groups were analyzed using open conceptual coding and a line by line analysis. Research team members were given two weeks to read the transcripts and do any initial coding that they believed to be relevant to the research questions. I suggested they underline, circle, or somehow mark comments, words, or sections that they believed helped to answer the research question and/or struck them as being important. Some members copied quotations directly from the transcripts under the two question headings: "Why did you initially come?" and "Why do you keep on coming?" All members kept a personal journal log and commented on their overall impressions of what was said during the focus group. Most of us pulled excerpts from the transcripts, discussed at length any common responses, and identified any potential themes that appeared to be emerging.

An interesting process emerged early during the analysis. Not only did the focus group participants widely utilize metaphors in their descriptions of their experiences, but also the members of the research team had an incredible ability to draw out metaphors from the transcripts and further expand these metaphors based on their own personal experiences. During the first analysis sessions, the rebirth metaphor emerged to describe the process of recovery that appeared to be taking place at NISA. In addition, a needs—drive, needs—met analytic category began to emerge that appeared to account for the reasons people initially came

to NISA and, more importantly, why they continued to come. A circular process of discussing, arguing, comparing, and expanding on ideas continued for a period of two months. This was a very personal process for each of the research members. Oftentimes, their input during analysis would factor in personal reflections or experiences, some of them being quite painful. In my opinion, this process of analysis was exhausting. Many times we would exit the analysis sessions feeling "brain dead," emotionally and intellectually exhausted. Prior to this experience, I had always struggled with data analysis on my own, with some assistance and a listening ear from a long-distance mentor. Now I had three research partners in the same room who came to the analysis with a different set of eyes and vastly different range of life experiences on which to draw. The only leading I did throughout the analysis process was to ensure that whatever analysis took shape or was brought to the table could be substantiated or found in the transcripts. I would simply ask that each of us check the transcripts prior to the next meeting to ensure that a particular train of thought could actually be traced to the transcript and direct comments made at the focus group.

Another method incorporated into the analysis process was one of taking notes or making a record of the analysis sessions. This proved to be very useful for two reasons. First, we had a record of the analysis for the purposes of the audit trail, and second, we had a written reminder of where to begin at the next analysis meeting. Some weeks it was hard to keep track of where we left off because of the intensity of these sessions. Although the analysis meetings were only a few days apart, as the analysis became more complex and involved, it became increasingly difficult to track where and from whom certain ideas originated. This written record was also helpful prior to the next focus group meeting with respect to providing focus group members with a summary of analyses to date. The research team would meet on a regular basis until we were satisfied that we had something worthwhile to present for feedback and/or we felt that we were at a crossroad and could not continue with any meaningful analysis until we had confirmed our present line of thought with the focus group members. At such times, the research team needed to ask further questions to begin the process of meaningfully categorizing the data. We were all a bit fearful and cautious; we did not want to force the data. We were also cognizant of outsiders viewing the process, and we wanted to ensure that we provided detailed descriptions of all stages of the research process. Mostly, we were aware that outsiders viewing a research team consisting of a somewhat novice lead researcher and three consumers of the mental health system might be sceptical of the trustworthiness of the study.

Focus Group Two: December 1998

We explained that it appeared from reviewing the data from the first focus group that certain themes were repeated by everyone present. We stated that people told us participants are driven by certain needs, which helped to explain why they initially came to NISA. These needs were: need for belonging, negative social identity, drive for recovery, and occupational void. In addition, we explained that several metaphors were developing around the experiences described in the first focus group that appeared to account for why people continued to come to NISA. These experiences appeared to describe the needs being met that were the primary forces driving people to NISA, that is, the needs that previously were being unmet were now being satisfied at the NISA program.

The focus group participants were given a handout to review that contained three columns describing what we felt were aspects of the person, environment, and occupations available, as well as an initial attempt at defining a needs—drive, needs—met model. In hindsight, this handout was too complicated and included too many details of the analysis. This was reflective of our desire to be totally open with the focus group members and also to ensure their confirmation of our analyses throughout the research. However, we recognized from the questions posed by the focus group members that it was too much information and could most likely have been presented in a simplified manner. This was corrected for the third focus group. The analysis at this time was limited. We asked the participants to tell us more about the three categories and whether this explained their own personal reasons for coming to and staying with NISA. The responses given were quite detailed, very personal, and provided the research team with a great deal of data to analyze for the next focus group. The transcripts were again typed and given to the research team in February. Analysis then resumed every Tuesday and Thursday until mid-May 1999.

The analysis that occurred between February and May 1999 became quite detailed and complicated, and I often wondered whether we would get anywhere. I personally struggled back and forth between an academic perspective and the very real, very personal viewpoints that my research colleagues brought to the table. I was so grateful to have them with me and to learn from them. At one point during my own personal analysis of the second transcript, I became unable to proceed. I could not view the transcripts without being reminded of an article I had read sometime during graduate school. This was an article by Renwick and Brown (1996) about quality of life and the three themes "being, belonging, and becoming" that they used to conceptualize this construct. I searched for the article, and then asked the team members to read it. "Being, belonging, and becoming" continued to resonate in my own mind as I analyzed the transcripts. I personally could see nothing in the transcripts that did not mirror the idea that NISA appeared to be fostering people's being, belonging, and becoming needs. *Belonging* and *becoming* had been words raised in the focus groups and could be found in the transcripts. *Being*, I thought, best reflected those expressed sentiments around rebirthing and recovery that continued to be raised in any meaningful dialogue about NISA. I explained to the research team that I was finding it extremely difficult to proceed with any further analysis of the transcripts without viewing the data within this framework. I declared my bias and asked each of them to read the article for comment at the next analysis meeting.

During the next few analysis meetings, we discussed the article, my declared bias or rather narrow occupational therapy vision, and what this meant for the research team and process. I was a bit concerned about influencing the research team with my "occupational therapy" viewpoints. Although I was only one member of the research team, it was obvious that the others looked to me for direction throughout the process. The other members of the research team read the article and came back with feedback as requested. One member spoke of forcing the data. Again, I spoke of my own bias and how I did not intentionally ask to view the transcripts with the themes of being, belonging, and becoming in mind. I also explained that these themes fit beautifully with what I heard and learned thus far in the research study but that I did not believe the definitions of the concepts by Renwick and Brown (1996) fit precisely with our data. As general themes or categories, being, belonging, and becoming helped to simplify and explain the data from the first focus group that we had provisionally placed under person, environment, and

occupation (also occupational therapy constructs). Further, I explained that in reading the second focus group transcripts with the great emphasis on belonging and on healing, recovery, and the importance of a safe and person-supportive environment, I could not get past viewing the transcripts within this framework. I believed that these themes made too much sense to me and fit the data so perfectly that, in my own mind, I could go no further until we had fleshed this out.

A second member of the research team agreed wholeheartedly with the use of the themes being, belonging, and becoming. She too felt that this helped her in the analysis at that point. She stated that the themes helped to clarify and structure what she believed was a huge amount of data into something that not only made sense to her, but also helped her to explain it to someone else. The third research team member felt that the themes fit the data but also expressed concern about forcing the data. The first member went over the definitions provided in the article and agreed that if we wanted to use these broad themes to help explain the data, this would be acceptable if we abandoned the definitions provided and just used the thematic concepts (names). We needed to develop our own definitions, based on what we learned and using words that could be traced to the transcripts. I reiterated that I was merely suggesting the use of the themes for the purposes of categorization. We agreed as a group that we would rereview all of the transcripts and analysis notes to date (including the first focus group, again) under these three themes to see if the data did fit, as I expected, or whether I was forcing occupational therapy constructs on the research process. If it was determined that the data were being forced into these broad themes, then we would abandon them and reconvene to plan next steps. We adjourned for a period of two weeks to rereview the data within this framework.

When we met again, we decided that the concept of "being" described the many personal and internal processes that were talked about by the focus group participants. The being needs would be those needs of the self and of the process of rebirth, and recovery that were articulated time and time again in the focus groups and by the members of the research team during analysis. What was initially described as a drive for self-identity and self-worth or a drive for self-acceptance was framed within the broader context of "being" needs. These needs are of the person, having to do with basic affirmation of one's self-worth and right to be regardless of the person's past, diagnoses, or whatever baggage the person brings to NISA.

The belonging needs would capture what we tried to explain about the environment at NISA and what people said about the importance of belonging. It was a huge theme that literally yelled at us from the transcripts. Right from the start of the first focus group, people spoke of their need to belong to something and the importance of having a place to belong to, something to call their own. People also spoke of the importance of a place of unconditional acceptance, a safe environment both physically and emotionally in which to recover and meet and address the "being" needs. This is where the metaphors of rebirth and recovery became prominent in the discussions. The "belonging" needs also fit with the metaphor of family, the nurturing and nourishment that supposedly comes from families but that was often missing in the lives of NISA members. The breaking of bread while joining like a family at potluck lunches was also determined to be important. Finally, the environment at NISA was also deemed to be important because it offered both personal space and common meeting space. It offered opportunities for both being by oneself and for visiting and gathering with others. We knew that belonging was crucial to meeting

members' needs and important to describing people's experiences at NISA.

The "becoming" theme helped to clarify and explain the doing or participation in occupation that occurred at NISA, although there was some discussion about whether NISA existed to provide people with opportunities to do meaningful things or to prepare people to reenter the competitive workforce. It became evident from the transcripts and from observations made between focus groups and at NISA on a daily basis that some members clearly wanted to improve their economic situation either by obtaining part-time work or by creating an employment opportunity that might eliminate their need for social assistance. The participants clearly indicated that the occupational opportunities at NISA assisted them in their journey of "being," helped to consolidate their reasons for "belonging," and gave them a means for "becoming." All three themes appeared to dovetail into the next, or support the growth of the other rather than any linear process.

An interesting point raised by one of the researchers was that sometimes people, himself included, were unable to actively participate in the program when they came to NISA. Thus, they spent a great deal of their time playing Free Cell or solitaire on the computer. During the second focus group, this point was raised and confirmed by everyone present. After much discussion, one of the participants suggested that this might account for the "being" needs being addressed. That is, if a great deal of internal healing work was being done within the person, this process would explain energies being directed internally versus externally through participation in one of the NISA programs. Indeed, we had evidence from members that they sometimes came to NISA merely to just be there, to feel safe, and to be around people. They personally did not feel pressured to do anything. Everyone at NISA was entitled to just be, exist, and be accepted for whatever they were feeling, what they wanted to do or not do, and just for being with us. This was an incredible insight for the research team. It should not matter to anyone at NISA whether a person was working on internal doing or was actively participating in a visible occupation because both, though different, were deemed essential to the person and recovery.

I wonder now if this helps to explain some of the hesitancy or inability to participate by some clients that I have witnessed over the years in mental health. I knew that a great deal of lack of participation had to do with the lack of a safe, affirming, and supportive social environment. I knew that part of it could be explained by the provision by professionals of prescriptions for doing rather than the provision of opportunity for doing. I knew that part of it could be explained by the lack of "real work" opportunities, the emphasis on arts and crafts and "make-work" projects. I also realized that people's need to manage stigma resulted in a great deal of energy being expended, oftentimes at the expense of occupation. But now, a new insight was evolving that made a great deal of sense to me. As an occupational therapist, I held strong beliefs that people were innately driven to action and participation in occupation. Previously, I would have lamented inaction or limited participation as a personal failure of myself as the occupational therapist. Perhaps I did not provide the right opportunities, or I challenged too much or too little. However, the revelation by the participants that they could not or were unable to participate because of healing or recovery work and that they were meeting "being" needs intuitively made sense to me based on what I experientially knew. That people could not participate and felt guilty about not participating (for, truly, those who could not do anything expressed guilt about their lack of contribution to the NISA program)

because they still had a lot of the internal healing or recovery work to be done made sense to me as a therapist. This was potentially the missing link to my understanding of the process of engaging in occupation as a means to recovery or health.

That occupation might need to be factored in at a later stage for some people was certainly an interesting clinical insight for me. I never thought that perhaps the most needed occupational work was required within the person and would be manifest in what might be perceived as "doing nothing." Now that I reflect on it, the result of this internal occupational work gradually does become manifest in some form of doing, whereas none could occur previously. I think about all of the NISA members who spoke of this process or phenomenon, about how troublesome it was for them to not be doing anything or fearing that others would comment or think poorly of them for participating less or not participating, but who nonetheless were still coming and participating in some capacity by just being present at NISA. I knew that any occupation needed to be self-directed, self-reflective, and self-benefiting. What I truly did not know was that this was sometimes, for certain people, a very internal process within the person, one that allowed healing (the rebirth metaphor), one that took whatever time was necessary for recovery ("being" needs), and one that would not occur (and had not to date for any of the members) except within the confines of a safe, affirming, supportive social environment ("belonging" needs) that by design also offered participants an opportunity to be involved in collective and individual occupations ("becoming" needs).

The third focus group was scheduled for mid-June 1999 and included participants who had not attended the first two focus groups but who had participated in the quality of life and member surveys in both August 1998 and February 1999. The research team believed that we were ready to share our analysis broadly. We desired a member check at this point before we ventured any further with our analysis.

By the time of the third focus group, the analysis had become quite complicated, and we decided not to make the same mistake with our handout that we had made prior to the second focus group. One member of the research team briefly summarized the analysis to date and provided a one-page summary of what we had learned thus far about "being, belonging, and becoming" needs. We also provided a brief definition of what the research team meant by each of these terms. Examples were provided to focus group members one week before the third focus group met.

We decided that the first half of the focus group would member check the "3 Bs," as they became coined, and ascertain whether there was agreement within the group that the "3 Bs" accurately reflected why the participants initially came to NISA and also why they kept coming. We asked focus group members one question during the first half of the focus group: "In your opinion, do the findings as presented accurately reflect your reasons as to why you initially came to NISA and why you continue to come?" We received a unanimous confirmation of the three themes. The second half of the focus group asked participants to reflect on their own personal experiences of the themes of being, belonging, and becoming, and to provide the research team with examples of how these themes were manifest in their lives and their participation at NISA.

Once again the participants spoke very deeply about their personal feelings and experiences and in great detail. At one point, all of us had tears in our eyes because we connected with the depth of the sharing that was taking place. I said to one of the members that my student, who was given permission to observe, would never practice

occupational therapy without recalling this focus group and this focus group would give her insight into the struggles, human feelings, and mental health that she might never have learned in school. This focus group was an incredible experience for me, and it is still very hard to articulate how I feel about the participants and the sheer strength of their experiences.

Reflections on the Journey Thus Far

I suppose that at this point in the research journey, I am less surprised by what I am learning and the insights of the people I work with than when I started. It only makes sense to me that I would learn (and continue to learn) a great deal about something like mental health, illness, and recovery from someone who has lived it. For me, going to the source, to the insider, makes a great deal of sense. Consumers/survivors are quite happy to share with professionals what works and what does not work. It becomes a matter of mutual respect, good listening, reciprocity, and a matter of asking the right questions.

The consumers with whom I have worked have been great collaborators in the research process. Their interest in research has been strikingly similar to mine. They have wanted to make a difference for the people who experience mental illness and for the system that is supposed to be there to help them. They have been less interested in academic theories but respectful that research methods must be followed and clearly articulated. They have not been interested in publication, although those with whom I have published have been extremely pleased with the accomplishment. They have hoped that their sharing and experiences can help someone else. Their giving has been without strings, but in the process of this giving, they have realized new benefits and insights about themselves. This has been helpful in their own journey.

The insights and knowledge that I have acquired have been crucial to who I am today as a person and an occupational therapist. I make no claims to be an expert at anything, let alone research or the theory of human occupation. I consider myself first and foremost an occupational therapist who works in mental health. I hold strong opinions with respect to the mental health system and have articulated some that are quite critical of occupational therapy practice (Rebeiro, 1998, 1999; Rebeiro & Allen, 1998). Nonetheless, these opinions factor into all that I do, including my research and clinical endeavors.

Although this journey is not yet complete and most likely will not be for some time, I have attempted to reflect on where I have been and where I am presently, and to speculate on where I might be in the future. Certainly I will never go back to a clinical practice that is informed solely by textbooks and classrooms. This knowledge may be useful for articulating practice and giving students some structure within which to frame their practice. However, I have found that clinical and educational academic knowledge can be limited and can be limiting to a clinician and researcher.

Applied theory in the clinic can be useful if done collaboratively with people, the consumers of the mental health system. Mental health consumers are well positioned to inform practice in terms of what works, what does not work, and what needs to be changed or adjusted. But if the consumers are not involved in the process of program planning, development, and review, then any intervention or evaluation becomes merely lip service, completed in a vacuum and with very little value or meaning for the people it is intended to help. I am hopeful about the future of occupational therapy practice in mental health as we share many beliefs and values with consumers/survivors. As a profession, we too are often misunderstood and undervalued by society. We too must fight for acknowledgment and recognition and for our place in society. We too struggle within a system in which we often do not seem to fit. People with a disability are logical partners for occupational therapists. Perhaps together we can figure out a way to make society more inclusive and accepting of all persons and viewpoints, whereas neither of us has been terribly successful on our own. Together, perhaps, we can make a difference.

References

Abbott, A. (1988). *The system of professions.* Chicago: University of Chicago Press.

Goffman, E. (1963). *Stigma: Notes on the management of spoiled identity.* New York: Simon & Schuster Inc.

McCracken, G. (1988). *The long interview.* Newbury Park, CA: Sage.

Meyer, A. (1922). The philosophy of occupational therapy. *Archives of Occupational Therapy,* (Vol. I, pp. 1–10).

Ministry of Health. (1988). *Building community support for people: A plan for mental health in Ontario.* Toronto, Canada: Queen's Printer for Ontario.

Ministry of Health. (1993). *Putting people first: The reform of mental health services in Ontario.* Toronto, Canada: Queen's Printer for Ontario.

Ministry of Health. (1999). *Making it happen: Implementation plan for mental health reform.* Toronto, Canada: Queen's Printer for Ontario.

Morgan, D. L. (1997). *Focus groups as qualitative research* (2nd ed.). Thousand Oaks, CA: Sage.

Rebeiro, K. L. (1998). Occupation-as-means to mental health: A call to research. *Canadian Journal of Occupational Therapy, 65,* 12–19.

Rebeiro, K. L., & Allen, J. (1998). Voluntarism as occupation. *Canadian Journal of Occupational Therapy, 66,* 279–285.

Rebeiro, K. L. (1999). The labyrinth of community mental health: In search of meaningful occupation. *Psychiatric Rehabilitation Journal, 23,* 143–152.

Rebeiro, K. L., & Cook, J. V. (1999). Opportunity, not prescription: An exploratory study of the experience of occupational engagement. *Canadian Journal of Occupational Therapy, 66,* 176–187.

Renwick, R., & Brown, I. (1996). The centre for health promotion's conceptual approach to quality of life. In R. Renwick, I. Brown, & M. Nager (Eds.), *Quality of life in health promotion and rehabilitation: Conceptual approaches, issues and applications* (pp. 75–86). Thousand Oaks, CA: Sage.

Townsend, E. (1998). *Good intentions overruled: An institutional ethnography of occupational therapy practices.* Toronto, Canada: University of Toronto Press.

PART

Qualitative Research Studies of Occupation, Occupational Therapists, and Client Experiences

These studies were all written by occupational therapists. Some are based on theses written as graduate students. Others are reports of ongoing programs of research. All of the studies were previously published in well-established, peer-reviewed journals and thus have met the requirements of scholarly rigor.[1,2]

The studies have been grouped according to their primary focus: issues concerning the nature of occupation; the practices, beliefs, and values of occupational therapists; and the experiences of clients. There is some overlap, as a number of the studies explored the concept of occupation in terms of client experiences. Therefore, the classification here is arbitrary but chosen to distinguish the varieties of research questions that are of interest and relevance to the profession of occupational therapy.

Many of the studies deal with issues of mental health and illness. This is not surprising as the subjectivity, ambiguity, and lack of clarity and certainty in this domain require a research approach that is open, flexible, not bound by predetermined hypotheses, and considers the actors' meaning and perspectives to be important to an understanding of phenomena. Qualitative research can provide a "voice" for persons who are most often the "object" of quantitative, statistical studies of such phenomena as incidence, diagnosis, and length of hospitalization. In providing that voice, qualitative studies can increase the knowledge base of the experience of mental health and illness and can contribute to more effective policies and programs. Most of the studies reprinted here discuss the implications of the findings for practice.

These research studies illustrate the variety of stimuli that lead to research questions. Some began with questions regarding "clinical irritations." That is, why is this happening, or why is that not happening? Others began as a response to and questioning of extant theory and research. Still others were stimulated by the scarcity of certain types of exploration and knowledge in the literature of the profession. Other studies developed because of intellectual curiosity and a coincidence of opportunity and life experience.

These studies also demonstrate the diversity of design, methods, and types of study described in Parts I and II of this text. This introduction provides a brief description of the studies in light of their inspiration, method, and type.

Studies of Occupation

D. Laliberte-Rudman et al.

In seeking to develop knowledge of the relationship between occupation and the subjective sense of well-being, particularly among senior citizens, this study explored the occupations and meanings attached to them by elderly persons living in the community. The chosen research strategies were semistructured, in-depth interviews and group member checking interviews. The study is an example of an exploratory inquiry with the purpose of developing grounded theory regarding the role of occupation in seniors' lives from their perspective, rather than that of the researcher.

R. Segal and G. Frank

Segal became intrigued with the changes in occupational routines in her own life after the birth of her first child. This led her to question the possible occupational adaptations of parents who have children with special needs. This interview study explored the manner in which families with children with a diagnosis of attention deficit hyperactivity disorder scheduled the routines of daily living to best accommodate the needs of their children. The study results contribute to the growing body of literature on the complexity of the concept of occupation, with particular attention to the areas of temporality and adaptation. As a descriptive and analytic type of study, this research has implications for the planning of intervention practices by therapists.

K. L. Rebeiro and J. Allen

This research study is an example of a single-case study of a particular occupation, that of volunteer. The methods used were sessions of observation followed by several in-depth, relatively unstructured interviews. The exploration of the meanings attached to the occupation of volunteer by the informant (J. Allen) and the analysis and interpretation of those meanings by the researcher (K. L. Rebeiro) provide collaborative insights into many aspects of productive occupation. The informant's description of the development of a valued and valuable self through meaningful occupation has implications for the therapeutic use of occupation as a means toward health and a sense of well-being.

R. Segal

This in-depth interview study of the purposes of daily occupations in families with children who have special needs continued the exploration of the intricacies and complexities of the concept of occupation. This research contributes to the theoretical base of the academic discipline of occupational science by proposing that people construct occupations to meet purposive, culturally determined values.

K. L. Rebeiro and J. V. Cook

This research study was stimulated by a clinical irritation. Why did a group of women who were diagnosed with a mental illness continue to attend an outpatient craft group for many years and remain out of the hospital during that time? Rebeiro asked the question: Is occupation a means to health, and if so, why? This research study employed the strategies of participant observation and in-depth interviewing. The results of the interpretative analysis of the data were confirmed through member checking groups. While exploratory in nature, Rebeiro's study developed a conceptual framework of the phases and implications of participation in personally chosen occupations. This conceptual framework provides the basis for a future grounded theory of occupational engagement. In addition, the analysis of the research data points to an incipient theory of the role of the sociocultural environment in enabling occupation and a sense of well being.

Studies of Occupational Therapists

M. F. Managh and J. V. Cook

Originally, Managh intended to examine the ability of a standardized mental health assessment (the BAFPE-R) to predict successful community tenure of clients after their discharge from inpatient therapy. Initial research inquiry based on examination of the clients' hospital records and their BAFPE-R protocols indicated that a different research question was required before the original question could be explored. Thus, Managh used indepth, semistructured interviews to discover why occupational therapists used the assessment, how they administered it, and the uses they made of it. Managh's results are intriguing in that they imply that some standardized assessments are incompatible with firmly held occupational therapy values. Hence, the assessments are often not administered according to the protocols of the standardized instructions. These findings have implications for the use of assessments in practice.

J. V. Cook

Cook was interested in how all the services once provided by large psychiatric institutions were being delivered in the community following the policy of deinstitutionalization. The case study describes how one new program in case management services came to fruition. Document analysis, in-depth interviews, and on-site, participant observation were the methods used to retrospectively reconstruct the development of the service innovation. Using existing sociological and organizational theory, Cook analyzed the actions of a single occupational therapist to illustrate how professional values and commitment contributed to the perseverance and leadership necessary to initiate a new program of services.

S. Moll and J. V. Cook

Believing that what distinguished occupational therapy as a profession was the value it placed on the therapeutic use of activity or "doing," Moll initially set out to gather evidence of the therapeutic outcomes of occupational doing. She used the strategies of observation and interviewing with occupational therapists working in the area of mental health and illness. In the interviews, therapists attributed a variety of therapeutic gains for clients to "doing" occupations or activities. However, based on both the observations and the interviews, it was apparent that the therapists primarily used verbally based or "talking" groups as interventions. This led to a change in the research focus and an analysis of therapists' beliefs about the value of occupation, rather than the outcomes of activity-based therapy.

Studies of Client Experiences

H. A. Emerson et al.

As an occupational therapist with many years of experience in mental health practice, Emerson's study was stimu- lated by Csikzentmihalyi's theory of "flow." In particular, Csikzentmihalyi's statement that "persons with schizophrenia cannot experience flow" led to Emerson's research question: Do persons with schizophrenia experience enjoyment, and if so, what are the contexts, conditions, and contents of such experi- ences? Emerson used audiotaped, in-depth interviews for data collection. Her analysis of the data suggests that enjoyment may be a broader concept than flow, that persons with schizophrenia do experience enjoyment, and that the conditions and contents of those experiences have implications for therapists in their activities to promote occupational engagement.

D. J. Corring and J. V. Cook

While exploring the concept of client-centred care in the litera- ture, Corring discovered that none of the articles or books exam- ined the concept from a client's perspective. Her research question was: "What are the characteristics of client-centred care from a client's point of view? She focused, in particular, on con- sumer perspectives of mental health services. Corring used the strategy of focus group interviews, facilitated by two former consumers, while she participated as an observer. The results of her analysis indicate that while the professional and consumer perspectives on client-centred care share many similarities, the importance of recognition of human identity, and its validation by service providers to persons with a mental illness, is the cen- tral, crucial characteristic that contributes to a sense of a valued self. This study also poignantly describes the often negative experiences of clients receiving services and includes their rec- ommendations for enabling positive experiences.

K. L. Rebeiro

In her continuing program of research into the role of occupation in the lives of persons with severe and persistent mental illness,

Rebeiro conducted a five-phase study using the strategies of a survey questionnaire, in-depth interviews, participant observation, and member checking group interviews. This study is both a case study of services in one city and an exploration and analysis of the experiences of persons seeking to engage in meaningful occupation. The interpretative conclusion that an emphasis on "problems within the person" precludes an examination of the sociocultural and physical barriers to occupation has important implications for policy and program development.

D. Laliberte-Rudman et al.

Using focus group interviews, Laliberte-Rudman and her colleagues sought to discover what conditions, experiences, and feelings contributed to and were important for enjoyment of life for persons with a serious mental illness. Many quality of life measures were developed by researchers who "assumed" the content issues. This study was designed to elicit the perspectives of consumers in order to develop a quality of life measure that reflected their issues of concern. The analysis indicates that measures of quality of life will be better developed when based on participants' perspectives. In addition, the descriptions of clients' lives, illustrated by quotations from the focus groups, give strong indication of the contribution occupation can make in improving quality of life.

Notes

[1] These journal articles are reprinted as originally published. Therefore, some of the authors' academic and clinical affiliations and titles may currently differ from those listed in the journal credits.

[2] All articles are reprinted with permission from the journals and authors. Royalties from this book are designated to a charitable foundation that supports occupational therapy graduate students and occupational therapy research. Therefore, the following journals agreed to waive or reduce their reprint fees:

- The Canadian Journal of Occupational Therapy
- The Journal of Occupational Science
- Psychiatric Rehabilitation Journal
- The Scandinavian Journal of Occupational Therapy
- The American Journal of Occupational Therapy

We thank the publishers of these journals for their support of research in occupational therapy.

Understanding the Potential of Occupation: A Qualitative Exploration of Seniors' Perspectives on Activity

The American Journal of Occupational Therapy

1997, 51(8): 640–650

Deborah Laliberte Rudman, Joanne Valiant Cook, Helene Polatajko

Deborah Laliberte Rudman, MSc, OT(C), is Lecturer, Department of Occupational Therapy, Faculty of Medicine, University of Toronto, 256 McCaul Street, Toronto, Ontario M5T 1W5, Canada. At the time of this study, she was Student, Master of Science in Occupational Therapy Program, University of Western Ontario, London, Ontario, Canada.

Joanne Valiant Cook, PhD, OT(C), is Assistant Professor, Department of Occupational Therapy, Faculty of Applied Health Sciences, Elborn College, The University of Western Ontario, London, Ontario, Canada.

Helene Polatajko, PhD. OT(C), is Professor and Chair, Department of Occupational Therapy, University of Western Ontario, London, Ontario, Canada.

KEY WORDS

- aging
- occupational therapy (profession of)

ABSTRACT

This article presents the results of a qualitative study that explored the characteristic and potential of occupation. Semistructured interviews with 12 seniors who live in the community followed by member-checking groups were used to explore informants' perspectives on the importance and role of occupation in their lives by asking them about their activities. Themes pertinent to the characterization of activity, the contributions of activity, and a condition allowing for the potential of activity emerged from the inductive analysis. These themes provide information about how occupation naturally functions in the lives of seniors and suggest a tentative conceptualization of the characteristics and potential of occupation. The findings have implications for research regarding occupation and for clinical practice aimed at enabling occupation.

Occupational therapy was founded on a belief in the fundamental importance of occupation (American Occupational Therapy Association [AOTA], 1995). Engagement in occupation is assumed to be an essential part of living and to have the potential to influence health and well-being (Polatajko, 1992; Yerxa, 1993). Research that addresses occupation and its contribution to well-being is required to develop an empirically based body of knowledge (AOTA, 1995; Christiansen, 1990; Wilcox, 1991).

Demographic projections and the increasing prevalence of disability associated with aging indicate that seniors will become an increasingly greater proportion of both the general population and the occupational therapy clientele (Carlson, Fanchiang, Zemke, & Clark, 1996). To meet current and future needs, it is essential that occupational therapists examine the potential of occupation in seniors' lives.

Although there is a general recognition that occupation is complex and relates to doing (Henderson et al., 1991; Wilcox, 1993), there is no consensus regarding the definition of occupation and its relationship to activity (AOTA, 1995; Henderson, 1996). Various definitions of *occupation* and *activity* have been proposed. In some cases, these definitions would suggest that *occupation* and *activity* are synonymous terms (Henderson, 1996; Yerxa et al., 1990). Other definitions of occupation, particularly more recent ones, suggest that activity is a subset of occupation. For example, Christiansen (1994) and Trombly (1995) delineate activity as one of the levels of occupation.

For the purposes of this study, the term *occupation* was conceived as referring to anything that people do in their everyday lives. Outside the occupational therapy profession, the term *activity* is typically used to express this concept. Thus, the literature on activity and aging was examined for its relevance to an understanding of occupation.

Although the relationship between activity and well-being has been a major focus of social gerontological research, the contribution of occupation within seniors' lives is not well understood. Research that has explored three major social gerontological theories, specifically activity, disengagement, and continuity theories, has primarily addressed the social dimension of activity (Lawton, 1985). Overall, this research has indicated that social activities have a positive, but weak, relationship with subjective well-being (Okun, Stock, Haring, & Witter, 1984; Zimmer, Hickey, & Searle, 1995).

The failure to address a range of types of activity and meaning is considered to be a factor that has contributed to weak findings regarding the relationship between activity and subjective well-being (Burbank, 1986; Zimmer et al., 1995). In particular, it has been hypothesized that the meaning seniors attach to activity has a vital influence on the contribution activity makes to subjective well-being (Jackson, 1996; Lawton, Moss, & Fulcomer, 1986–1987). Although the perspectives of persons who are engaged in activities need to be explored in order to fully understand the meaning of activities (Henderson, 1990; Lawton, 1985), the majority of studies addressing the meaning of activity for seniors have been guided by investigator hypothesis. Such studies have examined reasons for participation (e.g., Hersch, 1990; Ward, 1979), definitions of types of activity (e.g., Nystrom, 1974; Roadburg, 1981), and feelings and attitudes associated with activity (e.g., Gregory, 1983; Russell, 1987). Although some studies have found a positive, significant relationship between feelings and attitudes associated with activity and subjective well-being (Gregory, 1983; Smith, Kielhofner, & Watts, 1986), there is little consensus regarding what characteristics of activity are important and little exploration of seniors' perspectives.

Reseach examining the activities of persons who are not considered to be disabled can provide basic information about occupation that will contribute to theory development and that can be applied in clinical work (Gilfoyle & Christiansen, 1987; Polatajko, Miller, MacKinnon, & Harburn, 1989; Rogers, 1984). With reference to seniors, research investigating the activity of seniors living in the community would contribute to an understanding of how occupation naturally functions to influence well-being (Hasselkus & Kiernat, 1989; Rogers, 1981; Smith et al., 1986; Watson & Ager, 1991).

Therefore, this article reports the results of a study that explored seniors' perspectives about the meaning they attach to activity and the factors that influence their well-being. Although the study provided rich data about activity, well-being, and sociocultural factors, only the results most pertinent to the characteristics and potential of occupation are presented. Within this article, the potential of occupation refers to the possible affects that occupation can have in people's lives.

METHOD

Research Design

A qualitative approach was used because it is recommended to uncover the meaning of phenomena from informants' perspectives (Rowles & Reinharz, 1988). A major consideration in the design of a qualitative study is the issue of trustworthiness (Krefting, 1991). Trustworthiness refers to the extent to which the findings of a study can be viewed as worthy of confidence. The criteria used to assess trustworthiness include credibility, transferability, dependability, and confirmability (Lincoln & Guba, 1985). The criterion of credibility was addressed by using semistructured interviews and member-checking groups. A formal member check, which involves obtaining the original informants' viewpoints about the accuracy of results, is a powerful method to address credibility (Lincoln & Guba, 1985). Detailed descriptive information about informants and the setting of the study was compiled to address transferability. Dependability and confirmability were addressed through a field journal and through a partial audit of audiotaped interviews and transcripts by the first author's thesis committee members.

Informants

The principle of maximum variation (Lincoln & Guba, 1985) guided the selection of informants so that they were chosen to reflect as wide a variation in descriptive characteristics as possible within limits set by the inclusion criteria. The inclusion criteria were (a) 65 years of age or older, (b) living in the community, (c) not receiving intensive support services, and (d) able to participate in an interview. A sample size of 12 was deemed adequate on the basis of McCracken's (1988) estimate that qualitative, exploratory studies require 8 informants to obtain an adequate amount and range of information.

Three contact persons from different seniors' organizations located in a middle-sized city assisted with recruitment. The attempt to obtain informants who varied met with success for most variables, including gender, income level, educational level, and living arrangements. Of the 12 informants, 5 were men, and 7 were women. They belonged to four of five possible income categories, and their educational levels ranged from completion of elementary school to university. Living arrangements varied according to the type of persons informants lived with as well as the type of residence. Although all informants rated their health as at least the same as others their age, their ratings of their current health varied from very good to average. There were married, widowed, and single informants, but the distribution by gender was skewed because all the men but none of the women were married at the time of the study. The major limitations of the sample were that all informants were Caucasian and only ranged in age from 67 to 79 years.

Information Gathering

A semistructured interview guide consisting of open-ended questions and structured and unstructured probes was developed. Five major topics were addressed: (a) description of activities, (b) preferences for activities, (c) personal relevance of activities, (d) satisfaction with activities, and (e) well-being. To ensure that informants clearly understood that the intent was to explore the things they did in their everyday lives, it was decided to use the word *activity* rather than *occupation* during the interviews. This was done to avoid potential inferences on the part of the informants that occupation referred only to paid work. Before initiating data collection, the guide was pilot tested with three volunteers who were seniors. Interviews were conducted in the home for 10 informants and in the interviewer's office for 2. The length of the interviews ranged from 1 to 2 hr. All interviews were audiotaped and transcribed verbatim.

Two member-checking groups were conducted. During these groups, informants were shown the results of the analysis, and an interview guide consisting of open-ended questions and probes was used to facilitate group discussion. One group session included four of the original informants, and the other included three of the original informants. Both sessions lasted approximately 2 hr.

Analysis of the Information

The information collected during the interviews and member-checking groups was analyzed with techniques from the constant comparative method proposed by Glaser and Strauss (1967). The three techniques used included unitizing, categorizing, and forming themes (Lincoln & Guba, 1985; Strauss & Corbin, 1990). Essentially, transcripts were broken down into units of information and grouped into categories that, in turn, were grouped into themes. Several frameworks of relationships among the categories were tested against the data to obtain the framework that offered the best reconstruction of informants' perspectives.

INFORMANTS' PERSPECTIVES

Seven major themes pertinent to the characteristics and potential of occupation emerged from the study. One theme relates to the definition and characterization of activity, five relate to the contributions of activity, and one deals with a condition required for activity to fulfill its potential. The following interpretative analysis is illustrated by quotations from the informants' transcripts.

Defining and Characterizing Activity

The essential defining characteristics of activity that emerged is that activity involves doing. Informants described their activities in terms of the type or types of doing involved. These types include mental, physical, and social. Mental activity was characterized as activity that keeps one's "mind active." Physical activity was described as activity that involves exercising one's body. Activities that involve doing with other people were often labeled social activities.

It is apparent that any one activity can involve more than one type of doing. For example, when describing bridge, one female informant stated that "it's a mental stimulation and also social." Another female informant indicated that tai chi involved physical doing because "you're exercising every muscle in your body" and mental doing because "it's a great test of your memory because it's in sequence." Moreover, the types of doing associated with any one specific activity varied from informant to informant, as there were instances where they stressed different types of doing when describing the same objective activity. For example, some informants described golfing as a physical activity, whereas others stressed its social element.

It is evident that not all instances of doing are defined as activity. The extent of engagement associated with an instance of doing influences whether it is labeled an activity. For example, an informant in a group session stated that activity involves mental and physical exercise and that "sitting and watching television isn't what I'd call an activity, myself." The other three group members suggested that watching television is an activity if it involves being interested in what one is watching.

Contributions of Activity

Activity as a contributor to well-being. Informants indicated that activity contributes to one's sense of well-being and suggested several ways in which it can exert a positive influence. At the most fundamental level, activity contributes to well-being because doing activity is a basic need essential to one's continued existence and to the quality of that existence. For example, one female informant stated that if a person did not have activities, then "you'd

Chapter 11

only be a vegetable if you didn't [do activities]. You certainly wouldn't be alive mentally or whatever." This idea that activity is an essential need is reflected in stories informants told about persons they knew who had experienced a decline in activity, which, in turn, led to a decline in well-being. For example, one informant talked about his wife's friend:

L. [referring to his wife] has a friend who evidently was a concert pianist, and since her husband died, she won't touch the piano, which is sheer lunacy. She doesn't particularly like going out. Well, alright, I guess you carve your own grave if you keep that up. Guess you're gonna deteriorate, and that's it.

Another male informant stated that

most people have a job and that's the only thing, one job all their lives. And the trouble with them is that when they retire, they don't know what the hell to do with themselves. In 2 years, they usually get sick and die.

Informants stressed that physical, mental, and social activity are all important for well-being. With respect to mental activity, one informant stated, "You have to do something that's intellectual too. You've got to read and find an area of reading that you like, something that will . . . stimulate your mental process." Physical activity was described as having the potential to contribute to both physical and emotional well-being. One female informant discussed the effects of not engaging in physical doing:

I find if I don't [do physical activity] and just sit around, I don't feel as good. I feel better if I get out and do something, like even if I walk to the store, I don't feel as alive as if I do some physical activity.

Social activities contribute to well-being by providing a way to fulfill one's need for social contact. For example, when discussing the benefits she derived from participating in an exercise class, an informant stated that "you need that contact with people."

Activity may also influence one's sense of well-being through the feelings it promotes. Informants discussed a number of positive feelings that they derive from activities, including competence, increased mastery, being needed, belonging, doing something worthwhile, social recognition and approval, and escaping. Although the importance attributed to any one kind of feeling varied from informant to informant, an especially prevalent feeling was that of accomplishment. When asked what makes up a good day, one female informant stated, "I think accomplishment, if you accomplish something, even though it might be very small." A male informant stated, "When you've accomplished a lot, you feel good." In addition, the other contributions of activity described later in this article may reflect ways in which activity can exert a positive influence on subjective well-being.

Activity as a means to express and manage identity. Activity can be used to demonstrate aspects of one's identity, to describe oneself, and to achieve social recognition. Informants described numerous instances of how activity demonstrated some aspect of their identity. For example, several informants described how their activity choices reflected some aspect of their basic nature. One informant explained that she had baked cookies in preparation for the interviewer's visit instead of doing housework because "that's what I do, you see. I don't do the obvious, I'll do something a little extra. That's just my nature." Another informant explained that she travels because "I like to be out and meet people. That's my nature."

Activities related to a socially recognized role can be used to describe oneself. Informants often described themselves in terms of activities that involve helping others and that are part of a role that others recognized and acknowledged. Informants stressed that they are the type of persons who like "doing for others." For example, one informant who was a volunteer tutor compared himself with his friends who did not volunteer, stating that although he derived a great deal of satisfaction from helping others, his friends "were not that kind of person." This same informant talked about the "social goodies" and "social recognition" he receives as a result of doing income tax forms for persons living in a long-term-care institution and that this "social approval is very necessary for my happiness."

With respect to the management of identity, activity may contribute both to a sense of continuity of identity and to a sense of continued growth. Informants indicated that the basic structure of who they are had remained continuous over time. In the words of one female informant, "Just because you have so many birthdays behind you doesn't really, it changes you physically but it doesn't change you inside." It is apparent that activity can be used to promote this sense of continuity of identity. In addition to sometimes maintaining participation in the same objective activity over a long period, the maintenance of factors related to activity can promote a sense of continuity of identity. These factors include associations, likes and dislikes, interests, and skills.

For example, with respect to associations, informants described activities done with the same group of people for long periods, ranging from 8 years to almost 60 years, that appear to facilitate the maintenance of their identity as part of a group. One informant described his association with a group of friends as follows:

We started going to coffee back in the 1930s at the back of Metropolitan stores. And there was a whole group of people that I met with at that time, and the only ones left are B., J., and myself. All the rest of them died.

This informant continued to meet each morning for coffee with the remaining members of this group. Other informants used activity to retain associations with organizations that were and continued to be an important part of their lives and identities. For example, one informant stated that being in the air force is an important aspect of his life and that his involvement in a veteran organization allows him to maintain the connection because "you sort of have the feeling that

you're showing the flag, you're holding up your end of the thing. You're still . . . there representing the service."

Although informants suggested that they had basically remained the same person over time, they also indicated that they are continuing to develop. It is evident that activity, especially if it involves developing and improving skills or learning, can foster a sense of continued growth by promoting the development of personal characteristics and the discovery of new aspects of oneself. For example, one informant talked about how she had discovered aspects of herself through being a volunteer: "You start off gradually, and then you find that you have ability and talent that you didn't even know you had." Another informant reflected on how she had become more competent in her role as a fitness instructor:

And I can't believe it now because I get up, I don't have any written outline or plans, and I just go ahead and do it. And while we're doing the exercises, I've developed a way of telling stories, very much as ease, I've surprised myself.

It is also evident that activity can influence one's age identity. Several informants stressed that they did not feel old and differentiated themselves from negative stereotypical images of "old people" by describing aspects of their activities. For example, one informant who had stated several times that she does not feel old remarked that "I've got so many interests, probably more than most people my age" and "there are not many people at this age that are active."

Activity as a connector to people. The use of activity to establish and maintain social connections emerged as a major theme. Informants highlighted the need for contact with other persons and provided numerous examples of using activity to connect with others. One informant emphasized the importance of social contact and planned her activity to ensure this contact:

I like to be in touch with people too, that helps me. I like to see somebody every day. If the weather was bad or something and I [did not have] any plans, I would maybe go over to the mall and do my shopping and maybe meet somebody over there for coffee or something.

Another informant indicated that his connections with a group revolved around a specific activity: "I would never see any of those people except at curling or at the banquets that we have. And those are the things I see them at. I generally don't see them anywhere else."

The importance of this contribution is highlighted by the finding that the social contact facilitated by an activity can be one of the main reasons that a person decides to participate and can have a major impact on the enjoyment and satisfaction derived from the activity. For example, an informant stated that he belongs to a bridge group because "it's the sociability. Several of the characters that have been in, the men, say that if it wasn't for the sociability, they wouldn't bother being in it at all." Another male informant described being in a particular lodge as fun because "there's parties. There's, what do you call it, being with people."

It is also apparent that specific activities in a person's life facilitate contact with certain types of persons. A widowed informant indicated that one reason she liked volunteering in a gift shop was that she was "with a very nice type of ladies who all have the same thing in common, a lot of them are widows." Another informant remarked that she had contact with young families in her neighborhood through shared activities: "On my street, there are young families with children, and it's a street that gets together for various things. And each time there's a new baby, they all have a baby shower and so on."

Activity can be used to make connections with new persons and expand one's social network. One informant stated that if he had not become involved in a specific lodge, he and his wife would have a "much narrower group of friends and/or acquaintances." Another informant stated that he and his wife's "circle of friends" has enlarged because of his involvement in a service organization and a curling club.

Informants stressed the importance of friendships and indicated that part of the

definition of friendship is that a friend is someone with whom one shares numerous activities. One informant indicated that the persons he does one activity with are "casual" friends and that his closer friends are persons he does many activities with and sees more frequently. A female informant stated, "I've got a really good friend, she's in my arthritis class. And we do a lot of things together."

Overall, the findings indicate that the absolute amount of social activity a person does may be less important than how content he or she is with the level and quality of social contact facilitated by the activity and with the balance that exists between the time spent with others and the time spent alone. Although all the informants indicated that they have a need for contact with people, some stressed this need more than others. Informants' comments regarding the types of persons with whom activity facilitated contact and the distinctions made between activity done with acquaintances and that done with friends suggest that the quality of the social contact facilitated by activity is also important.

Activity as an organizer of time. Engagement in activity can affects one's perception of the passage of time, and it can be used to organize or manage one's time. Informants indicated that doing activity can promote the feeling that time is passing quickly. For example, one informant stated the following about gardening:

And the summers, of course, just go with the gardening . . . I spend many hours in the garden. I go out with my compost, and then I see, "Well, I better pick that, I'd better. Oh. there's a weed." And instead of being out there for 5 minutes, I'm out there for an hour . . . the time just flies, and it's gone, and there's always something else to do.

Activity can also be used to "take up" or "put in" time. For example, one informant talked about how activities throughout the day takes up the time: "You talk to your neighbors. There's . . . little blocks that take up 10 minutes here or 15 minutes there. [I] walk over to the drug store to get some stamps or to get my medication refilled."

In addition to structuring each day by doing certain activities at specific times, activity can be used to create a weekly schedule. Although there was variation in the degree to which informants scheduled activities on a weekly basis, all had some scheduled activity. Informants who stressed the importance of a schedule had scheduled activity to a greater extent than those who did not express this concern. For example, a female informant who has activities scheduled on 4 weekday mornings stated:

> Well, I think it's important when I've worked all my life. And I did. I worked from the time when I was 18 until I was 65. To suddenly stop and every morning get up and not have anything that you have to do that day is not good. At least it's not good for me.

Alternatively, a male informant who stated that the "opulence of free time" was part of what makes up a good day has activities scheduled for only 1 weekday morning and a few evenings a month.

Several benefits and drawbacks associated with using activity to organize time emerged. The benefits include having a sense of structure to one's day, having something to look forward to, feeling that one is not wasting time, and ensuring that one's days are not identical. Because scheduled activities are often done outside the home and involve social contact, the use of activities to organize time may provide a way to ensure that one has a reason for leaving one's home and has a way to fulfill one's need for social contact. As well, the creation of a weekly schedule may facilitate the experiencing of time in terms of weeks rather than just in terms of days. The drawbacks the informants described pertained to a decreased sense of control over one's activities and a decreased amount of free time because scheduling activities may lead one to feel obligated.

Activity as a connector to the past, present, and future. Activities can lead to a sense of connectedness with the past by facilitating the recall of experiences. One informant stated that he and his wife enjoy putting together slide shows of their previous travels "because it revives memories." Another male informant stated that the speeches presented during the meetings of an ex-officers' club are "sometimes it's pure, what do you call it, remembering back, the good old days sort of thing." Activity can also facilitate a feeling of connection with past familial generations. Some informants suggested that personal characteristics associated with activity had been passed down from previous generations. For example, one informant indicated that her approach to bridge had been passed down from her mother: "My mother taught me, my sister, and my husband before we were married. And she was a very competitive player, and we've all developed that same competitiveness in the game."

Certain activities can provide a way to keep "in touch" with and be knowledgeable about what is happening in the present. One informant stated that she reads the newspaper each morning because "I want to keep in touch with what's going on in the world. I think maybe I spend too much time doing that, but I don't want something to happen and I don't know about it." Another informant indicated that reading is one of his favorite activities because it "keeps you in touch with what's going on, if you read the right stuff."

Activities that provide something to look forward to can connect a person with the future. Numerous informants talked about looking forward to annual activities. For example, one informant talked about how she looks forward to an annual trip: "I look forward to going out west once a year and go out and see everybody [referring to family members]." Another informant talked about the enjoyment that she derives from an annual activity: "That's another thing I do every year is go to Point Pelee for the bird-watching for a week, which is really interesting." Activity that involves working toward a goal can also facilitate a future orientation. One informant talked about her goal of creating 100 cryptic crossword puzzles: "I have at the moment about 25 on file. I'm aiming for a hundred, if I ever get around to completing it. I just might get a publisher." Another informant talked about how she had participated in a project at her church that involved creating a special garden "so that some day, maybe 40 years down the road, kids will be bused from all over Ontario to the church."

Aspects of activity that are passed on to future generations provide a connection to the future. Informants suggested that members of the next generation possess characteristics associated with activity that they themselves possess. For example, one informant suggested that his desire to do some type of "social work" had been carried out by his daughter through her job: "And I often wonder. I think that what didn't come out in me might have come out in her."

Control as an Essential Condition for the Potential of Activity

The sense of control associated with activity appears to be an important mediator of the relationship between activity and well-being and an essential condition for the realization of other potential contributions of activity. The message conveyed by informants is that a person not only needs to be doing, but also needs to be in control of his or her activity. While giving advice on how to stay healthy, a male informant stated, "You should do what you want to do." Another male informant stated, "Doing all these things is good, but being a slave to them isn't the answer."

Informants talked about the negative effects of not feeling in control of their activities. One female informant suggested that the two things that make up a bad day are not feeling well and "if you can't do the things that you wanted to do." When a male informant was asked whether he thought it was important for his well-being to be able to do what he wanted, he stated, "I think that if you're doing things that you don't want to do, I can't think of anything more devastating than that." It is evident that a sense of control over activity can exist in a situation where a person has external factors impinging on his or her activities. Despite the fact that all informants mentioned factors in their lives that restrict their activities, they expressed that they feel in control of their activity. For example, an informant who had discussed how his arthritis periodically restricted his activities stated, "[I do] the things I do because I want to do them, not because I have to do them. So I'm free and easy. I can just pick and choose whatever I want to do." Another informant who had previously indicated that her health and fear of the night restrict what she does was asked whether there is anything she would like to be doing that she is not doing. She responded, "I don't know because if it were something that was possible to do and I wanted to do it, I don't see why I couldn't do something."

Thus, informants appeared to have a sense of control over their activity, and, in turn, activity appeared to make numerous positive contributions to their lives. The sense of control over activity the informants possessed in the presence of restrictions appears to be related to the existence of choice. Informants gave numerous examples of how they make choices about their activities. For example, one informant talked about her decision to go only to the plays that she is interested in rather than go to plays because of other persons' interests. She stated, "I'm going to pick and choose just the ones I want to go to because you can do that." Some informants arrange activities so that they would have the choice of when they would do them. For example, an informant stated that a positive feature of a bridge club that he and his friends had set up was that he and his wife could choose to play when they want to play: "It's a volunteer situation, there's no schedule. You just phone around and find a few couples that want to play on a certain night."

The need for control appears to be strong because informants were implementing strategies aimed at ensuring that they would maintain control over their activity in the future. An informant suggested that one of her reasons for becoming involved in bird-watching was to ensure that she would have something she is capable of doing if her physical health decreased: "I think I'm looking to the future, if maybe I couldn't get around all that well." A male informant indicated that the ability to maintain control is considered when choosing an activity:

> I wonder if we tend to take up activities in which we are in control and avoid those in which we aren't really, for any reason at all, whether . . . we never would have been or whether because of age we're no longer able to control.

REFLECTIONS

Overall, our study supports Yerxa et al.'s (1990) assertion that exploration of persons' perspectives about their everyday activities can contribute to an in-depth understanding of occupation. When these relatively healthy informants discussed their doing in terms of preferences for activities, personal relevance of activities, satisfaction with activities, and well-being, they talked about chunks of activity within a wide range of occupations. Informants rarely, if ever, talked about the common, basic self-care activities that tend to be the focus of much of occupational therapy practice. It appears that when healthy persons are asked to talk about what they do, the occupations that have meaning for them are rarely at the level of the basic occupations, such as grooming or dressing.

Our findings confirm, elaborate on, and question aspects of the existing literature in social gerontology and occupational therapy. The study provides information on how occupation naturally contributes to seniors' lives and, given the small sample size, provides a tentative conceptualization of the characteristics and potential of occupation.

Understanding the Potential of Occupation for Seniors

Activity theory, disengagement theory, and continuity theory each propose a different role for activity in seniors' lives (Burbank, 1986). The central hypothesis of activity theory is that

there is a direct, positive relationship between the amount of social contact facilitated by activity and subjective well-being (Havighurst & Albrecht, 1953). The central hypothesis of disengagement theory are that there is a mutual, inevitable withdrawal between seniors and society and that the need for social interaction decreases as one ages (Cumming & Henry, 1961). The findings support the importance of social contact but, contrary to disengagement theory, do not indicate that aging is associated with a declining need for social contact. It is also evident that occupation can make contributions other than social connectedness and can involve more than social doing. Moreover, the findings indicate that the need for social contact varies from person to person and that the quality of social contact may be as important as quantity. Thus, as indicated by Burbank (1986) and Lawton et al. (1986–1987), the central hypothesis of activity theory appears too simplistic to address the relationship between activity and subjective well-being for seniors.

With respect to the original version of continuity theory (Neugarten, Havighurst, & Tobin, 1968), the findings support the proposition that successful aging is an individualized process characterized by differing levels of social activity. Atchley (1983, 1989) proposed that successful aging involves having a sense of internal and external continuity. The informants in this study appeared to have a sense of internal continuity as well as a sense of external continuity that is related to their activities. The findings support two other propositions of Atchley (1989): (a) that it is necessary to examine seniors' perceptions to determine whether a sense of continuity exists and (b) that successful aging involves achieving a balance between continuity and change. Although informants expressed having a sense of continuity, they also talked about achieving personal growth. Overall, the study supports continuity theory and suggests that further exploration of seniors' perspectives could lead to a more in-depth understanding of the ways in which activity can be associated with a sense of continuity.

Numerous questions regarding the nature of occupation require investigation (AOTA, 1995; Clark et al., 1991). The findings suggest an essential aspect of the definition of occupation and call into question the categories of occupation traditionally used by occupational therapists.

Currently, various definitions of occupation can be found in the occupational therapy literature (Trombly, 1995). Doing that involves engagement emerged as the essence of occupation in this study. Several existing definitions emphasize that occupation is a doing process in which a person is engaged. For example, Clark et al. (1991) defined occupation as "chunks of culturally and personally meaningful activity in which humans engage" (p. 301), and Evans (1987) defined occupation as an "active or 'doing' process of a person engaged in goal-directed, intrinsically gratifying, and culturally appropriate activity" (p. 627).

Occupational therapists have traditionally categorized occupations into work, self-care (or self-maintenance), play, and leisure. It is thought that these categories are recognized across persons and across cultures, even though the specific tasks that make up each category may vary from person to person (AOTA, 1995). However, the informants did not spontaneously use these categories; instead, they chose to refer to activities in terms of social, physical, and mental doing. This suggests that the conventional categories used by occupational therapists may not always be relevant to their clients. It appears that occupational therapists need to be flexible when categorizing occupation in order to ensure that the categories make sense in the context of clients' lives. Moreover, the findings show that the assignment of any occupation to a categorical system is likely to vary from person to person. The need to consider the perspective of the individual when categorizing occupation has been recognized in the occupational therapy literature (Clark et al., 1991; Smith et at, 1986; Trombly, 1995).

This study responds to the need for empirical support for the assumptions that form the basis of occupational therapy. Overall, it suggests that occupation is a basic need essential to one's continued existence and the quality of one's existence. Thus, the study provides empirical support for two central assumptions of occupational therapy; (a) that humans have an occupational nature and that occupation is, therefore, a basic need essential to living (Polatajko, 1994; Wilcox, 1993; Yerxa, 1991) and (b) that occupations can positively influence health and well-being (Kielhofner, 1985; Polatajko, 1992; Reilly, 1962; Rogers, 1984).

Although numerous potential benefits or contributions of occupation have been identified in the occupational therapy literature, there is a need for research to substantiate many of these benefits (AOTA, 1995). This study indicates that occupation may exert a positive influence on subjective well-being in many ways. Beyond being a basic need, occupation may influence well-being through the other contributions it makes in peoples' lives. The contributions that emerged in the present study include means to express and manage identity; connector to people; organizer of time; and connector to the past, present, and future. Although further investigation is required to determine whether these contributions are specific to seniors, the findings suggest ways that occupation exerts an influence on subjective well-being.

Several of these contributions of occupation are not likely to be age specific because they have been proposed as general contributions within the occupational therapy literature. The idea that occupation can be used to express one's identity and can contribute to personal growth has been suggested by several authors (Christiansen, 1994; Nelson, 1988; Wilcox, 1993; Yerxa, 1994). In addition, both Wilcox (1993) and Yerxa (1994) asserted that occupation serves to facilitate social connections. The use of occupation to organize time was suggested

---

by Meyer (1922) and has been emphasized by Christiansen (1994) and Kielhofner (1985), among others.

Finally, the findings provide information pertinent to three characteristics of the potential of occupation. First, they suggest that the potential of any occupation is multidimensional and that these dimensions relate to the contributions of occupation. For example, one occupation may contribute by being a means to connect with people and to express one's identity. Several authors have proposed that occupation is multidimensional and have called for research to investigate its dimensions (AOTA, 1995; Canadian Association of Occupational Therapists [CAOT], 1994; Polatajko, 1994; Yerxa et al., 1990). Similar to the findings of this study, Nelson (1988) asserted that the purpose of occupational performance is multidimensional in that a person may be seeking more than one goal when performing a specific occupation.

Second, it is apparent that the potential associated with an occupation is individualized, as indicated by informants who described realizing different contributions from the same occupation. Several authors have also indicated that the meaning attached to occupation is determined by the individual person (Henderson et al., 1991; Trombly, 1995; Yerxa et al. 1990). In addition, Christiansen (1994) and Nelson (1988) asserted that the meaningfulness and purpose associated with an occupation is unique to each person. One reason that may explain why the potential of occupation is individualized is that the importance attached to any contribution varies from person to person.

Third, it appears that the potential of occupation is dynamic because its contribution to a person's life may change according to the context in which it is done and over time. Several authors have recognized the importance of the context (Henderson et al., 1991; Nelson, 1988; Yerxa et al., 1990), and some stress the importance of temporal context (Kielhofner, 1985; Nelson, 1988).

Understanding the Conditions That Allow for the Potential of Occupation

Yerxa et al. (1990) stated that

> *Some venerable assumptions of occupational therapy are that engagement in activity is wholesome, health influencing, and contributory to the significance and meaning of life. Yet the opposite is also true. Engagement in occupation can be frustrating, anxiety provoking, and/or boring. What is the difference? (p. 9)*

The findings suggest that control is one condition that differentiates occupation that positively contributes to subjective well-being from occupation that does not The message conveyed by the informants is that a person not only needs to be active, but also needs to be in control of his or her occupations.

The importance of having a sense of control over occupation has been emphasized in recent occupational therapy literature (CAOT, 1994; Polatajko, 1994; Yerxa, 1994). Both Gregory (1983) and Smith et al. (1986) conducted studies with samples composed of seniors that examined the importance of personal causation in effecting the relationship between occupation and life satisfaction. Gregory found that there was a significant, moderate correlation ($r = .37, p < .01$) between the sense of autonomy associated with occupational behavior and life satisfaction. Smith et al. measured perceived competence and found that it also had a significant, moderate correlation ($r = 39, p < .005$) with life satisfaction. The findings of the present study combined with those of Gregory and Smith et al. provide much needed empirical support for the importance of having a sense of control over occupation.

In addition, the findings inform about the nature of the sense of control associated with occupation. It appears that this sense of control can vary from situation to situation and is more complex than a feeling of wanting to do something versus a feeling of having to do something. For instance, activities and schedules that have flexibility and allow for varying decisions appear to facilitate a sense of control. Thus, the correlation that resulted in Gregory's (1983) study may not represent the extent of the relationship between a sense of control and life satisfaction because autonomy was measured by asking whether subjects did an activity because they wanted to do it or because they had to do it.

Another finding indicating that the sense of control associated with a occupation is not an all-or-none phenomenon is that it can exist even when there are factors negatively affecting a person's occupations. Although informants provided numerous examples of environmental and health factors impeding their ability to pursue certain occupations, they still expressed having a sense of control over their occupations. The essential element appears to be the existence of choice, that is, choice of what one does, when one does, with whom one does, how one does, and where one does.

Limitations

The major limitations of the study relate to the sample's limited age range and lack of cultural variation. The trustworthiness of the findings could have been strengthened by using other means of data collection, such as observation, to triangulate the findings. Overall, it is not claimed that the findings address all the characteristics or contributions of occupation. At the same time, the findings appear to be trustworthy and provide tentative hypotheses that warrant further investigation.

Implications

The findings suggest several variables that need to be addressed in future research in order to understand occupation and its relationship to subjective well-being. Studies need to examine the direct relationship between occupation and well-being as well as the indirect relationship that is mediated by the other contributions of occupation. It is also evident that the sense of control associated with occupation needs to be considered and examined as occurring on a continuum and as affected by context.

As well as demonstrating that exploration of persons' perspectives can contribute to an in-depth understanding of occupation, themes that emerged in this study may be useful for the development of grounded theory. Some of the key issues that warrant further investigation include:

- The contribution of occupation to identity, especially in terms of its relationship to a sense of continuity
- The function of occupation as both an organizer of time and a connector to time periods
- The extent to which the contributions of occupation comprise a dimension of occupation
- The multidimensional and individualized nature of occupation
- The dynamic nature of occupation and how this is influenced by time and context
- The complexity of the sense of control associated with occupation

With respect to clinical interventions aimed at enabling occupation, the findings provide empirical support for an individualized approach that offers clients choice and facilitates a sense of control. The findings suggest that occupational therapists must use an approach that considers the client's perspective because both the categorization and the contributions of occupation vary from person to person. The individualized nature of the potential of occupation means that it is not possible to assume the benefits a person derives from an occupation. The importance of exploring the level of occupation that has meaning for a client in his or her present context is also apparent. The need for an approach that involves client participation and facilitates a sense of control is supported by the finding that the sense of control associated with occupation can considerably affect the contribution of occupation to well-being. It is also evident that control cannot be viewed as an all-or-none phenomenon and that therapists can work to facilitate choice and promote a sense of control with clients of varying abilities and in varying contexts.

ACKNOWLEDGMENTS

This article was based on a thesis completed by the first author in partial fulfillment of the requirements for the master of occupational therapy degree at the University of Western Ontario. Thanks are extended to the 12 seniors who served as informants and to all members of the thesis committee, which include the second and third authors of this article as well as Gail Frankel, PhD, Department of Sociology, University of Western Ontario.

This article was presented, in part, at the 1993 CANAM Conference in Boston with the financial support of the Ontario Society of Occupational Therapists' Research Fund. The first author received financial support through an Ontario Graduate Scholarship.

References

American Occupational Therapy Association. (1995). Position paper: Occupation. American Journal of Occupational Therapy, 49, 1015–1018.

Atchley, R. C. (1983). Aging, continuity, and change (2nd ed.). Belmont, CA: Woodsworth.

Atchley, R. C. (1989). A continuity theory of normal aging. Gerontologist, 29, 183–190.

Burbank, P. M. (1986). Psychosocial theories of aging: A critical evaluation. Advances in Nursing Science, 9(1), 73–86.

Canadian Association of Occupational Therapists. (1994). Position statement on everyday occupations and health. Canadian Journal of Occupational Therapy, 61, 294–295.

Carlson, M., Fanchiang, S.-P., Zemke, R., & Clark, F. (1996). A meta-analysis of the effectiveness of occupational therapy for older persons. American Journal of Occupational Therapy, 50, 89–98.

Christiansen, C. (1990). The perils of plurality. Occupational Therapy Journal of Research, 10, 259–265.

Christiansen, C. (1994). Classification and study in occupation: A review and discussion of taxonomies. Journal of Occupational Science, 1(3), 3–21.

Clark, F. A., Parham, D., Carlson, M. E., Frank, G., Jackson, J., Pierce, D., Wolfe, R. J., & Zemke, R. (1991). Occupational science: Academic innovation in the service of occupational therapy's future. American Journal of Occupational Therapy, 45, 300–330.

Cumming, E., & Henry, W. (1961). Growing old. New York: Basic.

Evans, K. A. (1987). Nationally Speaking—Definition of occupation as the core concept of occupational therapy. American Journal of Occupational Therapy, 41, 627–628.

Gilfoyle, E. M., & Christiansen, C. H. (1987). Nationally Speaking—Research: The quest for truth and the key to excellence. American Journal of Occupational Therapy, 41, 7–8.

Glaser, B. G., & Strauss, A. L. (1967). The discovery of grounded theory. Chicago; Aldine.

Gregory, M. D. (1983). Occupational behavior and life satisfaction among retirees. American Journal of Occupational Therapy, 37, 548–553.

Hasselkus, B. R, & Kiernat, J. M. (1989). Nationally Speaking—Not by age alone: Gerontology as a specialty in occupational therapy. American Journal of Occupational Therapy, 43, 77–79.

Havighurst, R. J., & Albrecht, R. (1953). Older people. New York: Arno.

Henderson, A. (1996). The scope of occupational science. In R. Zemke & F. Clark (Eds.), Occupational science. The evolving discipline (pp. 419–424). Philadelphia: F. A. Davis.

Henderson, A., Cermak, S., Coster, W., Murray, E., Trombly, C., & Tickle-Degnen, L. (1991). The Issue Is —Occupational science is multidimensional. American Journal of Occupational Therapy, 45, 370–372.

Henderson, K. A. (1990). The meaning of leisure for women: An integrative review of the research. Journal of Leisure Research, 22, 228–243.

Hersch, G. (1990). Leisure and aging. Physical and Occupational Therapy in Geriatrics, 9(2), 55–78.

Jackson, J. (1996). Living a meaningful existence in old age. In R. Zemke & F. Clark (Eds.), Occupational science: The evolving discipline (pp. 339–363). Philadelphia: F. A. Davis.

Kielhofner, C. (Ed.). (1985). A model of human occupation. Baltimore: Williams & Wilkins.

Krefting, L. (1991). Rigor in qualitative research: The assessment of trustworthiness. American Journal of Occupational Therapy, 45, 214–222.

Lawton, M. P. (1985). Activities and leisure. *Annual Review of Gerontology and Geriatrics, 5,* 127–164.

Lawton, M. P., Moss. M., & Fulcomer, M. (1986–1987). Objective and subjective uses of time by older people. *International Journal of Aging and Human Development, 24,* 171–187.

Lincoln, Y. S., & Guba, E. G. (1985). *Naturalistic inquiry.* Newbury Park, CA: Sage.

McCracken, G. (1988). *The long interview.* Newbury Park, CA: Sage.

Meyer, A. (1922). The philosophy of occupation therapy. *Archives of Occupational Therapy. I,* 1–10.

Nelson, D. L. (1988). Occupation: Form and performance. *American Journal of Occupational Therapy, 42,* 633–641.

Neugarten, B. L, Havighurst, R. J, & Tobin, S. S. (1968). Personality and patterns of aging. In B. Neugarten (Ed.), *Middle age and aging* (pp. 173–177). Chicago: University of Chicago Press.

Nystrom, E. P. (1974). Activity patterns and leisure concepts among the elderly. *American Journal of Occupational Therapy, 28,* 337–345.

Okun, M. A., Stock, W. E., Haring, M. J., & Witter, R. A. (1984). The social activity/subjective well-being relation. *Research on Aging, 6*(1)45–65.

Polatajko, H. J. (1992). Naming and framing occupational therapy: A lecture dedicated to the life of Nancy B. *Canadian Journal of Occupational Therapy, 59,* 189–200.

Polatajko, H. J. (1994). Dreams, dilemmas, and decisions for occupational therapy practice in a new millennium: A Canadian perspective. *American Journal of Occupational Therapy, 48,* 590–594.

Polatajko, H. J., Miller, J., MacKinnon, J., & Harburn, K. (1989). Occupational therapy research in Canada: Report from the Association of Canadian Occupational Therapy University Programs. *Canadian Journal of Occupational Therapy, 56,* 257–260.

Reilly, M. (1962). Occupational therapy can be one of the great ideas of 20th century medicine, Eleanor Clark Slagle lecture. *American Journal of Occupational Therapy, 16,* 1–9.

Roadburg, A. (1981). Perceptions of work and leisure among the elderly. *Gerontologist, 2,* 142–145.

Rogers, J. C. (1981). The Issue Is—Gerontic occupational therapy. *American Journal of Occupational Therapy, 35,* 663–666.

Rogers, J. C. (1984). American Occupational Therapy Foundation, Inc.—Why study human occupation? *American Journal of Occupational Therapy, 38,* 47–49.

Rowles, G. D., & Reinharz, S. (1988). Qualitative gerontology: Theme and challenges. In S. Reinharz & G. D. Rowles (Eds.), *Qualitative gerontology* (pp. 3–33). New York: Springer.

Russell, R. V. (1987). The importance of recreation satisfaction and activity participation to the life satisfaction of age-segregated retirees. *Journal of Leisure Research, 19,* 273–283.

Smith, N. R, Kielhofner, C., & Watts, J. H. (1986). The relationships between volition, activity pattern, and life satisfaction in the elderly. *American Journal of Occupational Therapy, 40,* 278–283.

Strauss, A., & Corbin, T. (1990). *Basics of qualitative research: Grounded theory techniques and strategies.* Newbury Park, CA: Sage.

Trombly, C. A. (1995). Occupation: Purposefulness and meaningfulness as therapeutic mechanisms, 1995 Eleanor Clarke Slagle lecture. *American Journal of Occupational Therapy, 49,* 960–972.

Ward, R. A. (1979). The meaning of voluntary association participation to older people. *Journal of Gerontology, 34,* 438–445.

Watson, M. A, & Ager, C. L. (1991). The impact of role valuation and performance on life satisfaction in old age. *Physical and Occupational Therapy in Geriatrics, 10*(1), 27–62.

Wilcox, A. (1991). Occupational science. *British Journal of Occupational Therapy, 54,* 297–299.

Wilcox, A. (1993). A theory of the human need for occupation. *Journal of Occupational Science. 1*(1), 17–24.

Yerxa, E. J. (1991). Nationally Speaking—Seeking a relevant, ethical, and realistic way of knowing for occupational therapy. *American Journal of Occupational Therapy, 45,* 199–204.

Yerxa, E. J. (1993). Occupational science: A new source of power for participants in occupational therapy. *Journal of Occupational Science, 1*(l), 3–10.

Yerxa, E. J. (1994). Dreams, dilemmas, and decisions for occupational therapy practice in a new millennium: An American perspective. *American Journal of Occupational Therapy, 48,* 586–589.

Yerxa, E. J., Clark, F., Frank, G., Jackson, J., Parham, D., Pierce, D., Stein, C., & Zemke, R. (1990). An introduction to occupational science: A foundation for occupational therapy in the 21st century. In J. Johnson & E. Yerxa (Eds). *Occupational science: The foundation for new models of practice* (pp. 1–18). New York: Haworth.

Zimmer, Z., Hickey, T., & Searle, M. S. (1995). Activity participation and well-being among older people with arthritis. *Gerontologist, 35,* 463–471.

Chapter 12

The Extraordinary Construction of Ordinary Experience: Scheduling Daily Life in Families with Children with Attention Deficit Hyperactivity Disorder

Scandinavian Journal of Occupational Therapy

1998, (5): 141–147

Ruth Segal[1] and Gelya Frank[2]

From the [1]School of Occupational Therapy, Faculty of Health Sciences, University of Western Ontario, London, Ontario, Canada and the [2]Department of Occupational Science and Therapy and Anthropology, University of Southern California, Los Angeles, California, USA

KEY WORDS

- adaptation
- culture
- dinner
- free time
- homework occupations
- public time

ABSTRACT

Interest in the concept of occupation as a basic human phenomenon, and the establishment of the discipline of occupational science, are prompting a renewed appreciation among occupational therapists of the temporal dimension of patients' lives in and out of the clinic. Although most clinicians know that the orchestration of activities in daily life can support or hinder treatment, the organization of occupations into daily routines has not yet been studied extensively in occupational therapy or occupational science.

The present study examines the adaptation of families raising children with attention deficit hyperactivity disorder (ADHD) in terms of the extraordinary work they perform to construct daily schedules within the ordinary pattern of time use. Seventeen families with children with ADHD were interviewed about their daily schedules and routines. This paper focuses on parents explanations of their family's afternoon (i.e. after-school) schedules, particularly how the parents scheduled times for homework, dinner, and free time. Parents' scheduling considerations included their children's abilities to concentrate, the children's other physiological and emotional needs, and parental work schedules. The cultural relevance of the afternoon schedule and its importance for designing occupational therapy intervention at the homes of children with special needs is discussed.

INTRODUCTION

Interest in the concept of occupation as a basic human phenomenon, and the establishment of the discipline of occupational science, are prompting a renewed appreciation among occupational therapists of the temporal dimension of patients' lives in and out of the clinic [1, 2]. Although most clinicians know that the orchestration of activities in daily life can support or hinder treatment, the organization of occupations into daily routines has not yet been studied extensively in occupational therapy or occupational science. Reilly [3] recognized that the "natural social order to daily living" (p. 63) could be used as a guiding principle for developing the schedule of an occupational therapy program. Twenty-five years later, Hinojosa & Anderson [4] found that mothers with children with cerebral palsy followed home treatment programs only when the prescribed activities did not interfere with family schedules.

Schedules as social and cultural phenomena have been studied in other disciplines, such as anthropology and sociology [5–7]. According to Zerubavel [7], schedules "are one of the major dimensions of social organization along which involvement, commitment, and accessibility are defined and regulated" (p. 140) in Western cultures. He demonstrates, for example, how the socially established use of public time (i.e. work and school hours) regulates the separation between public time and private time. Although family time is private time, still it appears that the more communal or "public" occasions, such as dinner, also dominate family schedules. Dinner is made to take place when family members are most likely to be available [8]; along with other obligatory or fixed events, dinner regulates the boundaries of personal "free time." This point about the scheduling of dinner when people are available may seem at first self-evident and even circular. (It is like the naive observation: "Isn't it lucky how Christmas always seems to come at Winter Break?".) On closer inspection, however, it can be seen that even the most seemingly ordinary and natural events are constructed through carefully coordinated action. In fact, the more ordinary the event, the more highly coordinated and well-reinforced are the habitual actions that make it appear natural [9].

Schedules regulate the duration, frequency, pace and sequence of daily occupations in families ([10], p. 122). Such regulation of time use ensures that all family members come to family events, such as dinners. They also reveal family priorities or values [11]. For example, whether or not a child is allowed to watch television and for how long reveals his or her family's evaluation of that occupation [10, 12].

According to Daly [10], family schedules are internalized and continue unchallenged until a crisis calls attention to them. Raising a child with Attention Deficit Hyperactivity Disorder (ADHD) often provokes such crises. ADHD is a childhood disorder whose symptoms include inattention, hyperactivity, and impulsiveness [13]. In addition to these behavioural manifestations of the disorder, children with ADHD have difficulty attending to and completing tasks and occupations [13]. Such difficulties generally interfere with the family's schedule and disrupt the reliability and predictability of activities of ordinary daily life. Thus the family is frequently required to adapt.

MEDICAL MANAGEMENT OF CHILDREN WITH ADHD AND FAMILY ADAPTATIONS

Comprehensive interventions with children who have ADHD include the use of medications, parent training, and changes in family schedules [14–17]. The most frequently used medication is commonly known by the brand name Ritalin (methylphenidate). Ritalin is a short-acting medication (3–5 hours). While the medication is working, the children's symptoms decrease and their occupational performance improves. Insomnia and loss of appetite are the most common side effects. Commonly, children take the medication twice a day—in the morning and around noon. This regimen facilitates the children's school performance while ensuring that they eat dinner and sleep at night [18]. As the medication wears off in the middle to late afternoon, a rebound effect may occur in which the children's symptoms worsen [19]. Families, therefore, may not always achieve the full desired benefit from a two-dose regimen in terms of the child's improved occupational performance.

Training programs for parents of children with ADHD typically aim to educate them about the disorder, including how to use consequences to encourage appropriate behaviour and discourage inappropriate behaviour [17, 18, 20, 21]. Kelly & Aylward [17] alone, among the literature, suggest modifying the family's schedules and daily routines to adapt to the challenges of a child with ADHD. They suggest that (i) participation in prolonged and stimulating activities should be avoided (e.g. long shopping trips); (ii) schedules and daily routines should be predictable; and (iii) complicated tasks or activities should be broken into sub-components, and instructions for each sub-component be given separately [17].

From the standpoint of occupational science, adaptation has been defined by Frank [14] as "a process of selecting and organizing activities (or occupations) to improve life opportunities and enhance quality of life according to the experience of individuals or groups in an ever-changing environment" (p. 50). This conceptualization was influenced by the eco-cultural theory of family adaptation [15]. In eco-cultural theory, families are understood to construct their children's occupations and schedules based on the perceived needs of the children in the context of the family's cultural environment and unique values.

The present study examines the adaptation of families raising children with ADHD in terms of the extraordinary work they perform to construct daily schedules within the ordinary pattern of time use—which again, as Zerubavel [7] demonstrates, is regulated by the public sphere, consisting of work and school. Segal [16] interviewed 17 families with children with ADHD about their daily schedules and routines. This paper focuses on parents' explanations of their family's afternoon (i.e. after-school) schedules, particularly how the

parents scheduled times for homework, dinner, and free time. Parents' scheduling considerations included their child's ability to concentrate, the child's other physiological and emotional needs, and parental work schedules. The cultural relevance of the afternoon schedule and its importance for designing occupational therapy intervention in the homes of children with special needs will be discussed.

METHODS

Qualitative research methods were used to elicit descriptions from the research participants of their life experiences and to understand their explanations of their actions [22–24]. Qualitative research interviews [23] were the primary method selected for gaining access to the life experiences of the parents of children with ADHD. Using this approach, the researcher uses an interview guide to ask non-directive questions on topics relevant to the study, encouraging the participants to talk about any issue that they think is relevant to the topic that the researcher introduced [23, 25]. Although the data analysis is guided by the researcher's theoretical orientation, an attempt is made not to force or impose such constructs on the data. Once the interviews are recorded and transcribed, themes (or findings and interpretations) are inductively derived from the data through systematic and rigorous comparative analysis [26, 27].

Sample

Three local chapters of a nationwide support group, Children and Adults with Attention Deficit Disorder (CHADD), were identified and contacted in the Los Angeles area, in Southern California. The researcher [16] received permission to attend meetings on a regular basis in two of the chapters. On three occasions, she presented her research interests at meetings, asked for participants, and handed out flyers. Flyers were also mailed to the co-ordinator of the third chapter of CHADD. An occupational and physical therapy clinic was contacted and the clinic organized a mailing of flyers to all their current and previous clients. Potential participants had to initiate first contact with the researcher.

The inclusion criteria for study participants were that the children who had ADHD were between 6 and 11 years of age and that families could communicate in English. Of the 17 families participating in the study, 12 were two-parent families and 5 single-parent families. Only 3 fathers from the 12 two-parent families participated with their spouses. The single-parent families consisted solely of mothers and children. The participants were predominantly of European descent. Nine mothers, including the five single mothers, were employed. Three families had one child only and the rest had two to four children. Three families each had two children with ADHD. Data analysis coincided with data collection, and recruitment of new research participants ended when the researcher determined that the data set approached saturation. Saturation occurs when the analysis of new data does not add to the findings [26].

Collection and Analysis of the Data

Data collection consisted of one to four interviews with each family. The total time spent interviewing each family ranged from one-and-a-half to five hours. Parents were asked to tell the researcher their family story and to describe their daily schedules and routines. Family stories [28] were elicited to help provide a context for understanding parents' descriptions and explanations of their daily schedules and routines. Concerning their routines, parents were asked to describe a typical day, how scheduled activities were performed, and who was involved. They were also asked to describe the previous day and assess whether it was typical. If the previous day was not typical, parents were asked to discuss what was unusual about it.

All the interviews were audiotaped, and transcripts were produced by a professional transcriber. Data analysis began within two weeks after the second interview. In the initial phase of analysis, the interviews with each family were dealt with as a single case. When that process was completed, the researcher allowed a few weeks to lapse before reanalysing the transcripts. In the second phase, the transcripts were separated into family stories and descriptions of daily routines and occupations, and analysed again. The researcher coded the data according to meaningful conceptual units (categories or themes). The data under each theme were further analysed to identify the conditions, contexts, strategies and consequences—as perceived by the research participants—of their scheduling choices [27]. In the presentation of findings from this study, all names are pseudonyms.

ORGANIZING THE AFTERNOON SCHEDULE: FINDINGS AND INTERPRETATIONS

The afternoon schedules of families with children with ADHD seem at first indistinguishable from those of other Euro-North American families. In fact, this is the intent of the parents when organizing the family's time, and they view it as a sign of their success. The creation of these schedules, nevertheless, is uniquely constrained for parents of children with ADHD. When scheduling time for homework, parents in this study primarily considered their child's ability to concentrate and complete homework tasks, given the typical two-dose regimen of Ritalin. In addition, parents considered their child's other physical and emotional needs, such as the need for a snack or a break from school-based activities. The scheduling of dinner, which in two-parent families depended on the work schedule of the second parent, added an additional constraint. Free time (e.g. play or watching television) was scheduled between homework and dinner or between evening cleanup and bedtime. Because the family schedules appear so ordinary, the presentation of findings below focuses on the careful selection and orchestration of occupations that parents perform by which this apparent normalcy is achieved.

Homework

Parents of children who take Ritalin said that the medication improved their child's occupational performance. All parents (whether or not their child took medication) explained that they scheduled time to coincide with their child's ability to concentrate. One might expect that the scheduled time for homework would vary for children with different medication regimens. The data showed, however, that the time scheduled for homework, regardless of the child's medication regimen, was between 3:00 and 5:00 in the afternoon. Beginning homework at 3:00 p.m. gave the child time to change clothes and have a snack before settling into their main occupation for the afternoon—homework. The end time of 5:00 p.m. (if not earlier) usually left about an hour before dinner. If the child needed more time to finish homework, the remaining time before dinner could be used without interfering with the meal. Here is how some parents explain their scheduling of homework:

> If we don't grab [her] as soon as she's eaten, after she comes home—like by 3:30 or so—to start homework—or even 4:00—she falls apart . . . By 5:00 she's had it. (Donna, the mother of a 9-year-old girl who takes a Ritalin twice a day)

> He [my teenage son] will give Doreen her medicine at 4:00. They will come here and . . . they would watch TV and he'd help Doreen with her homework and that would all be hopefully done by the time I came home. That was because I was having trouble coming home from work, making dinner, and then having to help her with her homework because her medication has worn off. It just was not working that way. So I told him he needed to help her with her homework so that when I get home from work, I could help with whatever else needed to be done and the medication would already still be working—because it

> only lasts about 2–3 hours. That was kind of a problem for a while, but it seems to be better now. (Cheryl, the mother of a 7-year-old girl who takes Ritalin three times a day)

> I pick up the boys at 2:30, and we come home. This year we have had to implement doing homework right after school, or "You can take a half an hour break but then everything goes off [e.g. TV] and you have to come do your homework." We have to do it that way, because if we wait until after dinner, like last year, Don [the son who has ADHD] just will not lock onto homework—he still wants to play . . . We just decided it's homework first, and then: "You can have the whole rest of the night just to do what you want." And that makes him feel better. Or if he gets stuck on homework, we know we have time, instead of saying "Get it done because you have to get a bath and go to bed." (Mary, the mother of an 8-year-old boy who does not take Ritalin)

Only one family scheduled homework *after* dinner, a family in which the child took three doses of Ritalin, not two. Fostering her 7-year-old son's successful academic performance and emotional well-being was the main concern of the mother (Shannon). She provided her son with an educational consultant, a psychologist, and an occupational therapist as needed. Appointments with these various professionals therefore took up the time before dinner, but Shannon knew that her son would be able to concentrate on his homework because of the third dose of medication.

Dinner

Dinner as the family's time together each day was commonly scheduled so that all family members could be seated at once around the table. Since the work day is typically longer than the school day, dinner was scheduled to begin when the second parent arrived home from work, or up to half an hour later. Regardless of how the family defined the time when dinner should begin, it was scheduled between 6:00 and 7:00 p.m. Some parents discussed in great detail how they must attend to their child's hunger as the medication begins to wear off (one of Ritalin's side effects is appetite suppression). As the following comments by parents show, however, the timing of the medication's effects was not the primary factor determining when dinner was scheduled:

He has a [television] program he likes to watch around 5:00 and that's about the time I come in the kitchen and start to get dinner ready . . . Daddy gets home about 6:30—anywhere from 6:15 to 7:00 he comes home. We eat dinner together at the table, hang around and talk . . . I usually start the kids eating no later than 6:30. We try to wait for him [my husband]. He'd come at the tail end—maybe we'll have anywhere from 15 to 45 minutes together. (Naomi, the mother of a 9-year-old boy who takes Ritalin twice a day)

[Dinner] is as soon as I walk in . . . But I do get home on the late side because I do go to the gym . . . And I usually call from the car when I leave the gym and say I'm on my way home. (Robert, the father of a 7-year-old boy who takes Ritalin three times a day) [When my husband comes home at 5:30 or 6:00] everybody has a need. I need to get dinner, they [the children] need to get their homework done, he [my husband] needs to calm down and we've tried all kinds of things to try and work it. Like, [my husband needs to] have 30 minutes alone, and one of them doing piano, and one of them doing homework when he comes in [gives] him a break when he first comes home. (Sally, the mother of a 9-year-old boy who takes Ritalin three times a day)

At 5:00 the dinner has to be in the oven, whatever we are doing, because my husband gets home between 6:00 and 6:30. We eat together as a family. (Sharon, the mother of a 10-year-old boy who does not take Ritalin)

We get home around 6:45–7:00 in the evening. Right away . . . I pull out a portion [of cooked food from the freezer], defrost it in the microwave, and heat it up. That's their first meal of the night. (Sarah, the single mother of a 6-year-old and a 4-year-old who both take Ritalin three times a day)

In two families, dinnertime depended on when the child became hungry enough to want to eat. Both families described their experiences of raising their children who had ADHD as very traumatic: One of the parents said that in the past, she felt that the child was "devouring" her; the other mother described how in the past she often felt that she wanted to hit her child. In both cases, the parents went to therapy and parent training courses and seem to have concluded that the best solution would be to attend only to the needs of their children before and after school. They scheduled family time together for the weekends or just before the child's bedtime.

Free Time

Unlike homework and dinner, some afternoon activities are optional because they are less directly tied to performance in the public sphere. Free time activities, such as play or watching television or movies, occurred only after homework and any possible chores were done. Free time often serves, therefore, as a positive consequence, or incentive, for children to finish their homework quickly (so they can play before dinner) or their chores (so they can play before they are sent to bed). The fact that free time is conditional reveals that it is essentially a privilege that has to be earned by doing one's duties. Similar to dinner schedules, a child's regimen of medication did not appear to be a factor in how parents scheduled free time. Here is how parents described and explained how they decide whether or not to allow their child free time on a given day:

If he finishes [his homework] quickly he goes out and plays. (Naomi, the mother of a 9-year-old boy who takes Ritalin twice a day)

He has his homework, piano practice, and if there's any time before dinner, then he can have free time. If he gets all this done in that time, he knows he can either watch a video or whatever. (Sally, the mother of a 9-year-old boy who takes Ritalin three times a day)

They are not allowed eight o'clock TV until the family room is clean, and that's usually their mess. And so I make them clean it up, because that's kind of their work space and play space, and all. If it's not cleaned, nobody gets eight o'clock TV. Um, so then, it's usually cleaned up by 8:30, it makes its impression, so usually they get a program between 8:30 and 9:00. (Mary, the mother of an 8-year-old boy who does not take Ritalin)

I think that homework . . . it's important it be done early in the evening: we don't let it go late—certainly before general television is done or story reading. (Shannon, the mother of a 7-year-old son who takes Ritalin three times a day)

Two families scheduled free time in the same way they scheduled time for dinner and homework—as an occupation that regularly occurs. In both families, the time scheduled for this occupation was between school and homework (or between school and therapy), at the same times scheduled for optional free time. The two mothers, Donna and Shannon, who regularly scheduled free time, felt it was necessary to their child's emotional well-being. Each felt that her child tried very hard to behave appropriately and perform well in school and therefore needed a break (or reward) before he had to continue with other stressful occupations, such as homework or therapy.

As the preceding data show, parents' reasons for how they scheduled afternoon family time to include homework, dinner, and free time were expressed in the language of their unique life experiences. It can be seen how these unique life experiences were strongly affected by their child's ADHD, the medication taken by the child, and parental work schedules. The fact that the afternoon schedules of these disparate families are so remarkably similar indicates that something other than the effects of Ritalin and the diverse needs of the particular families serves as an overarching guide for their scheduling choices. This "something" is their participation in a shared culture.

DISCUSSION: FAMILY SCHEDULES AS CULTURAL ADAPTATIONS

At the outset of her study, the researcher [16] did not anticipate the degree of detail and elaboration that parents would offer in their descriptions and explanations of their family schedules. According to Daly [10], family schedules are internalized and taken for granted until there is a crisis that calls attention to them. During the course of the study, only one parent reported undergoing a current change in her family's afternoon. The highly detailed accounts given by the remaining families suggests that they did not need a current crisis to bring scheduling issues to mind. As the family stories indicated, they had already invested a lot of thought and planning in the organization of their schedules as prior crises were faced and adapted to. But in the end, despite the differences among families, their schedules looked remarkably alike, whether or not the child took Ritalin, and whatever the dosage.

The latter finding—that is, the consistency among the families' schedules—confirms ecocultural theory [15], which predicts that adaptations by families with children with special needs will necessarily tend to be oriented toward fitting the family and their child into the relevant cultural context. Since there are no studies of family schedules in the general population [10], one can only suggest that the afternoon schedules of the families that participated in this study conform to cultural norms. To shed more light on this issue, the researcher conducted an informal survey among several acquaintances with children about their afternoon schedules. These acquaintances reported, like the research participants in the study, that dinnertime depended on the parents' work schedules. There the resemblance ended. In the families whose children did not have ADHD, free time or extracurricular activities took place in the slot after school but before dinner, moving homework to the after-dinner and before television slot. The contrast between the groups, while anecdotal, suggests that subtle differences exist between the schedules of families with and without a child who has ADHD, but that both conform generally to the cultural value of work before play (i.e. homework has to be done before the next play occupation is allowed).

Dinner as a family time together is an important cultural ideal signifying the notion of family wholeness [10]. Organizing for family time together such as dinner requires planning, and is usually the responsibility of the mother [8]. In this study, dinner was commonly organized around parental work hours, because work schedules are anchored in public time over which individual families have little control [7]. The ideal of dinner as family time was maintained by members of the sample, even if a child was too hungry to wait and had already been given something to eat, indicating the value that parents placed on this family event.

The importance of scheduling homework so that the ADHD child could successfully complete it is another expression of the family's cultural values. As one parent of a child with ADHD explained, academic success was necessary not only for her child's future, but for his daily emotional well-being:

> My feeling is that every child, no matter how talented they are in other areas, they need to feel some academic success . . . I want him to feel good about himself and he can only have that in school, when he's there half of the day, if he has some academic success. (Sharon, mother of a 10-year-old boy who does not take Ritalin)

The importance of homework is further highlighted by the way it regulates free time. Only two mothers regularly scheduled free time for their children. But in the other families, free time was given only if spare time was left in the slot between homework and dinner or between chores and bedtime. Following Daly's [10] line of argument, the organization of these occupations reflects their relative value: homework, dinner, and bedtime are more important than free time. And, following Zerubavel [7], they are more important because they are anchored more closely to public time—that is, to the overarching culture.

CONCLUSION

Knowing which occupations are important for families with children with special needs is important for occupational therapists who devise home treatment programs for such children. Hinojosa & Anderson [4] demonstrated that mothers of children with cerebral palsy followed home treatment programs if activities could be integrated into their families' daily lives, and so that interactions with their children could remain enjoyable. That is, successful home treatment programs must take into account family schedules and family values. The current study supports this conclusion with data from families with children with a different disability, ADHD, a disorder whose symptoms have the potential to disrupt the smooth flow of ordinary daily life. A further contribution of this study, then, is its demonstration of how parents of children with ADHD orchestrate the occupations of their families to achieve a more satisfactory—i.e. more ordinary—cultural adaptation [14]. Finally, this study exposes the powerful impact of seemingly natural, taken-for-granted cultural norms of time use that guide family adaptations despite the differences among family structures, family stories, and family values.

ACKNOWLEDGMENTS

This research was supported by the American Occupational Therapy Foundation (AOTF) Center for Research on Adaptation and Occupation (1992–1995) at the Department of Occupational Science and Therapy, University of Southern California. Principal investigator Professor Florence Clark.

References

1. Yerxa EJ. Clark F. Frank G. et al. An introduction to occupational science, a foundation for occupational therapy in the 21st century. In: Johnson JA, Yerza EJ. eds. *Occupational science: the foundation of new models of practice.* New York: Howard Press, 1989; 1–17.

2. Clark FA. Parham D. Carlson ME. et al. Occupational science: academic innovation in the services of occupational therapy's future. *Am J Occup Ther* 1991: 45: 300–10.

3. Reilly M. A psychiatric occupational therapy program as a teaching model. *Am J Occup Ther* 1966: 20: 61–6.

4. Hinojosa J. Anderson J. Mothers' perceptions of home treatment programs for their preschool children with cerebral palsy. *Am J Occup Ther* 1991: 45: 273–9.

5. Fraser JT. *Time, the familiar stranger.* Washington, DC: Tempus Books of Microsoft Press. 1988.

6. Hall ET. *The dance of life: the other dimension of time.* Toronto, ON: Anchor Books. 1983.

7. Zerubavel E. *Hidden rhythms: schedules and calendars in social life.* Los Angeles, CA: University of California Press. 1981.

8. DeVault MJ. *Feeding the family: the social organization of caring as gendered work.* Chicago, IL: University of Chicago Press. 1991.

9. Bourdieu P. *Outline of a theory of practice.* Nice R. trans. Cambridge: Cambridge University Press. 1977.

10. Daly KJ. *Families and time: keeping pace in a hurried culture.* Thousand Oaks, CA: Sage. 1994.

11. Kantor D. Lehr W. *Inside the family: toward a theory of family process.* San Francisco: Jossey-Bass. 1976.

12. Broderick CB. *Marriage and the family.* 3rd ed. Englewood Cliffs, NJ: Prentice-Hall.

13. American Psychiatric Association. *A diagnostic and statistical manual of mental disorders.* 4th ed. Washington, DC: American Psychiatric Association.

14. Frank G. The concept of adaptation as a foundation for occupational science research. In: Zemke R. Clark F. eds. *Occupational science: the evolving discipline.* Philadelphia, PA: FA Davis Co. 1996: 47–55.

15. Gallimore R. Wiesner TS. Kaufman SZ. Bernheimer LP. The social construction of ecocultural niches: family accommodation of developmentally delayed children. *Am J Ment Retard* 1989: 94: 216–30.

16. Segal R. *Family adaptation to a child with attention-deficit hyperactivity disorder* [dissertation]. Los Angeles, CA: University of Southern California. 1995.

17. Kelly DP. Aylward GP. Attention deficits in school-aged children and adolescents. *Pediatr Clin North Am* 1992: 39: 487–512.

18. Hinshaw SP. *Attention deficit and hyperactivity in children.* Thousand Oaks, CA: Sage. 1994.

19. Barkley RA. McMurray MB. Edelbrook CS. et at. Side effects of methylphenidate in children with attention deficit hyperactivity disorder: a systemic, placebo-controlled evaluation. *Pediatrics* 1990: 86: 184–92.

20. Barkley RA. *Attention deficit hyperactivity disorder a handbook for diagnosis and treatment.* New York: Guilford Press. 1990.

21. Goldstein S. Goldstein M. *Managing attention disorders in children: a guide for practitioners.* New York: John Wiley Sons. 1990.

22. Bogdan RC. Biklen SK. *Qualitative research for education.* 2nd ed. Toronto, ON: Allyn & Bacon. 1992.

23. Kvale S. *Interviews: an introduction to qualitative research interviewing.* Thousand Oaks, CA: Sage. 1996.

24. Marshall C. Rossman GB. *Designing qualitative research.* 2nd ed. Thousand Oaks, CA: Sage. 1995.

25. McCracken G. *The long interview.* Newbury Park, CA: Sage. 1988.

26. Lincoln YS. Guba EG. *Naturalistic inquiry.* Newbury Park, CA: Sage. 1985.

27. Strauss A. Corbin J. *Basics of qualitative research: grounded theory procedures and techniques.* Newbury Park, CA: Sage. 1990.

28. Mattingly C. The narrative nature of clinical reasoning. *Am J Occup Ther* 1991: 45: 998–1005.

Voluntarism as Occupation

Canadian Journal of Occupational Therapy

1998, 65(5): 279–285

Karen L. Rebeiro, John Allen

Karen L. Rebeiro, M.Sc. O.T(C), is a Clinical
Researcher at Network North: The Community
Mental Health Group, 680 Kirkwood Drive,
Sudbury, Ontario, P3E 1X3. e-mail:
karenr@isys.ca
John Allen, is a mental health services consumer
who resides in Northeastern Ontario. John Allen
is a pseudonym by request.

KEY WORDS

- consumer attitudes
- exploratory research
- mental health
- occupation

ABSTRACT

*An exploratory, single-case design was con-
ducted to explore and describe the personal
experience of a voluntarism occupation for one
individual with schizophrenia who resides
within the community. Non-participant
observation and in-depth interviewing were
utilized to explore the voluntarism experience
of this individual. The findings suggest that
voluntarism is both a meaningful and purposeful occupation for this individual.
Volunteering is perceived to be a valued and
socially acceptable occupation which allows
for the individual to contribute to, and be a
productive member of society. In addition,
John (a pseudonym) perceived that his participation in a voluntarism occupation helped
him to construct a socially acceptable identity
and to maintain his preferred view of himself,
as a competent individual, not as a mental
health consumer. These findings suggest that
participation in a voluntarism occupation
may benefit some consumers of mental health
services. While these findings were based upon
the experiences of one person, occupational
therapists are encouraged to consider voluntarism as therapy and as a means of enabling
the occupational performance of their clients.
Implications for further research are suggested.*

The occupational therapy literature contends
that the use of occupation as therapy is what
distinguishes the profession of occupational
therapy from other professions. The literature
also suggests that the use of occupation is the
"domain of concern and the therapeutic medium of occupational therapy" practice
(Canadian Association of Occupational
Therapists [CAOT], 1997, p. 3). Occupation is
defined as "everything that people do to occupy
themselves, including looking after themselves,
enjoying life, and contributing to the social and
economic fabric of their communities" (CAOT,
1997, p. 3). Voluntarism is an occupation
which provides a means for people to contribute to their community, but which has
received little attention in the occupational
therapy literature. Certainly outside of occupational therapy other professions have advocated
voluntarism as an important occupation for
individuals with mental illness (Anthony &
Liberman, 1986; Estroff, 1981, 1989; Scheid
& Anderson, 1995). However, voluntarism
tends to be viewed as a means to paid employment, as opposed to a desirable occupation in
and of itself. This literature also tends to

emphasize paid work and productivity as the favoured outcome, whereas, the occupational therapy literature tends to emphasize a broader spectrum of "enabling occupation" to fulfill individual needs (CAOT, 1991, 1993, 1997). Since the ultimate goal of occupational therapy intervention is to "enable people to choose, organize, and perform those occupations they find useful or meaningful in their environment" (CAOT, 1997, p. 2), knowledge about voluntarism and its benefits should become integral to occupational therapy practice. Voluntarism is an occupation which appears to fit within an enabling philosophy, is a socially valued occupation within the larger community, and is a potentially valuable, untapped source of opportunity for engaging in occupation. To date, voluntarism has received little attention in the occupational therapy literature and in research.

A single case design was conducted to explore the personal experience of voluntarism for one individual with persistent mental illness who resided within the community. Specifically, this study sought to discover and describe the experience of voluntarism from the participant's perspective. Grand-tour questioning (Spradley, 1979), non-participant observation and in-depth interviewing (Holstein & Gubrium, 1995; McCracken, 1988) were the methods utilized to collect the data.

The purpose of this paper is to present the participant's perspective on voluntarism as occupation. The paper will be organized in the following manner. First, the reader will be provided with a brief overview of the occupational therapy literature to ground the theoretical basis for the study. Following that, the study design and methods will be described. The major findings of this study, which are that a voluntarism occupation can provide the means to staying well, to achieving a valued social identity, and to becoming a productive member of society, will be highlighted. Finally, in the discussion section of the paper, several issues of importance to the profession of occupational therapy will be raised. Although this paper is

based upon the experiences of one person, the findings provide insights that are relevant for clinical practice and future research.

LITERATURE REVIEW

Occupational therapists have traditionally employed a wide variety of therapeutic means within psychosocial practice. Historically, occupation has been considered as the medium of choice and central to the practice of occupational therapy (American Occupational Therapy Association [AOTA], 1979; Barris, Kielhofner & Hawkins Watts, 1983; CAOT, 1991). Recently, the literature has encouraged the enablement of occupational performance as the cornerstone of practice (CAOT, 1996, 1997). There have been several models proposed to address occupational performance and within which to "name and frame" occupational therapy practice (Polatajko, 1992). Law et al., (1996) for example, have proposed the Person-Environment-Occupation model of practice. In this Model, the authors propose that therapists need to attend to and understand the dynamic interaction of the person-environment-occupation in enhancing occupational performance outcomes. The Model provides a framework for both clinical and research interventions. In it therapeutic intervention is described as maximizing the fit between each of the constructs for optimal clinical outcomes. However, the Model does not explicate how occupation-as-means can enable a greater fit within the environment, nor which aspects of the environment might encourage enhanced occupational performance for the individual. According to Law et al. (1996) and Trombly (1995), the profession's understanding of each of the professional constructs of person-occupation-environment must be considered limited at this time. Subsequently, our understanding of how to apply this Model within clinical practice is currently evolving.

Similarly, the Enablement Model (Martini, Polatajko, & Wilcock, 1995), proposes that occupational competence is "the product of the dynamic interaction of the three dimensions of the individual, the environment, and occupation"(p. 16). In this model, the authors propose that an individual's capacity for occupational performance is contingent upon the interaction between the individual's characteristics (skills) and the environment. The Enablement Model (Martini et al., 1995) assumes that occupational competence is a precursor to choices. It seems logical to assume that enhanced skills will open up a greater spectrum of choices for the individual. However, this perspective conceptualizes therapy from the individual-out, meaning a focus on the individual will effect a change in an individual's interactions with the environment and result in greater occupational competence.

In contrast, a study by Rebeiro (1997) suggests that the opposite may also be effective. In this qualitative study, which explored the experience of engaging in occupations for individuals with mental illness, it was discovered that the provision of an accepting social environment, coupled with occupational choice and opportunity were essential to a positive outcome for the person. Rebeiro (1997) contends that an outside-in approach may result in enhanced occupational performance over time. An outside-in approach considers both the micro and macro environments and their capacity to facilitate and sustain occupational performance. In the Enablement Model (Martini et al., 1995), it is assumed that intervention at the level of the individual will enable competence. In the Person-Environment-Occupation Model proposed by Law et al. (1996), it is suggested that intervention may occur at the level of the person, the occupation, or the environment. The study by Rebeiro (1997) identified that intervention which focussed upon either the occupation or the environment resulted in a positive outcome for the person. Participants in this study suggested that an accepting social environment, and opportunity and choice to pursue individual occupational goals, resulted in enhanced occupational performance and ultimately, subjective well-being.

In Rebeiro's (1997) study, the provision of opportunity and choice in the environment enabled greater occupational performance and resulted in a positive outcome for the person without undue consideration of individual limitation or disability. In this conceptualization, choice is considered a precursor to occupational performance. The experience of engaging in occupations of choice then serves as a natural means to skill development, greater adaptation to the environment and ultimately, a greater sense of confidence, competence, and subjective well-being for the individual.

There has been speculation within the literature as to whether occupation should be the means of clinical intervention, the end or goal of therapy, or both. *Occupation-as-means* refers to occupation serving as the primary therapeutic medium towards enhanced outcomes for the individual (Rebeiro, 1997). *Occupation-as-ends* refers to the enablement or facilitation of occupational performance in the areas of self-care, productivity, and leisure as an outcome or goal of therapy which may be accomplished by a variety of therapeutic methods, of which occupation-as-means may be one method (Rebeiro, 1997). Rebeiro proposes that occupational performance is not necessarily an end, but is a cyclical and interactive process which serves as means to a variety of idiosyncratic ends, including, enhanced mental health. This study suggests that the provision of a "just right" social environment is the foundation of the process of occupational performance and collectively, the environment and the occupation contribute to a redefined sense of self over time. In addition, participants stated that they desired ongoing participation in occupation in order to sustain their enhanced sense of competence and well-being.

The recent literature describes a variety of theoretical approaches and models for potential application by occupational therapists. Empirical evidence to support the use of occupation as therapy, and which explains how to maximize occupational performance is presently evolving and largely grounded in professional beliefs and assumptions. Further, research which supports the use of voluntarism as occupation is limited at this time. Thus, for the purposes of this research, the professional belief in occupation-as-means to mental health serves as the theoretical basis and rationale for studying the benefits of voluntarism as occupation.

METHODS

Design

A qualitative, single-case design was chosen for this study for two reasons. First, the study is exploratory in nature and the phenomenon of occupation-as-means to mental health is not well understood. According to McCracken (1988), qualitative methods are ideally suited to the exploration of phenomena which are poorly understood. Second, mental health, and the converse mental illness, are often subjectively defined and expressed. As such, qualitative methods, especially the in-depth interview (McCracken, 1988; Holstein & Gubrium, 1995) appeared most appropriate to explore the meaning of the experience of voluntarism for an individual with persistent mental illness.

The study design was divided into three distinct, yet interrelated phases. In phase one, non-participant observation was employed to gain an overall impression of the environment and culture in which the voluntarism occurred. Spradley's (1979) grand tour questioning was utilized to guide the observations in phase I. In phase II, focussed observation and exploration of the voluntarism experience was conducted. Spradley's grand tour and descriptive questions were employed to explore the actual "doing" of the voluntarism, (i.e., "tell me about what you do as the librarian?"). In phase III, an in-depth interview was conducted with the informant. This interview served two purposes: to member-check (Lincoln & Guba, 1985) the information and interpretations of the first two phases and to explore in-depth and flesh out the main domain categories derived from the initial data analysis. The first author collected the data in this study.

Participant

The participant in this study, John, was recruited by the first author based upon a casual conversation in which John related his positive experiences in volunteering. John is known to the first author due to his attendance at the first authors' place of employment. However, he was not a client of the first author. John has a psychiatric diagnosis of paranoid schizophrenia and has had multiple drug trials and hospital admissions. John is on clozapine, and is currently unemployed. He experienced his first episode of schizophrenia at age 13, and describes his life and living with schizophrenia as a nightmare and as a struggle to this point. He is currently residing in the community with his family and considers himself in recovery. The pseudonym John is being used to conceal the informant's identity, and other identifying information has been altered to maintain anonymity. His volunteer experience is as a librarian. John is hopeful that his story will be helpful to others.

Data Collection

The primary data collection tool was the human instrument (Lincoln & Guba, 1985). According to Lincoln & Guba (1985), the human instrument has the adaptive and integrative qualities which are necessary in order to explore the lived experience and to analyse and integrate similarities and inconsistencies within the data. Data was collected by the first author during the three identified phases of the study through nonparticipant observation (general and focussed) and in-depth interviewing. Interview questions were both grand tour style and descriptive in order to verify the main domain categories and to expand and flesh out these domains (Spradley, 1979). In addition, extensive field notes, a method's log and a personal journal were maintained throughout the study for the purposes of triangulation (Lincoln & Guba, 1985). Field notes were initially written in condensed form and later expanded, as suggested by Spradley (1979).

Data Analysis

Data was analysed using Spradley's (1979) domain analysis. Data were categorized into preliminary domains based upon their apparent semantic relationships. The preliminary analyses were verified in the interview and the use of descriptive, structural and contrast questions were utilized to further clarify and expand existing domains. Domains which appeared to be linked by the same semantic relationship were organized into a taxonomy from which central or overarching themes could be identified. The overarching themes of this study constitute the basis of the interpretations and discussion in this paper. These findings were confirmed by John in a follow-up member-checking meeting. John also provided editorial assistance with this paper and is the second author.

FINDINGS

Occupation-as-Means

The experience of voluntarism was identified by John as a way to monitor his illness and ultimately, as a way to stay mentally healthy. John described his voluntarism as-means to: testing out his reality; proving himself and seeing what he could do; reducing schizophrenic relapses; and, doing something purposeful with his life. In describing the first purpose, John suggested that the occupation provided him with a tangible means of testing the limits of his illness: *"It's a test. I'm checking out my reality. And it's a test for me to see if I can handle this. Can I hack it?"*

In discussing the second purpose, John described the occupation as a means of proving himself and his competence:

"You have to prove yourself. Regardless of if it's paid work or unpaid work, and I believe I've done a good job at proving to them I'm competent, I'm punctual, you know, and I can take it seriously what I'm doing". "I can stand up and

say, look at me, look at what I can do. I am a part of the human race!"

The third purpose described by John concerned how volunteering served as a means to reducing the signs and symptoms associated with schizophrenia:

It cuts back on the auditory hallucinations to come here . . . it's relaxing . . . I don't feel threatened or scared here . . . Here, there is no pressure, but nothing I can't handle, that's why I like it here . . . Here there is no pressure on my mind, I don't have schizophrenic breakdowns or relapses.

The fourth purpose forwarded by John concerned occupation as-means to doing something productive and purposeful with his life and how this has affected how he feels:

I feel useful and I feel that I'm doing something right . . . volunteering gets me out and doing something beneficial . . . Voluntarism gives me something to do . . . you can't stare at the four walls of your house all day long . . . I have to get out and do something.

John described his personal reasons for volunteering and what he believed to be causal links to staying well:

"It gets my memory working and keeps my mind off of my personal problems. Volunteering gives me a bit of direction [and] allows me to use my mind".

VOLUNTARISM: A MEANINGFUL AND PURPOSEFUL OCCUPATION

The occupational therapy literature suggests that for occupation to have therapeutic value and to achieve desired outcomes, the occupation must be both meaningful and purposeful to the individual (Trombly, 1995). A second overarching theme which emerged from the data was that voluntarism was considered to be both a meaningful and purposeful occupation. John described his voluntarism occupation as "meaningful" because it afforded him an opportunity to accomplish, contribute, and to pay back society for the help he has received:

I'll use any means to make myself feel better . . . working as a volunteer . . . gives me strength and hope, you know, and encouragement . . . it makes me feel good like a functioning part of society . . . not just going along for a free ride. Feels great . . . I've actually done something and been recognized for it . . . and I feel good when I go home . . . fantastic, yes I did all that and people will benefit from my work.

In addition, John described his voluntarism as a "purposeful" way to stay well and to rehabilitate himself:

I try my hardest with the illness to get back on base . . . it's every psychosis, every episode, is worse and longer in years and it worries me very much . . . I'll use any means I can arrange to make myself feel better about myself . . . it's just a rough goal . . . it's a rough life dealing with this illness and, at least I'm not a sociopath who says there's nothing wrong because I know there's definitely something wrong . . . volunteering . . . working as a volunteer gives me strength and hope and encouragement.

In describing the personal meaning of voluntarism, John stated:

It makes me feel good. It makes me feel, like I said before, like a part of society. A functioning part of society. Not just going along for a free ride . . . I have been a patient of this hospital before and I've always thought with all the help that I received from the people around me, the staff and that, I feel that, in a sense, I'm saying thank you and let me help you.

John identified that his occupational choice was by no means random. He stated that the provision of just any volunteer position would not likely have resulted in the same outcome:

My choice was pretty clean cut and dried. Volunteering at [names place], it's strategic to me that it be [this place] because of the connection with the [hospital] and I don't like volunteering, like to volunteer at the [names another hospital], I wouldn't wanna do that. I've always felt comfortable with the [hospital] . . . No, I wouldn't take on any other type of volunteer work. This was specific. It was talked about a long time with the volunteer resources. It was a strategic role to hopefully rehabilitate myself.

SOCIAL IDENTITY AND PREFERRED SELF-IDENTITY

Throughout the interviews, comments were made in reference to social stigma, social identity and self-identity related to the experience of living with schizophrenia. One of the reasons forwarded by John for volunteering in the specific environment chosen was to "hang with the normals". Despite his belief that "all people are created equal", John recognized the impact of mental illness on both social and self identity: "People who suffer from mental illness aren't really clowns to be laughed at, they're human beings just like everyone else". In discussing his personal reasons for "hanging with the normals", John stated that being normal is a requirement of society. He suggested that hanging with the normals is one way to achieve social acceptance and ultimately, to fit into society:

I don't think anyone's normal. We all have pet peeves . . . We all have our hang ups, imagination, fantasizing thoughts, that's all normal . . . that's the human mind . . . I don't want to have schizophrenia. I don't like it at all. I don't like mental illness. I don't like the stigma. If you're acting weird in society, it's stigma. It's just you have to be normal in society . . . It's just required of people not to be doing bizarre things on the street. When I am constantly hanging around with people that suffer from a mental illness, it just brings me down. Working with people that have a little bit on the ball to me anyway, is helpful.

In further discussing the importance of social acceptance, John provided his perspective on how society views mental illness:

When you're suffering from schizophrenia, you feel pretty low . . . you feel like a non-person . . . you're a square peg trying to fit into a round hole . . . mental illness is something that society laughs at . . . if I broke my leg the neighbours would bring lunch over. If I told them I was schizophrenic, they'd move . . . We're all created equal, not a lower plane but just as a low in a person's life. A low point in their life . . . not to degrade a person, not to be degraded because they suffer from a mental illness. I have a wife and children who do not need to be stigmatized.

In discussing the attributes of his volunteer environment, "a nice niche," John suggested that "people not being appraised of the situation" was an important factor. John described his perception of the effects of stigma and how this would have affected his voluntarism occupation:

> I think it would be damaging if they were to know that I suffer from mental illness. Yeah, I think I'd be treated differently [if staff knew of his mental illness] . . . they'd talk behind my back and then they'd have to deal with you. They'd think I have to deal also with the schizophrenic in the [place of voluntarism] . . . even though they're professional people, people are only people. You're either gonna treat me like John the librarian, or you're gonna treat me, excuse the wording, John the head case.

In describing the meaning of the volunteer experience, John spoke of how volunteering allows him to assume a valued social identity, which in turn, helped him to maintain his own sense of self:

> I wear my ID tag and it makes me feel like a staff person. It makes me feel good that I'm doing something that's beneficial . . . I'm just another person, you know, that's helping a worthwhile cause.

Volunteering provided John with the opportunity to achieve a valued social identity, which in turn, complemented how he had envisioned himself and his life prior to the onset of schizophrenia:

> I want to come across to the clinicians as a guy that they can assign a project to and it will be completed . . . I seem to come across to them as, being alright and trustworthy . . . trustworthiness is another very important thing that I would like people to see in me. I get compliments from the team, I get affirmations. It makes me feel that I'm doing something right. . . . And fortunately for me, I am liked there. I've been told many times. A lot of affirmations, a lot of compliments. I've always been a people pleaser . . . that's how I wanna be with the clinicians at [names place] . . . quite a bit of thought goes into it.

There were three major findings in this study. The first finding was the identification of voluntarism as occupation-as-means to enhanced

mental health and to staying well. While these findings are preliminary, there appears to be some support for the use of occupation as therapy in the promotion of mental health and well-being. In addition, it is speculated that within an accepting social environment, the volunteer occupation afforded John the opportunity to confirm his competence. Collectively, the environment and the occupation contributed to John's desire to sustain his occupational performance over time in hope that it would sustain his sense of competency and enhanced mental health.

The second finding suggests that voluntarism is both a meaningful and purposeful occupation for one individual with a mental illness. John suggested that his volunteer occupation is meaningful in that it enables him to do something productive and to become identified in a social role commensurate with his preferred self-identity. John also suggested that his occupation is purposeful: it serves as a means to accomplishment, to demonstrating his competence and provides him the opportunity to pay back society for the help he has received. Voluntarism is not necessarily an end or outcome, but rather; is a means to a variety of personally meaningful goals.

The third finding concerns the construction of an acceptable social identity and the maintenance of a preferred self-identity. The data suggests that occupation as therapy, or more specifically in this study, the experience of voluntarism, provides a social context within which an individual with a mental illness can fulfill his/her belief that "all people are created equal" and can "normalize" their identity despite their belief that stigma and societal expectations do not facilitate such an identity. Voluntarism provided the means to establishing a valued identity within the community and larger society.

DISCUSSION

The findings of this exploratory study raise many issues of importance for the profession of occupational therapy. First, if occupational therapy is a profession concerned with the use and application of occupation as therapy towards enhanced mental health, then a greater understanding of the meaning and purpose of a variety of occupations is indicated (Trombly, 1995; Yerxa et al, 1990). This study provides some preliminary support that a voluntarism occupation can be a meaningful and purposeful occupation for an individual with a mental illness. Not only does the occupation serve as a means to stay well and to enjoy enhanced mental health, but also the volunteer occupation provides a means to become a productive and functioning member of society.

Second, the findings highlight attributes of the environment, "a nice niche", which was perceived to be enabling of occupational performance. For John, "a nice niche" entailed none of the time or fiscal pressures associated with his "making a buck". Previous goals of mental health reform and rehabilitation have advocated paid or sheltered employment as a desirable outcome (Anthony & Liberman, 1986; Estroff, 1981, 1989). This literature focusses upon the occupation, and less so upon the attributes of the environment which enable occupational performance. The findings of this study suggest that for one individual with a severe and persistent mental illness, employment or "making a buck" is not a desired outcome, and is in fact perceived to be an environment which facilitates schizophrenic breakdowns or relapses. In contrast, a specific, strategic and well thought out entry into voluntarism is perceived to produce many of the benefits of paid employment, specifically regarding self-identity and social worth without many of the deleterious effects of "making a buck". An environment which offered a meaningful and purposeful occupation and identity was more enabling of John's occupational performance than any financial reward. This finding highlights the importance of a client-centered practice, in particular, recognizing that people have their own reasons for becoming involved, and not necessarily for reasons obvious to the clinician.

Third, voluntarism is viewed as a purposeful means to fit into society, to construct or assume an acceptable social identity, as well as be a productive member of society. The sociological literature (Berger, 1963, p. 98) contends that identity is "socially bestowed, socially transformed and socially sustained". Goffman's (1963) treatment of moral careers focussed on the stigmatized person as he or she identifies with one's "own" or with "normals", the resultant social identity being largely tied to personal attributes, behaviours and occupation. Goffman (1963) refers to stigma as "an attribute that is deeply discrediting"(p. 3) and which highlights a discrepancy between an individual's virtual and actual social identity. John recognized society's perception of mental illness and purposely chose to conceal his label of schizophrenia. Instead, his occupation was strategic: it was chosen to complement John's preferred social-identity; afforded him the opportunity to transform what he perceived to be society's perception of an individual with mental illness; and, provided an environment which helped to maintain his preferred self-identity.

Many individuals (see Estroff, 1981, 1989, 1991; Goffman, 1963; Leete, 1989; Shaw, 1991) have written about the impact of stigma upon identity, productivity and opportunity. Estroff (1989), for example, stated: "schizophrenia, like epilepsy and hemophilia, is an I am illness, one that is joined with social identity and perhaps with inner self, in language and terms of reference" (p. 189). Estroff (1991) also stated that "more than any other enduring affliction, mental illnesses implicate identity and the self as both the primary locus and the casualty of the disorder" (p. 337). Similarly, Shaw (1991) stated that "stigma is not merely a label applied to people but rather a social construction of self and the other" (p. 303). Goffman's (1963) thesis is that individuals who are stigmatized actively manage or control for identity information in order to avoid being discredited and to reduce the perceived discrepancy between virtual and actual social identity.

In John's case, he recognized the stigma of mental illness within society and actively managed and controlled information about his illness within his chosen environment. Identity control allowed him to "hang with the normals". Identity control also allowed John to work in an environment which he valued, engage in an occupation which he believed made a valuable contribution to society, and ultimately, to sustain a self-identity commensurate with how he previously viewed himself prior to the onset of his schizophrenic illness. His voluntarism occupation gave John a place to belong. According to Estroff (1989), "belonging in a normative way to a larger group or groups both conveys and constitutes a sense of self, provides an identity in relation to others and by virtue of others' acknowledgement of us" (p. 192). Engagement in voluntarism allowed John an identity as a contributing member of society and his renewed sense of self gave him hope that "all people are created equal":

> Consumer survivors are people and they're capable of working and they're capable of not being aggressive and they're just people with problems. That's as basic as I can put it. You know we're no different than anyone else except we've got an illness, which, in today's day and age, it isn't fully understood . . . it's a very wonderful era we live in and hopefully some day there will be a cure for my illness.

CONCLUSION

This paper presented the results of an exploratory study which sought to explore and describe the personal experience of voluntarism for one individual with schizophrenia. The findings of this single-case design illustrate that a voluntarism occupation can provide the means for an individual with a mental illness to become a productive member of society, to stay well and to construct an acceptable social identity.

The continued use and application of occupation as therapy and the enablement of occupational performance as the basis of professional practice requires that occupational therapists continue to generate empirical evidence which can be used to substantiate and justify our unique contribution to human health and well-being. Only through ongoing, rigorous and systematic investigation of the phenomenon of occupation, can occupational therapy empirically support, identify and describe how meaningful and purposeful occupation, such as voluntarism, can contribute to or limit occupational performance for individuals with a mental illness. Single-case designs provide a means for clinicians to contribute to this knowledge base.

ACKNOWLEDGEMENTS

The first author would like to extend thanks to Dr. Ruth Segal for her support during this study and to John, for his honesty, insight and generosity. This paper was written while the first author was a graduate student at The University of Western Ontario.

References

American Occupational Therapy Association. (1979). Resolution D (532–79): Occupation as the common core of occupational therapy. *American Journal of Occupational Therapy, 33,* 785.

Anthony, W.A., & Liberman, R.P. (1986). The practice of psychiatric rehabilitation: Historical, conceptual and research base. *Schizophrenia Bulletin, 12,* 542–559.

Barris, R., Kielhofner, G., & Hawkins Watts, J. (1983). *Psycho social occupational therapy: Practice in a pluralistic arena.* Laurel, MD: RAMSCO.

Berger, P.L. (1963). *Invitation to sociology: A humanistic perspective.* Garden City, NY: Doubleday.

Canadian Association of Occupational Therapists. (1991). *Occupational therapy guidelines for client-centred practice.* Toronto, ON: CAOT Publications ACE.

Canadian Association of Occupational Therapists. (1996). Profile of occupational therapy practice in Canada. *Canadian Journal of Occupational Therapy, 63,* 79–95.

Canadian Association of Occupational Therapists. (1997). *Enabling occupation: An occupational therapy perspective.* Ottawa, ON: CAOT Publications ACE.

Canadian Association of Occupational Therapists, & Health Canada. (1993). *Occupational therapy guidelines for client-centred mental health practice.* Toronto, ON: CAOT Publications ACE.

Estroff, S.E. (1981). *Making it crazy: An ethnography of psychiatric clients in an American community.* Berkeley, CA: University of California Press.

Estroff, S.E. (1989). Self, identity, and subjective experiences of schizophrenia: In search of the subject. *Schizophrenia Bulletin, 15,* 189–196.

Estroff, S.E. (1991). Everybody's got a little mental illness: Accounts of illness and self among persons with severe, persistent mental illness. *Medical Anthropology Quarterly, 5,* 331–369.

Goffman, E. (1963). *Stigma: Notes on the management of spoiled identity.* New York, NY: Simon & Schuster.

Holstein, J.A., & Gubrium, I.E. (1995). *The active interview.* Thousand Oaks, CA: Sage.

Law, M., Cooper, B., Strong, S., Stewart, D., Rigby, P., & Letts, L. (1996). The Person-Environment-Occupation model: A transactive approach to occupational performance. *Canadian Journal of Occupational Therapy, 63,* 9–23.

Leete, E. (1989). How I perceive and manage my illness. *Schizophrenia Bulletin, 15,* 197–200.

Lincoln, Y.S., & Guba, E.G. (1985). *Naturalistic inquiry.* Newbury Park, CA: Sage.

Martini, R., Polatajko, H., & Wilcock, A. (1995). The proposed revision of the international classification of impairments, disabilities and handicaps (ICIDH): A potential model for occupational therapy. *Occupational Therapy International, 2,* 1–21.

McCracken, G. (1988). *The long interview.* Newbury Park, CA: Sage.

Polatajko, H. (1992). Muriel Driver Lecture: Naming and framing occupational therapy. A lecture dedicated to the life of Nancy B. *Canadian Journal of Occupational Therapy, 59,* 189–200.

Rebeiro, K.L. (1997). *Opportunity, not prescription: An exploratory study of the experience of occupational engagement.* Unpublished master's thesis. The University of Western Ontario, London, Ontario.

Scheid, T.L., & Anderson, C. (1995). Living with chronic mental illness: Understanding the role of work. *Community Mental Health Journal, 31,* 163–176.

Shaw, L.L. (1991). Stigma and the moral careers of ex-mental patients living in board and care. *Journal of Contemporary Ethnography, 20,* 285–305.

Spradley, J.P. (1979). *The ethnographic interview.* Orlando, FL: Harcourt Brace Jovanovich College Publishers.

Trombly, C.A. (1995). Occupation: Purposefulness and meaningfulness as therapeutic mechanisms. *American Journal of Occupational Therapy, 49,* 960–972.

Yerxa, E.J., Clark, F., Frank, G., Jackson, J., Parham, D., Pierce, D., Stein, C., & Zemke, R. (1990). An introduction to occupational science: A foundation for occupational therapy in the 21st Century. In, J.A. Johnson (Ed.) & E.J. Yerxa (Co-Ed.), *Occupational Science: The Foundation for New Models of Practice,* (p. 1–17). Birmingham, NY: The Haworth Press.

Chapter 14

Doing for Others: Occupations within Families with Children Who Have Special Needs

Journal of Occupational Science

1999, 6(2): 53–60

Ruth Segal, Ph.D., OT(C), OTR

Ruth Segal, Ph.D., OT(C), OTR,
Assistant Professor, School of Occupational
Therapy, The University of Western Ontario,
London, Ontario N6G 1H1, Canada
Phone: (519) 679-2111, ext 8984
Fax: (519) 661-3894
Email: rsegal@julian.uwo.ca

KEY WORDS

- ADHD
- experiences
- physical disabilities
- commitment
- individualism

ABSTRACT

Family occupations are carefully scheduled and constructed. Some family occupations, commonly dinner and leisure activities, provide families with the space and time to be together. In Western culture, such family time together is a source of idealized family images that are embedded in the experiences of togetherness and good relationships. Although actual experiences during such occupations often do not reproduce these idealized images, parents continue to construct and engage in them. The purposes of family occupations among families with children who have special needs are presented in this paper. These purposes are: being together; sharing; and affording learning opportunities. It is suggested in the discussion that these purposes motivate parents to construct family occupations. It is also suggested that the purposes of such engagement in family occupations are phenomena shared by all the families within a culture.

Occupations are defined in occupational science as "chunks of culturally and personally meaningful activity in which humans engage that can be named in the lexicon of our culture" (University of Southern California, Department of Occupational Science and Therapy, 1989 as cited in Clark, et al., 1991, p. 301). Family occupations are culturally meaningful chunks of activities—they are studied in professional literature, discussed in the popular media and described by each participant in the two studies discussed in this paper. Family occupations occur when the whole family is engaged in an occupation together. However, the shared engagement in the occupation may not be parallel or equal among family members and their purposes and experiences may be different.

One commonly studied family occupation is family dinner. For example, DeVault (1991) describes the work that women invest in preparing family dinners. That work extends beyond cooking and includes activities such as attention to the tastes and wishes of individual family members, shopping within budget constraints, maintaining supplies, and scheduling dinner so that all members can attend. In her discussion, DeVault suggests that the work of feeding the family is, in effect, the work of creating the time, space, and an atmosphere that are conducive for constructing the family.

An example of the difference between occupations that involve one individual and occupations that involve more individuals can be seen in the following example from DeVault's (1991) discussion of one of her participants: "When she is home alone, during the day, she eats casually, and she talked about how difficult it is, when her husband occasionally works at home, to prepare a 'really decent lunch'" (p. 147). This suggests that lunch alone and lunch with a spouse are different occupations.

Family leisure occupations have also been studied. Shaw (1992), for example, reviews the images of family leisure in the popular media and concludes that only the benefits from such activities are addressed. However, in her own study, she found that when families identify a family occupation as leisure, women often identify their individual experiences during such occupations as work. According to Henderson and Allen (1991), these experiences occur in the context of the activity, time, and interaction with others. As long as women feel obligated to care for others, they cannot experience leisure. Orthner and Mancini (1990) extend this notion and suggest that the interdependency of the family system functions as a constraint on family members' experiences during family leisure.

It is clear from this and other literature that family occupations are purposefully constructed. Family occupations provide families with the space and time to be together (DeVault, 1991; Orthner & Mancini, 1990). In our culture, this time and space is supposed to re-create the experience of togetherness and good relationships or the idealized family images in our culture (Daly, 1994). Although such experiences commonly do not occur for families as a

whole and for some family members, these idealized images still guide the behaviour of families (Daly, 1994; Shaw, 1992).

Bellah, Madsen, Sullivan, Swidler, and Tipton (1985) deal with similar issues in more abstract and general terms. In their book, *Habits of the Heart,* Bellah et al. discuss the concept of love and family in the United States in the contexts of individualism and commitment. They define love in the context of commitment as "placing duty and obligation above the ebb and flow of feeling, and, in the end, finding freedom in willing sacrifice of one's own interests to others" (pp. 95–96). This definition seems to generalize mothers' work and experiences to any role of commitment. This idea can be used as an explanation for mothers' construction of family leisure even though they do not experience leisure during these occupations. However, this idea does not give a reasonable explanation for the continued engagement in family occupations when the family experience during these occupations does not reproduce the idealized images of family experience.

The purpose of this paper is to elucidate the purposes of family occupations. It is assumed that the purposes of family occupations motivate parents to construct and engage in family occupations regardless of their family's and their own experience. Although this paper is based on two studies of families with children who have special needs, it is assumed that families with children who have special needs are ordinary families. This assumption is based on the current approaches to families with children who have special needs (Gallimore, Weisner, Kaufman, & Bernheimer 1989; Seligman & Darling, 1989). In particular, Gallimore et al. (1989) suggest that such families are more similar to other families in their culture than to families with children who have special needs in other cultures.

BACKGROUND OF THIS PAPER

This paper is based on two qualitative interview studies whose purpose was to explore and describe the daily experiences and adaptations of families with children who have special needs. The first study was the author's dissertation and the participants were families with children who have attention deficit hyperactivity disorder (ADHD) (Segal, 1995). At that time, the researcher was fascinated with the work that parents invested in scheduling and constructing family occupations. It was assumed that this parental work and attention were embedded in the nature of their children's special needs. The second study was with families with children who have physical disabilities. It began a couple of years after the first study was finished. The research question of this study was similar and the purpose was to find out whether the daily experiences and adaptations among families with children who have physical disabilities are similar to those among families with children who have ADHD. During the initial analysis, it was obvious that daily experiences and adaptations among families with children who have physical disabilities are different from the daily experiences and adaptations among families with children who have ADHD. However, in both studies the parents paid a great deal of attention to the construction of family occupations.

This observation prompted a review of the literature that is discussed in the introduction, reinterpretation of the theme of family occupations in the study of families with children who have ADHD, and the interpretation of the theme of family occupations from the study of families with children who have physical disabilities. These findings and interpretations are presented in this paper.

METHODS

Qualitative research interviews were used to explore descriptions of the life experiences of families with children who have special needs. The interview format followed the classical format of qualitative research interviews wherein the researcher asks the participants an open-ended general question about the issue that the researcher wants the participants to describe.

Their responses are followed up with questions that are constructed from the participants' initial responses (e.g., McCracken, 1988; Patton, 1990; Spradley, 1979).

The Participants

Recruitment. The method of recruitment was different for each study. The families with children who have ADHD were recruited from support groups and an occupational and physical therapy clinic in a large urban area in Southern California, USA. For details about this recruitment procedure see Segal (1998) and Segal and Frank (1998).

The families with children who have physical disabilities were recruited through a children's treatment and rehabilitation centre in Ontario, Canada. The centre serviced both urban and rural areas. A representative from the centre talked with prospective participants to secure their agreement to receive a letter of information and consent forms by mail from the researcher. The researcher called the potential participants about a week after mailing the information to find out whether they would like to participate in the research, to answer any questions, and, if appropriate, to set a time and a place for the interview.

Characteristics of the participants. The inclusion criteria for study participants were that the children with special needs were between 6 and 11 years of age and that families could communicate in English. The 25 families who participated in the two studies were predominantly from European descent. This group consisted of single and dual parent families from urban and rural areas in Canada and the United States.

Of the 25 families who participated in the two studies, 17 had children with ADHD, three had children with spina bifida, two had children with myotonic muscular dystrophy, one had two children with Duchenne muscular dystrophy, one had a child with atypical muscular dystrophy, and one had a child with a congenital amputation.

Overview of the children's special needs. At the time of data collection of the two studies, none of the children received interventions at home. Three of the children with ADHD had therapy after school and the rest of the children that needed interventions received them at their schools.

Children with attention deficit hyperactivity disorder (ADHD) may suffer from one or more of the following three categories of symptoms: short attention span, impulsive behaviour, and hyperactivity (American Psychiatric Association, 1994). These symptoms are associated with impaired occupational performance in areas such as self care (e.g., dressing and eating), school work, and personal responsibility (e.g., chore performance, homework) (Barkley, 1998). The children whose parents participated in the first study (Segal, 1995), had difficulties in their overall occupational performances.

Duchenne's muscular dystrophy is transmitted as a male sex-linked recessive trait. It begins in childhood and affects mostly the pelvic girdle and shoulder muscles. The muscles weaken progressively and commonly by the age of 12 the children are confined to an electric wheelchair. Death occurs in late adolescence or early twenties due to pulmonary and cardiac complications (Anderson, Anderson, & Glanze, 1997). The two children whose parents participated in the second study were confined to electric wheelchairs at the time of data collection.

The symptoms of the child with atypical muscular dystrophy in the second study were similar to the symptoms of Duchenne's muscular dystrophy. He was not diagnosed with Duchenne's muscular dystrophy because the laboratory findings did not confirm this disease. At the time of data collection this child was able to walk.

The child with congenital amputation whose parents participated in the second study was born without her right forearm.

Myotonic muscular dystrophy is an autosomal dominant disease (i.e., it affects males and females). Its common form is acquired and the age of the onset may be anytime in the first five decades of life. It progresses slowly and there is a great variety in the severity of its symptoms. The symptoms are muscle weakness to the face, feet and hands. People with this disease need more sleep, and may suffer from developmental delays and some emotional blunting. The two children with this disorder whose families participated in the second study suffered from the rare form of congenital myotonic muscular dystrophy. The common features of this disorder are minimal muscular control ("floppy infants"), difficulties sucking and nursing, respiratory distress and severe developmental delays (Roses, 1989). The children in the second study suffered from all these symptoms. Additionally, one of them had difficulties swallowing and choked on her food quite commonly.

Spina bifida is "a failure in the closure of the spinal column due to defects in the development of vertebrae" (Chutorian, 1989). Severity of symptoms depends on the location of the defect on the spinal column and whether the neural tube itself is damaged. Hydrocephalus may also occur. The range of symptoms among people with spina bifida may range from no symptoms to severe developmental delays and cognitive limitations, lack of bowel and bladder control, and inability to walk (Anderson, et al., 1997). Two of the three children with spina bifida in this study did not have hydrocephalus. All of them had manual wheelchairs but did not use them consistently and none of them had bladder control.

DATA COLLECTION AND INTERPRETATION

According to Kvale (1996), developing and finalizing the interview questions is the first step of the data interpretation because these questions shape the general topic of the interview. The participants were asked to: (a) tell the researcher their family story and (b) describe their daily schedules and routines. For the purpose of this paper, only the interview about daily routines was used. During this interview, parents were asked to describe a typical day, how scheduled activities were performed, and who was involved.

All the interviews were audiotape recorded and transcripts were produced by a professional transcriber. After the audio tapes were transcribed, the researcher listened to tapes to ensure the accuracy of the transcriptions. For this paper, the data about family occupations was grouped together as a category and analyzed to discover the motivation for constructing family occupations. The data about family occupations, therefore, was subject to the methods of grounded theory analysis, particularly to the phase of axial coding in which the category is coded for contexts, consequences, strategies, and conditions (Strauss & Corbin, 1990).

TRUSTWORTHINESS

The main strength of the findings and interpretations of this paper comes from the variety of its participants. The participants came from large and small urban areas and from an agricultural area. They also consisted of a variety of family structures (single and dual-parent families, employed and stay-at-home mothers, a grandmother, a house husband, and adoptive parents). Such great variety of participants contributes to the credibility, dependability, and confirmability of the findings (Krefting, 1991). In addition, the use of two types of interviews (family story and family schedule), and the variety of children's special needs contribute to the same issues.

Generalization in qualitative research is the prerogative of the reader (Lincoln & Guba; 1985). However, it is the responsibility of the researcher to give the reader enough information (dense description) to make sound decisions. In this case, the means that were described in the previous paragraph as well as the detailed descriptions of the participants at the end of each quote and a great variety of data excerpts constitute the dense description. In the following presentation of the findings, all names are pseudonyms.

THE PURPOSES OF FAMILY OCCUPATIONS: FINDINGS AND INTERPRETATIONS

Families constructed and selected shared occupations purposefully. These purposes or functions of family occupations were the desired consequences of such occupations. Some occupations were selected in order for the family to be together, some occupations were constructed so that family members could share their personal lives with each other, and other occupations were selected or constructed to provide learning experiences for the children.

Being Together

Occupations whose purpose was for the family to be together commonly were occupations that were fun for the children. The activities performed during these occupations were things that the children liked to do and the interactions during such occupations were relaxed and non-demanding. That is, there was no onus to make a conversation, sit properly at the table for dinner, or to learn. Parents selected the activities of such occupations carefully to ensure that being together was a pleasurable experience.

Well, we do one family thing together [on the weekend]. We either maybe go to the mall and go in the Disney store or go to the library or we all wash the cars together—something like that. We do one family thing. Whether it's getting ice-cream or the library. (Naomi, the married mother of a 9-year-old son with ADHD and a 2-year-old daughter).

We cuddled and all had our snack together watching something on TV for half an hour or so (Dawn, the married mother of an 8-year-old son with ADHD).

We usually, our favourite past-time is watching Star Trek. Any one of the series. (Veronica, the single mother of a 9-year-old son with ADHD).

Friday night is usually family night. That means we do something as a family . . . we watch a

Disney movie here. (Shirley, the married mother of a 9-year-old son with ADHD and a 7-year-old daughter).

After supper, you know, . . . if there's nothing going on, then we'll take them for a ride or whatever, you know, start wrestling downstairs or whatever. Play with the gerbil, or you know bounce on the beds or something. . . . You know, we try and spend time, the four of us together if we can. (Joyce, the married mother of a 7-year-old daughter with spina bifida and a 3-year-old son).

We get up Sunday. We take our good old time, do whatever it is. We play a few [video] games or whatever. We take our time dressing, take our time eating, play a [video] game, go for a ride. They (the boys) don't like riding too much, so usually we are home, go for a walk, drag them outside, then come back. It is just kind of an easy day. (James, the married father of two boys (12 and 10-year-old) with Duchenne muscular dystrophy and an 8-year-old daughter).

Sharing

Sharing usually occurred during family meals. The food and the eating were secondary to the interactions that were expected during these occupations. Here, unlike the "being together" occupation, there were clear behavioural expectations from the children. They were supposed to sit for the whole occupation, talk, and share their day. Similar to the previous kind of occupations, the focus was on the children. Parents may not always share their own day at the family meal, but children were always expected to do so. The method of sharing varied and the amounts of help given to the children in order to participate in these interactions depended on each child's special needs. Regardless of how this sharing occurred, it was considered an important and enjoyable family occupation.

[At dinner] We talk about what went on in their day . . . You know, it's like quality time. (Irene, the married mother of a 9-year-old son with ADHD and a 7-year-old daughter with autism).

[On Saturdays] we go out and sit down and have breakfast. That's the only really peaceful family time because its morning; it's not dinner when his medication is wearing off . . . we'll go around and everybody will get a chance to share on what they've done that week. (Sharon, the married mother of a 11-year-old son with ADHD and a 9-year-old daughter).

[On Sunday dinner] We go around the whole family and say one thing nice about everyone in the family and then also we have to say something nice about ourselves—something good that we do. (Brenda, the married mother of four boys (aged 16, 14, 11, and 5) whose 11-year-old has ADHD).

She also said that,

Sometimes I just read to them out of the Readers Digest at dinner time. The last one I read to them was about the Ben Carson story who is the top pediatric neurosurgeon in the world . . . So I read that to them because I have a son who wants to go into medicine. So any of their interests, you know.

I think the best time is at the dinner table at night when we can sit around and talk. I make it a point of talking to Allison [granddaughter] about her day at school and of course trying to talk to Carl [grandson] about his day at school too, you know, so the way we do that is I will get his communication book and I will read it and then I will talk to him about things that happened in school, you know, stuff like that. And then Sally [daughter], if Sally and Allison are up here, of course we have our conversations about the day, what they did that day and you know I like it when we are all together. That is actually the best part of the day for me. (Angela, the grandmother and legal guardian of her 9-year-old grandson who has congenital myotonic muscular dystrophy. Her daughter and granddaughter live with her as well. Both of them suffer from myotonic muscular dystrophy, acquired and congenital respectively.)

The best part of the day? Probably our family time at night because that's kind of when everybody sits on the couch and we either talk or you know tell how the day went. Dinner times are good too because we go over what went on at school and, you know who has had a bad day, who has had a good day, that kind of stuff. That's the time I enjoy most, is the communication, you find out what has been going on in their lives, what is bothering them, what is making them happy. That is the best time. (Jenny the single mother of three daughters (aged 9, 8, and 6-year-old) whose oldest daughter has spina bifida. Jenny also has spina bifida.)

Providing Learning Opportunities for the Children

Lastly, some family occupations were used to convey to and share with the children the family's religion, ethnic and family background, or hobbies. The information that is shared during these occupations is as important as their experiences. Similar to the occupations selected for "being together," the activities or the contents of these occupations were important. Similar to the previous two categories, the children were the focus of these occupations. The purpose was that the children would learn something. That something, however, depended on the interests and values of the parents. The content of these occupations was something that the parents wanted the children to embrace.

[After coming home from Church] We have lunch, we change our clothes, get relaxed. We usually have family home evening. Either my husband prepares a lesson or I prepare . . . but it's got to be fun. We have only 30 minutes. They have to sing songs, pray. We have a short lesson and then [we] usually have refreshments. (Brenda, the married mother of four boys (aged 16, 14, 11, and 5) whose 11-year-old has ADHD).

We're into some of [our] Scottish background. So, like, over Labour Day, we went up to the Scottish games in Santa Rosa . . . Or, . . . whatever history they [the children] are studying about. My son Allen did the Gold Rush Country, so last year, last summer, you know, we did a vacation up in the Gold Rush Country. So, so, it kind of, you know, reestablished itself, not just in the book, but actually real learning. (Mary, the married mother of three sons (aged 9, 7, and 4) whose 7-year-old has ADHD).

Saturday is time for us to visit some of the sites. . . . Like this weekend, we are going to Camp [. . .]—we are going to go through the amphibious assault area. Richard, at 6 [years of age], he's been in a tank, . . . He's seen fighter air craft up close. He's seen just about everything that can be seen . . . He's even flown a helicopter simulator . . . just about any place you can imagine military wise. (Sandra, a military officer and a single mother of a 6-year-old son and a 4-year-old daughter both with ADHD).

As a family—see that picture up there? [A picture of her family standing next to a teepee]—that's called a rendezvous. And what we do is we go out four or five times a year as a family and we all get dressed up like that and we do a living history in our teepee and we cook like this—the blacksmith made us the cook[ing] stuff. Chris [her son] gets all dressed up like a little mountain boy, you know. So that's something we've all worked together as a family . . . Chris has never been real interested in it but he's been coming along with us on it. I think later he'll kind of—he's getting into it now—he's getting into it now. (Dawn, the married mother of a 9-year-old son with ADHD).

Sometimes I have to drag them to a museum . . . I'll purposefully whip through and just concentrate on things that they can relate to. I make the visits very short—you know. I take them to art galleries and what have you and we just concentrate on one section. And I'll ask them questions like "What's your favorite and why do you like it?" and that type of thing. (Peggy, the married mother of a 7-year-old daughter with ADHD and a 5-year-old son).

I get out hunting, so they see me cleaning my rabbits or cleaning the deer, bringing some deer home. So they have seen all of that. They get to see a lot of things. They realize where things come from, rather than some people, I think they imagine these things come from nowhere. But these guys have seen where stuff comes from, what happens. (James, the married father of two boys (12 and 10 years-old) with Duchenne muscular dystrophy and an 8-year-old daughter).

I really like our meal times. I really like that we eat together as a family. We always end our meal with Bible reading and prayers and we usually talk about what we've read and I like, especially when the kids are engaged, I enjoy those discussions. (Anne, the married mother of an 8-year-old daughter with a congenital amputation and a 10-year-old son).

This last quote is also an example for how a single family occupation can be constructed as an opportunity for sharing as well as providing learning opportunities for the children.

DISCUSSION

In this paper, families with children who have special needs identified three purposes for family occupations: being together, sharing children's life experiences and providing learning opportunities for the children. These purposes were similar among families with children who have ADHD and families with children who have physical disabilities. The descriptions of how family occupations were selected or constructed to achieve these purposes show that parents constructed these occupations for their children. That is, the purposes of family occupations were the construction of particular experiences for the children and to socialize them into social-cultural and familial values.

Although many parents identified family occupations as the best part of the day indicating that they enjoyed these family occupations, their enjoyment cannot be fully explained in terms of the principle of individualism (Bellah et al., 1985). In the context of individualism, loving relationships occur when there is a "full exchange of feelings between authentic selves" (Bellah et al., 1985, p. 102), and continue to develop as long as there are individual benefits such as personal growth (Bellah et al., 1985). Therefore, activities such as sharing during dinner with children who have autism or are unable to communicate cannot be understood in terms of the principle of individualism. However, this enjoyment can be better understood in terms of the principle of commitment (Bellah et al., 1985). The principle of commitment in the context of love, marriage and family means that there is an obligation to sacrifice one's needs for the

well being of other family members. The enjoyment and happiness of the individual come from the happiness and well being of the other family members and from the practice of such occupations (Bellah et al., 1985).

Attention to the needs and desires of the children was evident among the parents who participated in the studies reported here. However, the purpose of children's experiences during family occupations was to facilitate their engagement rather than the actual performance of these occupations. The parental obligation to children is to prepare them for life. As Bellah et al. (1985) suggest, families, the main setting of a life of commitment and obligation in our culture, are also the main setting that prepares children to live in the world of individualism. The purposes of family occupations illustrate how this happens.

Family occupations whose purpose was "being together" were selected or constructed in order to create a temporal and social space for the family's experiences of togetherness and the construction of the family (Daly, 1994; DeVault, 1991). Similarly, an occupation whose purpose was to provide learning opportunities for the children indicates the parents desire to socialize their children into the family's interests and religious and cultural values. However, in providing learning opportunities related to the children's academic work they embody both individualism and commitment. On the one hand, they enforce the idea of individual excellence as a way to successful life which is an aspect of individualism (Bellah et al., 1985), and on the other hand, their orientation to the child's interests embodies parental commitment.

Sharing as a purpose of family occupations commonly consisted of asymmetrical participation of parents and children because parents did not share their day with the whole family. Therefore, these occupations embodied parental commitment. However, sharing one's personal life embodies the essence of relationships in the context of individualism where "love means the full exchange of feelings between authentic selves, not enduring commitment resting on binding obligation" (Bellah et al., 1985, p. 102). Since sharing one's life is an important aspect of love relationships, such family occupations enable the children to learn and practice this essential skill.

CONCLUSION

Family occupations are different from individual occupations in the purposes they serve. The expected experiences from participating in those occupations are different for different participants or family members. From the parents' point of view, family occupations are about *doing for the children*. The purposes of such occupations are the construction of the family and preparing the children for life. Parental enjoyment derives from the children's enjoyment, growth and success.

The discussion of occupations in this study is an example of the complexity of human occupations. In particular, this study suggests that occupations may consist of the engagement of a number of individuals whose participation is not parallel or equal and their experiences and purposes are different. In addition, this study suggests that the traditional categories of productivity, leisure and self care may not be helpful in understanding the experiences of individuals in family occupations. This research established the need for further study of the occupations of groups as a separate phenomenon in occupational science. In particular, studies of family occupations among families with ordinary children and studies of the experiences of children during family occupations are needed.

Lastly, all the families took it for granted that family occupations must be selected and constructed—none of them considered eliminating such occupations because of the children's special needs. Family occupations were perceived as essential features of the commitment and obligation to the family. Further, it seems that parents suspended the dominating ideology of individualism in favour of the ideology of commitment in the context of raising their children.

ACKNOWLEDGMENTS

I am grateful to Professor Gelya Frank for our discussions and her valuable advice during and after my dissertation work. I am also grateful to Professor Joanne Cook, my colleague and friend, for her advice, support and editorial work on this manuscript.

This paper was supported by the following grants:

- American Occupational Therapy Foundation (AOTF) Center for Research on Adaptation and Occupation (1992–1995) at the Department of Occupational Science and Therapy, University of Southern California. Principal investigator: Professor Florence Clark.
- The University of Western Ontario VP Research grant R2670A01.

References

Anderson, K. N., Anderson, L. E., & Glanze, W. D. (1997). *Mosby's medical, nursing & allied health dictionary.* Toronto: Mosby.

American Psychiatric Association. (1994). *Diagnostic and statistical manual of mental disorders* (4th ed.). Washington, DC: Author.

Barkley, R. A. (1988). *Attention-deficit hyperactivity disorder: A handbook for diagnosis and treatment.* New York: Guilford Press.

Bellah, R. N., Madsen, R., Sullivan, W. M., Swidler, A., & Tipton, S. M. (1985). *Habits of the heart: Individualism and commitment in American Life.* Los Angeles: University of California Press.

Clark, F. A., Parham, D., Carlson, M. E., Frank G., Jackson, J., Pierce, D., Wolfe, R. J., & Zemke, R. (1991). Occupational science: Academic innovation in the service of occupational therapy's future. *American Journal of Occupational Therapy, 45,* 300–300.

Chutorian, A. M. (1989). Spina bifida and cranium bifidum. In L. P. Rowland (Ed.), *Merritt's textbook of neurology* (8th ed., pp. 475–480). Philadelphia: Lea and Febier.

Daly, K. J. (1994). *Families & time: Keeping pace in a hurried culture.* Thousand Oaks, CA: Sage.

DeVault, M. L. (1991). *Feeding the family: The social organization of caring as gendered work.* Chicago: The University of Chicago Press.

Gallimore, R., Weisner, T. S., Kaufman, S. Z., & Bernheimer, L. P. (1989). The social construction of ecocultural niches: Family accommodation of developmentally delayed children. *American Journal on Mental Retardation, 94,* 216–230.

Henderson, K. A., & Allen, K. R. (1991). The ethics of care: Leisure possibilities and constraints for women. *Society & Leisure, 14,* 97–113.

Krefting, L. (1991). Rigor in qualitative research: The assessment of trustworthiness. *American Journal of Occupational Therapy, 45,* 214–222.

Kvale, S. (1996). Interviews. Thousand Oaks, CA: Sage.

Lincoln, Y. S., & Cuba, E. A. (1985). *Naturalistic inquiry.* Beverly Hills, CA: Sage.

McCracken, G. (1988). *The long interview.* Newbury Park, CA: Sage.

Orthner, D. K., & Mancini, J. A. (1990). Leisure impacts on family interaction and cohesion. *Journal of Leisure Research, 22,* 125–137.

Patton, M. Q. (1990). *Qualitative evaluation and research methods* (2nd ed.). Newbury Park, CA: Sage.

Roses, A. D. (1989). Progressive muscular dystrophies. In L. P. Rowland (Ed.), *Merritt's textbook of neurology* (8th ed., pp. 709–720). Philadelphia: Lea & Febier.

Segal, R. (1995). *Family adaptation to a child with attention deficit hyperactivity disorder.* Unpublished doctoral dissertation, University of Southern California, Los Angeles, CA, USA.

Segal, R. (1998). The construction of family occupations: A study of families with children who have ADHD. *Canadian Journal of Occupational Therapy, 65,* 286–292.

Segal, R. & Frank, G. (1998). The extraordinary construction of ordinary experiences: Scheduling daily life in families with children with attention deficit hyperactivity disorder. *Scandinavian Journal of Occupational Therapy, 5,* 141–147.

Seligman, M. & Darling, R. B. (1989). *Ordinary families, special children: A system approach to childhood disability.* New York: Guilford Press.

Shaw, S. M. (1992). Dereifying family leisure: An examination of women's and men's everyday experiences and perceptions of family time. *Leisure Science, 14,* 271–286.

Spradley, J. P. (1979). *The ethnographic interview.* Toronto: Harcourt Brace Jovanovich College Pub.

Strauss, A. & Corbin, J. (1990). *Basics of qualitative research: Grounded theory procedures and techniques.* Newbury Park, CA: Sage.

Chapter 15

Opportunity, Not Prescription: An Exploratory Study of the Experience of Occupational Engagement

Canadian Journal of Occupational Therapy

1999, 66(4): 176–187

Karen L. Rebeiro, Joanne V. Cook

Karen L. Rebeiro, M.Sc.O.T., B.Sc.O.T.(C) is a Clinical Researcher at Network North: The Community Mental Health Group, 680 Kirkwood Drive, Sudbury, Ontario P3E 1X3. This paper was written when the first author was a graduate student at the University of Western Ontario. J.V. Cook, Ph.D., O.T. (C) is Associate Professor at the School of Occupational Therapy at the University of Western Ontario, London, Ontario. Canada.

KEY WORDS

- models, occupational therapy
- mental health
- occupation
- purposeful activities

ABSTRACT

Occupational therapy practice is based upon the belief that the use of occupation-as-means can promote the health and sense of well-being of individuals with disability. Despite a firm commitment to the construct of occupation by the profession, little empirical evidence has been generated which supports the basic tenets of practice. In the psychosocial literature, no studies could be located which directly investigated the use of occupation-as-means to mental health. An exploratory study was conducted with eight participants of an occupation-based, women's mental health group. In-depth interviews and participant observation were utilized to explore the meaning of occupational engagement for these women. The experience of occupational engagement is presented in the form of a conceptual model named occupational spin-off. *Occupational spin-off represents conceptually the experience of occupational engagement for the participants in the research study and describes a process of occupation-as-means to mental health. The processes of affirmation, confirmation, actualization, and anticipation collectively contribute to and maintain occupational spin-off. The process of occupational spin-off contributes to an understanding of why these participants have remained out of hospital, and why they are feeling better. Implications of this process model for clinical practice and future research are suggested.*

The occupational therapy literature indicates that the use of occupation as therapeutic means has been central to the practice of occupational therapy in mental health (Barris, Kielhofner & Hawkins Watts, 1983), and that the use of occupation constitutes the common core of occupational therapy practice (American Occupational Therapy Association [AOTA], 1979; Canadian Association of Occupational

Therapists [CAOT], 1991, 1997). Reilly (1962), Fidler and Fidler (1978), Rogers (1984), Clark et al. (1991), Trombly (1995) and Yerxa (1967, 1991) have all postulated that the use of occupation is what distinguishes occupational therapy from other health care professions. The literature states that "the oldest and most central role of occupational therapists is that of directly engaging people in occupations as treatment" (Barris et al., 1983, p. 289). However, the occupational therapy literature is surprisingly limited in empirical support of this role. Fossey (1992) stated that "eighty years of clinical experience have provided a wealth of opportunities for occupational therapists to observe the direct and indirect effects of occupations on health", and yet, "much of the research data needed to support this claim remains uncollected" (p. 149).

There has been significant philosophical discussion in the profession's literature about occupation and its relationship to health over the last several decades. While few tested theories have been articulated regarding the relationship between occupation-as-means and health, the profession has put forth several speculative, relational assumptions (Trombly, 1995; Wilcock, 1993; Wood, 1993; Yerxa et al., 1990). In the psycho social literature, the area of practice with the longest tenure in occupational therapy, no studies could be found which provided evidence in support of a role for occupation-as-means to mental health. Further, no studies addressed the questions: does the use of occupation-as-means promote mental health and if so, why and how? These questions helped to guide the research.

The gap between the use of occupation-as-means and a research/knowledge base to support its continued use in mental health practice was the focus of this study. Reilly (1962) once said that occupational therapists have more medical knowledge than they need to apply in practice, and practice more the use and application of occupation than they have knowledge to support. Research which facilitates a better understanding of the impact of engaging in

occupations for individuals with disability will assist occupational therapists in the use and application of occupation-as-means, instill confidence that their "simple, operating procedures" are of worth to those whom they serve (Fidler, 1981), give the profession what Reilly (1971) calls 'face validity', and help to build knowledge on core professional constructs.

This paper will provide a brief overview of the occupational therapy beliefs and assumptions regarding occupation in order to ground the research study. The reader is directed to Rebeiro (1998) for a more thorough review of the use of occupation as therapy in mental health practice. The research methods and design will be described with the findings of the study presented in the form of a conceptual, process model. The discussion section will highlight the implications of this exploratory study for occupational therapy education, clinical practice and future research.

LITERATURE

The profession of occupational therapy has historically employed occupations as therapeutic means (Barris, et al., 1983; Kielhofner, 1992; Kielhofner & Burke, 1977). Therapists engaged individuals in a variety of occupations in order to provide a purposeful outlet for their mental and physical energies (Jackson, 1993; Kielhofner & Burke, 1977; Meyer, 1922/77). Therapists believed that diverting one's thoughts to the occupation was beneficial to the individual and that engaging in a daily rhythm of occupations which mirrored that of normal society would assist individuals to both recover from their ailments and to reintegrate them into larger society (LeVesconte, 1935/1986; Meyer, 1922/77).

The use of occupation as therapy was founded in the moral treatment era. Occupation was perceived to be a humane and effective method of treating mental illness (LeVesconte, 1935/1986). Occupation, both as a treatment modality and as a goal of treatment, found support in society during the early twentieth century since productive work and self-support were, and continue to be, valued by society (Ambrosi & Barker-Schwartz, 1995). The literature states that "the oldest and most central role of occupational therapists is that of directly engaging people in occupations as treatment" (Barris et al., 1983, p. 289).

The conceptualization of occupation-as-therapy has been discussed by occupational therapists since the profession was formally organized in 1917 (Diasio, 1971; Dunton, 1918; LeVesconte, 1935/1986; Woodside, 1971; Yerxa et al., 1990). Therapists philosophized about the vital need that occupation has historically and developmentally played, not only in human's health and well-being, but also, in the person's quest for personal meaning and self-actualization throughout the lifespan (Diasio, 1971; Fidler & Fidler, 1978; Johnson, 1971; Kielhofner & Burke, 1977; Reilly, 1962, 1966, 1971; Rerek, 1971; Shannon, 1977; West, 1984; Woodside, 1971).

In 1962, Reilly challenged the profession to identify which need the profession served in society. She suggested that occupation has, and will continue to be, a basic and vital need in the health of man. Reilly postulated that "man [sic] through the use of his hands as they are energized by mind and will, can influence the state of his own health" (p. 2). She directly challenged the use of activity for diagnostic and psychoanalytic purposes and advocated research and the generation of knowledge on the human need for occupation. This knowledge, she contended, would secure a place for occupational therapy in the health care forum and provide a scientific basis for the use of occupation as therapy for those with disability.

The use of occupation as treatment appears to be based upon four broad beliefs about the therapeutic value of occupation: first, that engaging in occupations provides a positive focus for one's attention and thinking; second, that engaging in occupations provides a structure or balance to one's day and normalizes one's sleep and wake cycles; third, that engaging in occupations is a means to mental and physical health; and, fourth, that occupation provides a sense of purpose and meaning to one's existence (Breines, 1989; Kielhofner & Burke, 1977; Meyer, 1922/77; Mosey, 1971; Reilly, 1962; Wilcock, 1993; Yerxa et al., 1990). These beliefs, based upon observation, remain the primary basis of support for the practice of occupational therapy in mental health (Barris et al., 1983; Trombly, 1995). Although the theoretical literature lacks consensus regarding the meaning of occupation (Englehart, 1977; Rogers, 1984), its definition (Nelson, 1988; Christiansen, 1991, 1994), whether to call it occupation or activity (Christiansen, 1994; Cynkin & Robinson, 1990; Yerxa et al., 1990), and its methods of scientific inquiry (Carlson & Dunlea, 1995; Mosey, 1989; Ottenbacher, 1992; Yerxa, 1991), there does appear to be agreement regarding the beliefs about occupation which the profession is prepared to uphold and defend. These beliefs, in the absence of empirical evidence in support of the use and application of occupation-as-means to mental health, provide the basis for the present study (Fossey, 1992; Rebeiro, 1998; Reilly, 1962; Yerxa, 1991).

METHODS

Design Rationale

A qualitative design was selected for the study for two reasons. First, mental health is subjectively experienced and often self-defined. A qualitative approach using interviews and participant observation permits the researcher to investigate the occupation-as-means experience from the participants' perspective (DePoy & Gitlin, 1994). Second, occupation is a construct which to date remains poorly defined and understood (AOTA, 1995; Trombly, 1995). The long interview (McCracken, 1988) is a qualitative technique designed for the exploration of a phenomenon which is not well known or understood, and "participant observation is especially appropriate for scholarly problems when little is known about the phenomenon" (Jorgenson 1989, p. 12).

Participants

According to Jorgenson (1989), the strategy for obtaining participants can depend on "opportunity, common sense, and theoretical logic in selecting a setting for observation and phenomenon to observe within the setting" (p. 51). In this study, the selection and recruiting of informants were based upon all three of Jorgenson's criteria. The group chosen was one of convenience, in that there was opportunity to study The Women's Group at the researcher's place of employment. The rationale to study The Women's Group was based upon the researcher's experiential evidence and common sense that something appeared to be helping these women. Theoretically, it was assumed that the occupational engagement might contribute to these observations, as occupation was the factor which distinguished The Women's Group from other mental health programmes in the region.

Historical Description of the Group

The Women's Group is an outpatient, women's mental health group that was developed in 1990 by the department of occupational therapy at a Northeastern Ontario mental health facility. The group was developed in response to the significant number of women who were readmitted to hospital on a regular basis, were suicide risks and/or did not appear to benefit from more traditional, verbal-based therapies.

The original objectives of The Women's Group were to provide a place where the women could meet on a weekly basis for support and the resolution of issues, and to cooperatively participate in an occupation-based project. A quilt was prescribed as the occupation of choice for the group because it offered a long-term project in which each of the women could participate and was conducive to both cooperative and parallel work.

Description of the Participants

There were eight members of The Women's Group who participated in the interviews and eleven members who were present during the participant observation phase. All members of The Women's Group are consumers of mental health services in Northeastern Ontario and have had at least one admission to an adult inpatient psychiatric unit. Most participants are attended to by a psychiatrist and most, but not all, participants are on some form of medication. All participants have a history of psychiatric difficulties which extend beyond a ten-year duration. Each participant has been given a pseudonym for the purposes of anonymity.

Data Collection Phases and Techniques

The study design consisted of four distinct, yet interrelated, phases for the purpose of data collection. These were: orientation and overview, including pilot interviews; focussed exploration through the use of in-depth interviewing; participant and non-participant observation for a duration of 25 weeks; and member-checking. Thus, the study utilized several data collection techniques in order to address the rigour of trustworthiness as proposed by Lincoln and Guba (1985). A variety of trustworthiness strategies were employed to ensure that the findings were credible, transferable, dependable and confirmable (Rebeiro, 1997).

Data Analysis

The constant-comparative method of data analysis as proposed by Glaser and Strauss (1967) was utilized in the study. All interview transcripts, field notes, and journals/logs were openly reviewed and coded using preliminary categories. Categories were then compared with each other to ensure that all categories were externally distinct and yet were consistent between all cases. A negative case was identified and incorporated as an integral aspect of the analysis and findings. In this study, there were two main sources of information which came to bear on the results. Some of the results were generated from non-participant observation and from participant observation. Some of the results were generated from in-depth interviews with the members. However, most of the results were generated from both; i.e., interview data were confirmed or elaborated by participant observation.

RESULTS

The results of this exploratory study generated three analytic themes and ten analytic categories which collectively reflect the experience of occupational engagement for members of The Women's Group (Fig 1). These themes and categories are expressed in the form of a conceptual process model named occupational spin-off. The model of occupational spin-off conceptually portrays the experience of engaging in occupations, and how this process serves as a means to enhanced mental health and well-being for eight women with a severe and persistent mental illness. The results are illustrated by quotations from the participants transcripts.

Figure 1

Analytical themes and categories

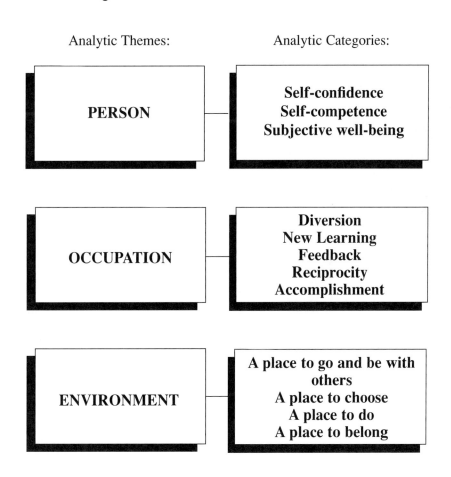

The Model of Occupational Spin-off

Occupational spin-off is presented as a hierarchy, with the social environment conceptualized as the foundation to the model (Fig 2). In this social environment, the individuals are given affirmation by other group members of their basic worth as human beings which subsequently enables engagement in occupations. Occupational engagement comprises the next stage which is interdependent with the affirm-

ing environment. In this stage, the individuals receive confirmation of their competency, through direct involvement in and feedback from the occupation and others. Collectively, the environment and the occupation interact and impact the individual through the stages of actualization and anticipation. The participants described enhanced self-confidence, competence and subjective well-being as a result of their engagement in occupations. Further, the participants began to anticipate that their ongoing engagement in occupation would serve as means to sustaining this actualized sense of self. Participants' anticipation of feeling better contributed to enhanced occupational performance. Occupational spin-off conceptualizes the experience of engagement in occupation and hypothesises that ongoing participation in occupation will contribute to the maintenance of the actualized self and of subjective well-being over time.

Figure 2

The Model of Occupational Spin-off

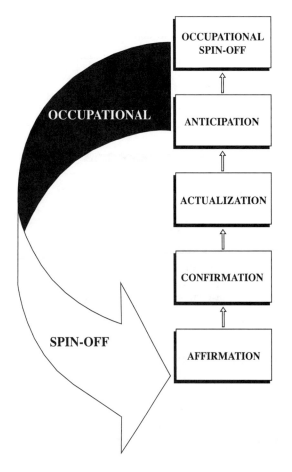

The Affirmation

The model of occupational spin-off begins in the social environment in a place with "the own" (Goffman, 1963, p. 20). It was in the social environment of The Women's Group that the members were first given positive declarations about, and thus affirmations of their selves. These affirmations were experienced in two ways: first, members were accepted as worthy persons; and second, they were encouraged as competent persons. The social environment was described by participants as being supportive, accepting and facilitating a sense of belonging. The social environment, they said, provided an affirmation of the individual as a worthy human being. Being affirmed was extremely important to the members' motivation to engage in occupations.

A "useful module" (Becker, 1986, p. 144) from the sociological literature on the social construction of identity can help explain the importance of affirmation to the experience of occupational engagement for the members. According to Berger (1963), "identity is socially bestowed, socially sustained and socially transformed" (p. 98). The informants in this study described being socially bestowed an identity as individuals of worth. Joan stated, "at least here you have somebody, and you feel like somebody and you are a somebody." In addition, the act of affirmation contributed to a sense of acceptance and belonging. Jane explained, "there was always a part of us that, in society, they want to be accepted. Like regardless of what our problems have been or what we've had in the past or what our illnesses have been."

The members described the social context of the group largely in terms of its membership. Goffman (1963) uses the concept of "the own" to describe "sympathetic others" who, "knowing from their own experience what it is like to have this particular stigma . . . provide the individual with a circle . . . to which he [sic] can withdraw for moral support and for the comfort of feeling at home, at ease, accepted as a person who is really like any other normal person" (p. 20). Being with "the own" meant gathering with women who had similar mental illness difficulties. The social context was largely described as understanding and caring. The group members were understanding because "they had been there". The group members were caring because they listened. The act of being listened to, they said, implies that the individual is important.

In The Women's Group, members were affirmed first as a worthy person. Many of the members of The Women's Group described their belief that in the larger society they were identified first by their mental illness, and second, by their humanness. As Phyllis stated, *it helped me to realize that I was not some sort of freak of nature.* Being affirmed by the other group members as a human being allowed the members to define themselves foremost as an individual of worth in this place with "the own".

The Women's Group also instilled a sense of belonging. This sense of belonging served several purposes, the most powerful being that it provided affirmation that the members were "loved", "cared for", "someone of worth" and

"someone of importance". In response to the question, why do you come to The Women's Group, Julie stated: *I wanted to have a sense of belonging to something, like be a part of something . . . they make me feel important . . . feel like I'm part of them.* Similarly, Edith stated: *I think it gives you a sense of belonging because you're with people that are like, as you, have similar problems . . . so you know, we can understand each other more that we have these highs and then we have these little downs . . . we belong there and that it's our group.*

Goffman (1963) analyses and describes the cost for the stigmatized in the management of identity and control of information in situations of possible stigmatization. Since the members of The Women's Group could be themselves with "the own," they did not have to expend energy in the form of interpersonal tension management with "normals" or worry that an unsuccessful performance would be ascribed to their mental illness or worse, that it would reflect upon their very humanness. Instead, the affirmed knew that it didn't matter if they were unsuccessful or needed help. They knew firsthand that the others would not only understand, but that they would help them through it and support their doing. The absence of the necessity for stigma management may also help to explain why the members described the environment as relaxing, safe and comfortable. As such, members could be both honest about themselves and about their difficulties without the fear of being "judged" by their families and friends, or only "saying what they want to hear" with professionals. For many, being affirmed was instrumental to their occupational performance within the group since it allowed each of them to move beyond a focus on their illness and towards a focus on doing something about it. Most of the members suggested that they could not even try to do an occupation until they were able to move past their perceived sense of failure and incapacity as a person with mental illness. As Edith suggested, *I wouldn't even try any of those things . . . I couldn't see the point in trying because I knew I couldn't do it.* For the members of The Women's Group, the social act of affirmation allowed them "a different way out." This different way out was realized as a result of directly engaging in occupations.

The Confirmation

While it is the affirmation by the other members that one is valued and of worth that enabled many of the members to actually engage in the occupation, to experiment and try novel doing, it is the occupational engagement itself and the accomplishments realized through the doing which confirmed their evolving identity. Whereas the affirmation encouraged "they think I can, therefore, maybe I can", the confirmation facilitated more "I did it and therefore, I can". By directly engaging in the occupations, members found that they could begin to move beyond their illness. Occupational engagement facilitated this process in several ways, the first of which was by the provision of diversion.

Diversion helped the members to focus on what they could do instead of what they could not do. Kelly, for example spoke of working on needlepoint as an opportunity to focus on what she could do instead of what she couldn't:

> It gave me something else to, to focus on. I had my mind off of my problems basically and my feeling of being a nobody and I could focus on doing this and it was something that I'm learning to do and that I can do it and . . . it was a step I took to self-confidence.

Further, diversion offered members respite from their negative thinking and worries, and allowed them to experience first-hand what it felt like not to be consumed with what was wrong in their life. Heather, in discussing her reasons for being involved in the group, described how occupation provided the opportunity to focus on her strengths and not her difficulties. She stated:

> Because if I don't [do something], I'll start thinking about suicide, I think about what my life is going to be in the future . . . and I'm trying not

to focus so much on what I can't do and that's why I'm trying to find something to do.

Edith also commented on how focussing on what she was doing helped provide diversion from a focus on problems.

> I go there and I don't think of anything but what I'm doing there, where the rest of the time, no matter where I am, I'm thinking about all the things that are going on in my life. I just relax and I think about what goes on in group and what I'm doing, and what the other ladies are saying.

Edith offered a contrast between being in the group to being at home:

> If you're sitting by yourself, you have a lot of time to think and worry . . . where when you're in the group, no matter what, there's always something going on in the group . . . somebody's talking or somebody's made a mistake in their knitting and she's helping them with it . . . you're always doing.

Diversion contributed to members' "feeling good", and confirmed that they could focus on something other than their problems, and accomplish tasks they previously would not have attempted. Participation in novel occupations was something that members did not feel confident in doing outside of the group prior to becoming a member. Julie, for example, stated:

> Before, I would never try something by myself at home. Like a new craft or whatever because I did not have the confidence and to me, The Women's Group gives me the opportunity to try out new things and develop talents . . . I can have a chance to learn and feel confident.

Edith also believed that she would not have had the confidence to try something on her own due to her prior self-assessment:

> I wouldn't have [tried something on my own] because before I started in the group, I thought I was stupid and I didn't think there was any sense in trying because I wasn't gonna be able to do it.

A second aspect of confirmation is the occupations' inherent capacity to provide feedback regarding competency. A sense of competency is confirmed by the act of accomplishment. The members spoke about how completing their project served to confirm their affirmed self-identity. Integral to this was an element of surprise or discovery that members really could do something with their hands. As Edith explained, *I realized that I could do a lot more than I thought I could.* For Jane, the occupation not only confirmed that she could do things, but more so, that maybe she could do more: *It made you feel good. I thought, Oh boy, I can do this . . . then maybe I can do the banking or make myself a decent meal . . . it grows from there.*

The members suggested that their completed projects confirmed an evolving sense of self-competence, and over time further supported and sustained their identity. Edith, in discussing the paper tole hanging on her wall, stated: *I look at it and realize that I did it and think if I can do this, maybe I can do other things too.* The product of the occupation afforded an objective, tangible means of feedback which members could not easily refute. The accomplishment served as a visible means to verify and corroborate their competency. The occupational product provided the initial confirmation to the individual, and the social group corroborated this confirmation of competency.

Confirmation not only sustained the affirmed identity of basic worth, but also appeared to contribute to a transformation of identity. Not only could members say to themselves *they think I can, therefore maybe I can, but instead, I did and they confirmed for me that I did.* Joan commented on the confirmation of competence and the resultant benefit:

I learn to make things, things that I would never have done before and never even thought of doing or being able to do. The feeling of incompetence is there, and then all of a sudden, you've come to this place and you achieve something and you have a real feeling of self-worth.

The impact of confirmation appeared to transform the members' self-identity beyond that of a mental illness and verify for them what had been affirmed by "the own". Members voiced a sense of confidence about themselves and their capacities that was vastly different than before they started the group. Their accomplishments confirmed for them that they were competent and this was further corroborated by the others. Joan stated:

It's a feeling of accomplishing. Something I've done. Not that you've done, not that anybody's done, and it's something that I've done and it's important . . . to me to learn something and for my mind to be able to absorb it because I have problems with my mind . . . for me, to accomplish this, is a big, big thing. That I can accomplish something. That I can start something and I can finish it.

The process of confirmation appeared to assist the members to recognize at a more personal level their future potential to do, and to instill a sense of confidence to try other things. The very social process of identity transformation as suggested by Berger (1963) becomes realized, confirmed and ratified through occupation. Collectively, the analytic categories associated with the occupation appear to contribute to a process of actualization of the individual.

Actualization

The collective impact of both the social environment and the occupation appears to actualize or make real for the person that they are valued, competent and productive individuals. The defining and redefining of the self appeared to result from a new-found confidence in themselves. The redefined self is socially sustained by acts of occupational engagement. Edith illustrates:

I used to think I was stupid, but now I know that I can do more than I thought I could . . . it gives me the incentive to try other new things because you realize you can do these things that you thought you could never do . . . before I didn't have the confidence to even attempt to do stuff like that.

Essentially, the affirmed individuals who speculated *maybe I can* received confirmation through their doing that *I can*. When both the affirmation and the confirmation came together, they collectively contributed to an actualization of *I am*. The actualized individuals tended to view both their situation and their mental illness through different lenses; they not only felt better about themselves and their situation, but also were hopeful about the future. Members expressed that they "looked forward" to the next group, towards activities that they need to do in preparation for the next group, and to further occupational engagement. The actualized individual began to anticipate and to be hopeful about the future.

Anticipation

For the members of The Women's Group, actualization contributed to a "looking forward to" future events. Phyllis, for example, stated "Really, you kinda look forward to Wednesday . . . it would make you feel better." Similarly, Joan discussed her anticipation of future groups: "I look forward every week to coming. Like when I go home after I'm finished, it's like, oh well, I gotta wait another week."

An actualized sense of self encouraged members to anticipate that if they did more of the same thing, they could continue to feel better. Phyllis in describing why she wanted to do more paper tole stated: "I know that after I did the wolf, I wanted to do more of that so I did have the feeling again." Julie provides a good illustration of how the group affected her sense of self and her perceived subjective well-being:

> There is a big difference in my mood . . . like when I come home from Women's group, like I'm always cheerful, and I'm always, I don't know, I'm bubbly and I'm full of life and like, I'm very positive and like other days of the week, like especially if I don't do housework or anything like that, it's like I'm not as much, I'm like more negative and he [spouse] notices a big difference . . . it recharges me for a while . . . it's like a booster . . . it's boosting me . . . You're boosting

> my will to live . . . it's something to look forward to . . . it elevates my mood . . . it's like a lift . . . it like, re-energizes me.

The members described two aspects of anticipation: a looking forward to being with "the own"; and a looking forward to further occupational engagement. They said that being with the other group members made them feel relaxed, comfortable and important. Being with "the own" seemed to enable the members to move beyond the labels and stigmas they perceived in larger society. In addition, members anticipated that continued occupational engagement would sustain their transformed identity, sense of confidence and subjective well-being.

The process of occupational engagement became essential to maintain and sustain the actualized self. The anticipation of the occupational engagement, in combination with one's anticipation of continuing to feel better as a result of the engagement, served as an ongoing and cyclical means of maintaining participants' sense of subjective well-being. This cyclical process is conceptualized as occupational spin-off.

Occupational Spin-off

The term, *occupational spin-off,* is a conceptualization based upon the members' descriptions of their experience of occupational engagement. Occupational spin-off explains a process of occupational engagement over time and attempts to explain the importance of the social environment to this experience. Occupational spin-off seems to motivate these women to continue to attend the group, to maintain themselves out of the hospital, and it appears to contribute to an enhanced sense of well-being. Occupational spin-off is the collective impact of being affirmed, confirmed, actualized and then in a position to anticipate (Fig 3).

The findings of this exploratory study suggest that members perceived a connection between what they did in The Women's Group and how they perceived themselves and their mental health. The idea of spin-off suggests that occupation is not necessarily an end, but instead, serves as means to confirmation of self and to maintenance of self over time. The members of this group clearly indicated that occupations were means to many personal goals, whether this be to give a gift to someone or for the sake of accomplishing something that was considered a challenge. However, it did not end there; occupation also served as means to feeling better, feeling more competent or more confident over time. Thus, the concept of spin-off infers that occupational engagement is a means to other and further occupational engagement which is driven by the individual's desire to continue feeling better.

The idea of spin-off resulted from the members' discussions of the progressive and gradual nature of their recoveries. Jane illustrates:

> *You have to start with something little and you get better, and better and better. You know, when you start something new, a craft that you haven't finished, you start small. Then your next could be a little more difficult . . . it starts small and it grows and grows and grows. It leads to doing more and there's more discussion, more talking because people are praising the one little, small thing that was accomplished by that individual and the praise is giving me, me like and everyone, a huge, a great aura of self-esteem.*

The affirmed individual in the group derived a sense of belonging, friendship and being cared for by the other members. The confirmed individual through engaging in occupations came to redefine their sense of self-confidence and competence. However, it was through the continued and varied occupational opportunities available to the members over time which sustained the actualized individual and which enabled spin-off into a variety of other occupations. This spin-off provided an ongoing means of actualization of self and capacity. Jane explained:

> *From accomplishing the first step, from the accomplishment that you feel when you've accomplished the first little step . . . to outside activities, outside doing, working, whatever, you name it . . . other volunteer work. It applies to life and living and dealing with depression.*

Occupation, in this sense, served as means to other occupation which served as means to continued support of the actualized individual. The ongoing and cyclical spin-off encouraged members to anticipate future occupations and to anticipate that this future engagement would provide the ongoing means for sustaining the transformed self, including their sense of subjective well-being:

> *Doing leads to more and it leads to accomplishing our goals . . . doing, I'm thinking of the word, occupation, it makes us, it makes me more mentally healthy, emotionally healthy. [Jane]*

DISCUSSION

Implications for Clinical Practice

This study suggests that the creation of a social environment based upon homogeneity is likely to encourage acceptance of the individual, and subsequently, result in greater participation by the individual. In this study, gathering with "the own" was essential to the social environment. Traditionally, therapists have based group composition upon pragmatic considerations such as the physical location of the client (e.g., in-patient versus out-patient, ward or unit), the purpose of the group (stress management versus community living skills), or by referral (doctor's order versus team recommendation). The informants in this study stated that gathering with individuals who are the same (diagnostically and according to gender) creates a social environment that is safe and accepting, and that is conducive to their engaging in occupations.

A second implication concerns client-centredness and relinquishing some of the decision-making power that we consider to be our right and obligation as professionals. Therapists need to create partnerships with

Figure 3

Application of the Model of Occupational Spin-off

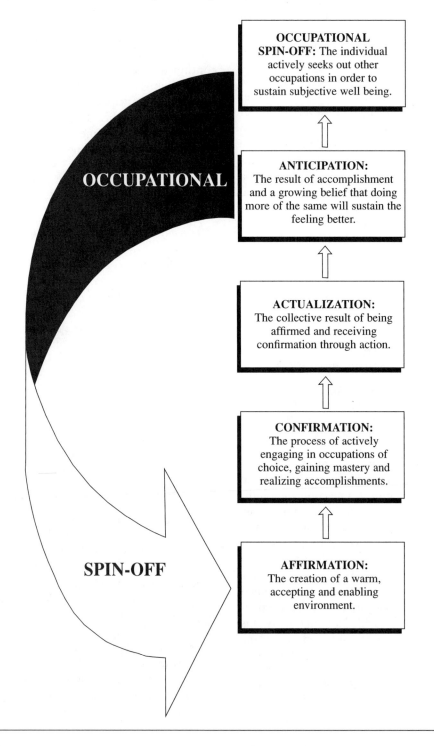

their clients that foster and enable their control of the therapy through the provision of opportunity and choice. This study suggests that the provision of a supportive environment which provides opportunity and choice can help enable both initial and continued occupational engagement. As clinicians, we can support our clients by listening to them, by providing them with the power and right to choose occupations which are meaningful to them, and by collaboratively setting goals which are based upon client-expressed occupational needs and goals.

This study suggests that the creation of a "just right" environment and the provision of occupation based upon client-expressed needs will have an impact upon clients' confidence to engage in occupation(s), as well as their desire to maintain occupational engagement into the future. The informants suggested that there were several elements of this "just right" environment which contributed to it being relaxing, safe and comfortable. In general, the social milieu was largely a result of the provision of opportunity and choice in a place with "the own". A focus on client strengths rather than upon any assessed deficits or limitations imposed by their disability is essential. Acknowledgement of the importance of a "just right" environment to engaging in occupations will encourage therapists to identify and to address those aspects of the hospital and community environments which pose a social handicap to the person and thus limits occupational engagement. The provision of opportunity will enable therapists to better address individual human needs and to create individual road maps which can guide the therapeutic process. Opportunity, not prescription, will give the client authority in occupational therapy practice.

The members stated that the provision of opportunity and choice gave them an environment conducive to experimentation and trying. This, they said, ensured that their individual needs were met. The stimulation of interest through the provision of choice was felt to be important to whether one would initially engage in the occupation and also whether one would continue the occupation towards completion. LaMore & Nelson's studies (1993) have shown that choice enhances participation. This study implies that the provision of choice is likely to stimulate greater interest in what the client works on, facilitate engagement in the occupation until completion and ultimately, result in a greater impact upon the person.

Implications for Education

The findings of this study suggest that theoretical knowledge of the person, occupation, and environment, and of the transactional nature of these theoretical constructs in the promotion of occupational engagement is important. A primary understanding of the social environment and how the provision of choice and opportunity affects occupational engagement is essential to understanding how occupation affects the person.

A second implication for education is that students gain a broader understanding of the environment. Knowledge of the environment should not be limited to the physical barriers to access and integration, but should also include consideration of the social handicaps which may limit occupational engagement for those with disability. Anthony and Liberman (1986), suggest that "handicap is a crucial aspect of psychosocial rehabilitation when disabilities put the individual at a social disadvantage relative to others in society" (p. 548). A broader knowledge of the environment might assist therapists to create occupational opportunities within the greater social environment which facilitate acceptance and do not banish those individuals with disabilities to "back places" (Goffman, 1963) or limit them in occupational choice. A greater understanding of stigma (see Goffman, 1963; Shaw, 1991), social policy, and health policy (see Renwick & Brown, 1996) would assist occupational therapists to intervene at the level of social handicap in partnership with their clients. Furthermore, a broader understanding of the social and cultural issues which impact occupational engagement would assist the therapist in identifying and providing the opportunity to engage in culturally appropriate and meaningful occupations for all clients.

A third implication for education concerns knowledge of the construct of self-identity. The discipline of sociology has a great deal of knowledge which could assist the occupational therapist in understanding how engaging in occupation impacts one's sense of self and one's social identity (see Estroff, 1989, 1991).

A fourth implication for education suggests a more comprehensive understanding of human occupations, their meanings and purposes in society and their implications in human health and well-being across the lifespan. Occupational therapy education has historically emphasized medical knowledge of impairment and disability applied to the idea of occupation (Reilly, 1966). This study indicates that a greater emphasis be placed upon knowledge of human occupation across the lifespan and of the environment. While it is recognized that published, empirical research on the phenomenon of human occupation and health is limited at this time, educators are encouraged to seek out non-published works, including master's level theses to share with their students (see Corring, 1996; Emerson, 1996; LaLiberte, 1995; MacGregor, 1995). In addition, there are many research endeavours outside of the occupational therapy literature which explore the meaning of work and leisure for individuals with disability (see Lilley & Jackson, 1993; Scheid & Anderson, 1995). The use of occupations as therapy and the enablement of occupational engagement over time require that occupational therapy educators, clinicians and researchers have an appreciation of the many factors which influence human occupation. To do this effectively, we must broaden our knowledge and understanding of human occupation in the larger society and of how individuals with disabilities can "make the world their home" (Reilly, 1962).

Implications for Research

The findings of this study raise as many questions as answers. The need to test the applicability of the model of occupational spin-off across gender, socio-cultural and diagnostic groups in a variety of environmental settings is obviously warranted. Is the process of occupational spin-off similar for men, for individuals with schizophrenia or those with a spinal cord injury? Are there idiosyncratic variations to the process within specific disabilities and for each individual? If therapists focussed upon the provision of occupational opportunities within the community, would this result in greater participation by individuals with a disability? How does affirmation of clients impact their performance regardless of their disability?

These questions are merely a beginning in an attempt to understand better the meaning of occupation in human life, its use as a therapeutic medium and its subsequent impact upon the health and well-being of individuals with disability. It is imperative that occupational therapists explore further these phenomena through empirical research, and continue to contribute to what is known about occupation for it to be applied in therapy with confidence.

CONCLUSIONS

A qualitative study which sought to explore the personal experience of occupational engagement for members of a women's, occupation-based, mental health group indicated that the social environment of the group was extremely important to both initial and continued engagement in occupations. Being affirmed in the therapeutic setting enabled the members to move beyond a focus on their perceived limitations and to anticipate their potential through occupational engagement. The provision of opportunities, rather than the prescription of therapy, enabled participants to meet their own occupational needs and to move through the process of occupational engagement at their own pace. The provision of occupational opportunities in the "just right" social environment enabled participants to become actualized as individuals through their accomplishments. The actualized persons came to anticipate and desire further engagement in occupations based upon their belief that further occupational doing would sustain their new-found confidence and maintain their sense of feeling better.

Occupational spin-off is a conceptualization of the experience of occupational engagement for the members of The Women's Group. The descriptions of their experiences indicate that occupational therapists need to attend to both the environment and to the occupation, in order to impact the person, their client. The provision of opportunity, not prescription, enabled members to engage in occupations of choice which positively affected their sense of subjective well-being and mental health.

ACKNOWLEDGEMENTS

The authors would like to acknowledge Dr. J. Polgar for her assistance during the thesis process, and The Canadian Occupational Therapy Foundation for its financial support of this study.

References

Ambrosi, E., & Barker Schwartz, K. (1995). The profession's image, 1917–1925, part II: Occupational therapy as represented by the media. *American Journal of Occupational Therapy, 49,* 828–832.

American Occupational Therapy Association. (1979). Resolution D(532-79): Occupation as the common core of occupational therapy. *American Journal of Occupational Therapy, 33,* 785.

American Occupational Therapy Association. (1995). Position paper on occupation. *American Journal of Occupational Therapy, 49,* 1015–1018.

Anthony, W.A. & Lieberman, R.P. (1986). The practice of psychiatric rehabilitation: Historical, conceptual and research base. *Schizophrenia Bulletin, 12,* 542–559.

Barris, R. Kielhofner, G. & Hawkins Watts, J. (1983). *Psychosocial occupational therapy: Practice in a pluralistic arena.* Laurel, MD: RAMSCO.

Becker, H.S. (1986). *Writing for social scientists.* Chicago, IL: University of Chicago Press.

Berger, P.L. (1963). *Invitation to sociology: A humanistic perspective.* Garden City, NY: Doubleday.

Breines, E. (1989). The issue is. Making a difference: A premise of occupation and health. *American Journal of Occupational Therapy, 43,* 51–52.

Canadian Association of Occupational Therapists. (1991). *Occupational therapy guidelines for client-centred practice.* Toronto, ON: CAOT Publications ACE.

Canadian Association of Occupational Therapists. (1997). *Enabling occupation: An occupational therapy perspective.* Ottawa, ON: CAOT Publications ACE.

Carlson, M., & Dunlea, A. (1995). The issue is: Further thoughts on the pitfalls of partition: A response to Mosey. *American Journal of Occupational Therapy, 49,* 75.

Christiansen, C. (1991). Occupational therapy intervention for life performance (pp. 1–43). In C. Christiansen & C. Baum (Eds.), *Occupational therapy: Overcoming human performance deficits.* Thorofare, NJ: Slack.

Christiansen, C. (1994). Classification and study in occupation. A review and discussion of taxonomies. *Journal of Occupational Science, 1*(3), 3–21.

Clark, F.A., Parham, D., Carlson, M.E., Frank, G., Jackson, J., Pierce, D., Wolfe, R.J., & Zemke, R. (1991). Occupational science: Academic innovation in the services of occupational therapy's future. *American Journal of Occupational Therapy, 45,* 300–310.

Corring, D. (1996). *Client-centred care means I am a valued human being.* Unpublished master's thesis. The University of Western Ontario, London, ON.

Cynkin, S., & Masur Robinson, A. (1990). *Occupational therapy and activities health: Toward health through activities.* Boston, MA: Little, Brown.

DePoy, E. & Gitlin, L.N. (1994). *Introduction to research: Multiple strategies for health and human services.* St. Louis, MO: Mosby.

Diasio, K. (1971). The modern era—1960 to 1970. *American Journal of Occupational Therapy, 25,* 237–242.

Dunton, W. R. (1918). *Occupation therapy: A manual for nurses.* Philadelphia, PA: W.B. Saunders.

Emerson, H. (1996). *Enjoyment as described by persons with schizophrenia.* Unpublished master's thesis. The University of Western Ontario, London, ON.

Englehart, T. H. (1977). Defining occupational therapy: The meaning of therapy and the virtues of occupation. *American Journal of Occupational Therapy, 31,* 666–672.

Estroff, S.E. (1989). Self, identity, and subjective experiences of schizophrenia: In search of the subject. *Schizophrenia Bulletin, 15,* 189–196.

Estroff, S.E. (1991). Everybody's got a little mental illness: Accounts of illness and self among people with severe, persistent mental illness. *Medical Anthropology Quarterly, 5,* 331–369.

Fidler, G. (1981). From crafts to competence. *American Journal of Occupational Therapy, 35,* 567–573.

Fidler, G. & Fidler, J. (1978). Doing and becoming: Purposeful action and self-actualization. *American Journal of Occupational Therapy, 32,* 305–310.

Fossey, E. (1992). The study of human occupations: Implications for research in occupational therapy. *British Journal of Occupational Therapy, 55,* 148–152.

Glaser, B.G., & Strauss, A.L. (1967). *The discovery of grounded theory.* Chicago: Aldine.

Goffman, E. (1963). *Stigma: Notes on the management of spoiled identity.* New York, NY: Simon & Schuster.

Jackson, M. (1993). From work to therapy: The changing politics of occupation in the twentieth century. *British Journal of Occupational Therapy, 56,* 360–364.

Johnson, J. (1971). Consideration of work as therapy in the rehabilitation process. *American Journal of Occupational Therapy, 25,* 303–308.

Jorgenson, D. L. (1989). *Participant observation: A methodology for human studies.* Newbury Park, CA: Sage.

Kielhofner, G. (1992). *Conceptual foundations of occupational therapy.* Philadelphia, PA: F.A. Davis.

Kielhofner, G., & Burke, J.P. (1977). Occupational therapy after 60 years: An account of changing identity and knowledge. *American Journal of Occupational Therapy, 31,* 675–689.

LaLiberte, D. (1995). *An exploration of the meaning seniors attach to activity.* Unpublished master's thesis. The University of Western Ontario, London, ON.

LaMore, K.L., & Nelson, D.L. (1993). The effects of options on performance in an art project in adults with mental disabilities. *American Journal of Occupational Therapy, 47,* 397–401.

LeVesconte, H.P. (1935). Expanding fields of occupational therapy. *Canadian Journal of Occupational Therapy, 3,* 4–12. [Reprinted (1986) In: *Canadian Journal of Occupational Therapy, 53,* 9–15.]

Lilley, J., & Jackson, L.T. (1993). The value of activities: Establishing a foundation for cost-effectiveness—a review of the literature. *Activities, Adaptation & Aging, 18,* 49–65.

Lincoln, Y. & Guba, E. (1985). *Naturalistic inquiry.* Beverly Hills, CA: Sage.

MacGregor, L. (1995). *An exploration study of the personal experience of occupational deprivation.* Unpublished master's thesis. The University of Western Ontario, London, ON.

McCracken, G. (1988). *The long interview.* Newbury Park, CA: Sage.

Meyer, A. (1922). The philosophy of occupational therapy. *Archives of Occupational Therapy, 1,* (pp. 1–10). [Reprinted (1977) In: *American Journal of Occupational Therapy, 31,* 639–642.]

Mosey, A. (1971). Involvement in the rehabilitation movement—1942–1960. *American Journal of Occupational Therapy, 25,* 234–236.

Mosey, A.C. (1989). The proper focus of scientific inquiry in occupational therapy: Frames of reference. *Occupational Therapy Journal of Research, 9,* 195–201.

Nelson, D.L. (1988). Occupation: Form and performance. *American Journal of Occupational Therapy, 42,* 633–641.

Ottenbacher, K.J. (1992). Confusion in occupational therapy research: Does the end justify the method? *American Journal of Occupational Therapy, 46,* 871–874.

Rebeiro, K.L. (1997). *Opportunity, not prescription: An exploratory study of the experience of occupational engagement.* Unpublished master's thesis. The University of Western Ontario, London, Ontario.

Rebeiro, K.L. (1998). Occupation-as-means to mental health: A review of the literature and a call to research. *Canadian Journal of Occupational Therapy, 65,* 12–19.

Reilly, M. (1962). Occupational therapy can be one of the great ideas of 20th century medicine. *American Journal of Occupational Therapy, 16,* 1–9.

Reilly, M. (1966). The challenge of the future to an occupational therapist. *American Journal of Occupational Therapy, 20,* 221–225.

Reilly, M. (1971). The modernization of occupational therapy. *American Journal of Occupational Therapy, 25,* 243–246.

Renwick, R., & Brown, L. (1996). The centre for health promotion's conceptual approach to quality of life (pp. 75–86). In R. Renwick, I. Brown, & M. Nager (Eds.), *Quality of life in health promotion and rehabilitation: Conceptual approaches, issues, and applications.* Thousands Oaks, CA: Sage.

Rerek, M. (1971). The depression years—1929 to 1941. *American Journal of Occupational Therapy, 25,* 231–233.

Rogers, J.C. (1984). Why study human occupation? *American Journal of Occupational Therapy, 38,* 47–49.

Scheid, T.L. & Anderson, C. (1995). Living with chronic mental illness: Understanding the role of work. *Community Mental Health Journal, 31,* 163–176.

Shannon, P.D. (1977). The derailment of occupational therapy. *American Journal of Occupational Therapy, 31,* 229–234.

Shaw, L.L. (1991). Stigma and the moral careers of ex-mental patients living in board and care. *Journal of Contemporary Ethnography, 20,* 285–305.

Trombly, C. (1995). Occupation: Purposefulness and meaningfulness as therapeutic mechanisms. *American Journal of Occupational Therapy, 49,* 960–972.

West, W.L. (1984). A reaffirmed philosophy and practice of occupational therapy for the 1980's. *American Journal of Occupational Therapy, 38,* 15–23.

Wilcock, A. (1993). A theory of the human need for occupation. *Occupational Science: Australia, 1*(1), 17–24.

Wood, W. (1993). Occupation and the relevance of primatology to occupational therapy. *American Journal of Occupational Therapy, 47,* 515–522.

Woodside, H. (1971). The development of occupational therapy 1910–1929. *American Journal of Occupational Therapy, 25,* 226–230.

Yerxa, E.J. (1967). Authentic occupational therapy. *The American Journal of Occupational Therapy, 21,* 1–9.

Yerxa, E.J. (1991). Occupational therapy: An endangered species or an academic discipline in the 21st century? *American Journal of Occupational Therapy, 45,* 680–685.

Yerxa, E.J., Clark, F., Frank, G., Jackson, J., Parham, D., Pierce, D., Stein, C., & Zemke, R. (1990). An introduction to occupational science: A foundation for occupational therapy in the 21st century (pp. 1–17). In J.A. Johnson (Ed.) & E.J. Yerxa (Co-Ed.), *Occupational science: The foundation for new models of practice.* New York, NY: Haworth Press.

Chapter 16

The Use of Standardized Assessment in Occupational Therapy: The BaFPE-R as an Example

The American Journal of Occupational Therapy

1993, 47(10): 877–884

Mary F. Managh, Joanne Valiant Cook

Mary F. Managh, MSc, OT(C), is Senior Occupational Therapist—Research, Clarke Institute of Psychiatry, 250 College Street, Toronto, Ontario, Canada M5T 1R8.
Joanne Valiant Cook, PhD, OT(C), is Assistant Professor, Department of Occupational Therapy, University of Western Ontario, London, Ontario, Canada.

KEY WORDS

- professional practice
- qualitative method
- values clarification

ABSTRACT

Before 1970, most assessments administered by occupational therapists were informal and nonstandardized. Since the 1970s, the use of scientifically sound instruments has increased. One such standardized assessment, the Bay Area Functional Performance Evaluation (BaFPE), was developed to measure the functional performance of psychiatric clients. This study was designed to explore the use of a revised version of BaFPE as an example of standardized assessment in occupational therapy.

The BaFPE was selected as an example of an assessment extensively used in psychiatric occupational therapy practice. A qualitative study that used in-depth semistructured interviews was conducted with a convenience sample of occupational therapists.

The occupational therapists who were interviewed described and explained making several adaptations and modifications to the recommended administration and scoring of the BaFPE. An analysis of the interview data suggested that standardized assessments are valued as indicators of professional status. However, the interview responses also suggested that the demands of test standardization were incongruent with the values that guide occupational therapy practice.

The findings of this study suggest that the future development and use of standardized instruments should be consistent with the values of the profession. In particular, assessments that recognize the diverse nature and needs of individual clients are required.

A person's ability to perform the tasks required to function successfully in his or her daily life is of fundamental concern to occupational therapists (Kielhofner, 1992). Traditionally, many occupational therapists have used homemade assessment tools such as checklists to assess function (Leonardelli Haertlein, 1992; Smith, 1992; Stein, 1988). Before 1970, most assessments administered by occupational therapists were informal and nonstandardized (Stein, 1988). Since the 1970s, however, scientifically sound instruments have been developed in an attempt to document client status and change more accurately, as well as to demonstrate treatment effectiveness (Watts, Brollier, & Schmidt, 1988).

The trend in the profession toward the use of standardized assessment has been followed by occupational therapists specializing in mental health (Hemphill, 1980; Moyer, 1984; Thibeault & Blackmer, 1987; Watts et al., 1988). The Bay Area Functional Performance Evaluation (BaFPE) was one of the first standardized instruments developed by occupational therapists for use with psychiatric clients (Bloomer & Williams, 1978; Watts et al., 1988). According to the test developers, the BaFPE was designed to measure some behaviors that persons must exhibit to carry out activities of daily living (Bloomer & Williams, 1978). The original version of the BaFPE was revised and a second edition (BaFPE-R) was published in 1987 in an attempt to improve its standardization and clinical utility (Houston, Williams, Bloomer, & Mann, 1989). This revised version is widely used by occupational therapists in psychiatry (Mann, Klyczek, & Fiedler, 1989). For the purposes of clarity, the revised BaFPE will be referred to as the BaFPE-R in this paper.

The BaFPE-R consists of two subtests, the Task-Oriented Assessment (TOA) and the Social Interaction Scale (SIS). The TOA is designed to assess general ability to act on the environment in specific goal-directed ways, and the SIS is designed to assess general ability to relate appropriately to people within the environment. Interrater reliability and internal consistency of the BaFPE-R has been established and some evidence of the validity of the instrument has been published (Williams & Bloomer, 1987).

Leonardelli Haertlein (1992) and Smith (1992) in the United States, Eakin (1989) in Britain, and Fricke and Unsworth (1992) in Australia have reported that the modification of standardized assessments in occupational therapy practice is widespread. During discussions with clinicians about the clinical use of the BaFPE-R, the principal investigator learned that there were often variations in the purposes for assessment use, methods of administration, and interpretation of the results. In an article dealing with current issues in occupational therapy assessment, Smith (1992) asserted that "we have not addressed the most critical questions pertaining to how occupational therapists collect data and what occupational therapists do with it" (p. 3). With these issues in mind, an exploratory study examining the clinical use of the BaFPE-R by an available sample of occupational therapists was conducted in 1991. The selection of the BaFPE-R as an example of standardized assessments was based on its reputation in the literature. Mann et al. (1989) have documented its extensive use and Leonardelli Haertlein (1992) described it as one of the assessments "setting the current standard for occupational therapy evaluation" (p. 952).

The study consisted of chart audits of occupational therapy department records and semistructured interviews with occupational therapists who used the BaFPE-R. The purposes of the research were to describe the demographic characteristics of both the clinicians who used the BaFPE-R and the assessed clients, to explore why and how the assessment was administered, and to determine how the assessment results were interpreted and used.

This paper focuses on three aspects of the study to provide (a) a classification of the therapists' descriptions of their administration of the BaFPE-R and their analysis and use of the assessment results, (b) an interpretive analysis of the therapists' descriptions, and (c) a discussion of the implications for the development and use of standardized assessment in occupational therapy.

METHOD

Sample

Thirty occupational therapists in four cities were interviewed. Each therapist was practicing in psychiatry and had used the BaFPE-R during the previous 2 years. The interviewees were graduates of nine different occupational therapy programs, both domestic and foreign. The sample included 18 (60%) therapists who were graduates of the same university program. Twenty-one (70%) of the therapists were employed at provincial psychiatric hospitals and 9 (30%) were employed in psychiatric units of general hospitals. On average, the therapists had been practicing occupational therapy for 7.5 years and had been practicing in psychiatry for almost 6 years. The mean length of employment at the therapists' current facility was 4.4 years.

Procedure and Instrument

Face-to-face, in-depth, semistructured interviews were used because of the exploratory nature of the study. This research method allows the interviewer to establish a "peer" relationship with the respondents (Lincoln & Guba, 1985, p. 269) and provides opportunities to ask questions relating to context and meaning (Schatzman & Strauss, 1973; Spradley, 1979). All interviews were conducted at the therapists' place of employment and recorded on audiotape by the first author. The length of the interviews ranged from 30 to 80 min. Typically, the interviews were "more like conversations than formally structured interviews" (Marshall & Rossman, 1989, p. 82). Using this technique, "the researcher explores a few general topics to help uncover the participant's meaning perspective, but otherwise respects how the participant frames and structures the responses" (Marshall & Rossman, 1989, p. 82).

The interview questions were based on the first author's personal use of the BaFPE-R and on a review of the literature about standardized assessments, including the BaFPE-R. The interview guide was elaborated and refined after pilot trials. Eight topic areas were covered in the interview: demographic and clinical information, use of the assessment, perceptions of the purposes of the BaFPE-R, administration of the assessment and analysis of the assessment results, assessment of clients' reactions to the BaFPE-R, therapists' knowledge of the BaFPE-R, evaluation of the strengths and weaknesses of the assessment, and attitudes toward standardized assessments in general (see Appendix).

Analytic Procedures

The taped interviews were transcribed by the first author and analyzed according to the methods described by Marshall and Rossman, who stated that

> analytic procedures fall into five modes: organizing the data; generating categories, themes, and patterns; testing the emergent hypotheses against the data; searching for alternative explanations of the data; and writing the report. Each phase of data analysis entails data reduction as the reams of collected data are brought into manageable chunks and interpretation as the researcher brings meaning and insight to the words and acts of the participants in the study (1989, p. 114).

In accord with these conventions of qualitative data analysis, the therapists' responses were organized into categories of patterns and themes. Sets of interrelated responses were compared logically, theoretically, and empirically with other findings (Polgar & Thomas, 1988). The interpretation of the patterns and themes was derived from the literature on the profession of occupational therapy and its values (Kielhofner, 1992; Shannon, 1977; Yerxa, 1983).

The emergent analysis and interpretation of the study results were examined by academic peers and members of the occupational therapy profession, including some who were involved in the study. The purpose of this examination was to assess the trustworthiness of the research (Guba, 1981; Krefting, 1990; Lincoln & Guba, 1985).

RESULTS

Reasons for the Use of the BaFPE-R

The categories of reasons that therapists provided for using the BaFPE-R, in order of frequency of responses, were (a) departmental procedure, (b) time efficiency, (c) screening function, (d) attitudes of multidisciplinary teams, (e) support for other assessments, (f) therapeutic medium, and (g) evaluation of task performance. Examples of these reasons, selected from the interview transcripts, follow.

Departmental procedure. The most commonly reported rationale for use of the BaFPE-R was that it was the standardized assessment that the occupational therapy department had decided therapists would routinely use.

Respondent 2: It is our standard tool . . . we made the decision that [it] was the tool we were going to use as a standard assessment for assessing task skills.

Respondent 1: All our patients, other than those with dementia or those who are illiterate or have poor English, get the test because it's part of our assessment process.

Time efficiency. The second most frequently cited reason for using the BaFPE-R rather than alternate assessments was that the BaFPE-R could be administered and scored in less time.

Respondent 17: It's a very quick turnover [on the unit]. They're allowed to stay 6 weeks, but they don't stay that long. And this is why the BaFPE [-R] is very useful. Because you do a quick one-shot assessment. That's why I'd use it, because time is a factor on admission units.

Respondent 9: It [the BaFPE-R] was probably meeting my needs, because I had to have something done quickly with [patients], because they likely weren't going to be in that long and at least this gave me some quick and dirty observations that I could get into a clinical note.

Screening function. Therapists reported that the BaFPE-R was often used for two screening

purposes. As the following statements suggest, therapists found the BaFPE-R helpful in establishing the clients' level of functional performance to determine whether occupational therapy intervention was required:

Respondent 13: It can also be an indicator of [whether] OT is required. . . . If they do super well [on the BaFPE-R], there may not be a need for extensive OT involvement.

Respondent 17: Sometimes they're very functional so I don't want them in OT because I don't feel they need it.

The second screening function was to identify difficulties in specific functional performance component areas. The recognition of these impairments then justified placement of the client in a particular occupational therapy group.

Respondent 18: I find it's very good as far as highlighting organization, memory, kinds of activities they do best on, structured versus unstructured . . . it helps me to pick the kind of activity that I would probably give them.

Attitudes of multidisciplinary teams. Many of the therapists interviewed indicated that their use of the BaFPE-R was influenced by the multidisciplinary team with which they were affiliated. Most explained, in some way, that their multidisciplinary team preferred standardized assessments to nonstandardized assessments.

Respondent 15: For the initial assessment, they prefer that it be a standardized test. . . . If they didn't know about it [the BaFPE-R], and if they didn't want me to use standardized tests, I might not tend to use it as much.

Respondent 2: Our psychiatrists challenge the OTs about the test [BaFPE-R]. They place a lot of importance on traditional standardized psychological tests such as the MMPI . . . they always felt we [OTs] didn't have a lot of basis in scientific method because we didn't have a standardized assessment. . . . The main expectation that psychiatrists have of the OT on the team is [providing] information about the patient's functioning. Psychiatrists are concerned with pathology, while [the] OT is the team member that accentuates the strengths of the patient. The OTs' initial concern, when the test was first used, was that it reflected the medical model of psychiatrists, rather than the client-centered model [of occupational therapy]. . . . Psychology is particularly interested in the BaFPE[-R] results. OT and psychology [testing] results often correlate. . . . Nursing has focused more on subjective information, while OT now has objective information instead of relying on observation.

Several of the therapists interviewed reported publicizing the BaFPE-R in grand rounds or inservices at their facilities. One respondent explained as follows:

Respondent 17: Most of them [the team] are [familiar with the BaFPE-R] because I've done an inservice on it. In fact, we flaunt it around here.

Supportive purposes. Therapists reported that the BaFPE-R was used to support clinical observations and to complement other life skills assessments.

Respondent 25: The BaFPE[R] gives me [a] back-up as to why they're not able to do certain things, like if they can't follow [the] directions of a complex task, can't concentrate, [or] are poorly organized. It gives me reasons why they're dysfunctional in those areas.

The BaFPE-R as a therapeutic medium. In addition to evaluating clients' current level of functioning, the BaFPE-R was used as a therapeutic medium. Therapists recounted that the feedback clients received from the BaFPE-R results often improved client self-esteem and self-confidence.

Respondent 7: One lady said "I can't concentrate, I can't do anything." I had something to show her. [I said that] "even though you're feeling that way, you scored 20 out of 20 on Attention Span, [and] your Memory for Instructions was 20." I can show her that, when she did this formal test . . . [her attention span] wasn't a problem area.

Respondent 6: [If the patient has] functional difficulties, [if he is] unable to cope with dependency and his world has become very small because of his illness, I might do the BaFPE[-R] to give [him] some concrete feedback.

Evaluation of task performance. Five therapists stated that the principal strength of the assessment was that it is task-based. They reported that they preferred the BaFPE-R because it requires the client to "perform" specific actions rather than merely respond to verbal or written questions. The following quotation represents this view:

Respondent 13: The biggest strength, as far as I'm concerned, is that it's task based. That is, to me, tremendously significant. As opposed to other standardized interviews, self-report questionnaires, [that ask] "how do you do in . . .?" [the BaFPE-R] is task based . . . I believe, certainly for the population that we deal with in the provincial system, I question the validity of self-report questionnaires [that ask] "do you have problems with . . .?"

In summary, the clinicians who used the BaFPE-R provided numerous rationales for their use of the assessment. These rationales included the influence of departmental policy, the time efficiency of the assessment, its screening function, the influence of the multidisciplinary team, its usefulness as an adjunct to other assessments, its therapeutic value, and its emphasis on task performance.

Variations in Assessment Administration and Analysis of Assessment Results

The developers of the BaFPE-R provided specific guidelines for the administration of the assessment and for the interpretation of the results (Williams & Bloomer, 1987). Therapists interviewed in this study reported varying degrees of deviation from the guidelines described in the assessment manual. Some of these variations in the administration of the assessment and in the interpretation of the results were consistent with the assessment guidelines. Conversely, some of the adaptations and modifications described did not conform to the developers' specifications. Many of these adaptations were explained in terms of the value therapists placed upon the therapeutic alliance and what they considered to be in their clients' best interests. The interview responses indicated three main areas where variations in therapists' use of the BaFPE-R were common: (a) exclusion of the Social Interaction Scale (SIS), (b) exclusion of the Qualitative Signs and Referral Indicators Section (QSRIS), and (c) modifications to the administration and scoring of the Task Oriented Assessment (TOA).

Exclusion of Social Interaction Scale. The most common form of variation in the administration of the BaFPE-R was the exclusion of the SIS. Twenty-six (86.7%) of the clinicians interviewed stated they had not used the SIS in the past 6 months. The assessment developers emphasized that the evaluation of functional performance should include both the task performance and social interaction scales (Williams & Bloomer, 1987). Therefore, clinicians who had only used the TOA can be said to have assessed task performance rather than functional performance using the BaFPE-R.

Therapists offered various reasons for not using the SIS. One frequently cited reason was that other therapists were not observed using the scale. Others reported that the SIS was not used because social interaction was routinely assessed by the observation of clients in therapy groups. Of most concern to therapists was the length of time required to rate the SIS. As one therapist stated:

Respondent 27: I used [the SIS] once, some time ago, but I just found that the amount of time that I had to put into the paper work wasn't conducive. As far as I can remember, I think that the areas that it covered were quite relevant. It's just that I felt I had an awareness of that sort of summary through my observations. It was more of a paper task that wasn't revealing something unusual to me that I wasn't aware of [already].

Exclusion of the Qualitative Signs and Referral Indicators Section. According to the assessment developers, the QSRIS is an optional component of the TOA that may provide information about possible organic involvement (Williams

& Bloomer, 1987). Six of the therapists interviewed stated they had not used the QSRIS at all. Of those therapists who reported that they had used the section occasionally, 11 therapists said that the QSRIS was only used if the client had previously exhibited organic signs. Some therapists who had not used the QSRIS stated that, with experience, they had learned to identify signs of organic involvement independently through observation of the client in other situations.

Respondent 13: Organicity is something . . . you can just tell, and yet the screening factors [on the QSRIS] wouldn't pick it up any more than with any schizophrenic who has the same kinds of problems of inability to abstract. . . . It was usually with clinical observation that you [could] say "there's something wrong here."

Adaptations and modifications in the administration and scoring of the TOA. When asked during the interview if they had ever adapted or modified the assessment administration, most therapists said they had not. However, in explaining their experience and use of the assessment, 21 therapists (70%) described some modifications they had made and their reasons for doing so. The majority of reasons given for the adaptations related to therapist's perceptions of clients' needs. Although therapists provided many examples of deviations from the assessment protocol of the TOA, three variations were most commonly described: (a) alteration of task completion time, (b) deviation from the protocols for scoring and analysis of results, and (c) modification of the verbatim instructions.

With regard to the first variation, 19 therapists (63%) stated that the guidelines for task completion time on the TOA were not always followed. Five therapists reported that additional important information about clients' task functioning could be gained if the client was permitted to complete the task rather than stop when the allotted time had expired. Several therapists explained that clients were allowed to complete tasks on the TOA to maintain their self-esteem. One of these therapists reported as follows:

> Respondent 6: *I don't want them to think I'm setting them up for failure. They get a certain satisfaction from completing it.*

Other therapists were concerned about the negative effect that timing the task had on client performance.

> Respondent 9: *It puts pressure on them that they can't tolerate, knowing that they're timed, so they probably don't function as well as they can. It affects performance.*

With regard to the second variation, deviations from the TOA scoring protocol and the guidelines for analysis of the results were made almost as often as the time allotted for assessment completion was altered. Nineteen therapists (63%) reported that they did not use the norms published in the BaFPE-R manual (Williams & Bloomer, 1987). None of the therapists interviewed had ever used the norms published by Mann et al. (1989) and Mann and Klyczek (1991). Therapists at one provincial psychiatric hospital reported that neither the scoring format nor the norms for the TOA were used. Conversely, therapists at a general hospital stated that they used the scoring protocol outlined in the manual. However, instead of comparing these scores to the norms, they used other methods of interpreting the scores.

Many therapists provided more than one reason for their decision to alter the scoring or the protocols used for analysis of the assessment results. Some reported that the length of time taken to score the assessment deterred them from using the formal scoring protocol. Other therapists made observations of performance while the client was completing the TOA. These observations were described as more useful than the actual task scores. Ten therapists (33%) expressed concerns with the scoring criteria for the TOA. Some said that they questioned the reliability of the scoring procedures. Three therapists did not score the TOA because of these concerns.

Therapists discussed their differing reservations about comparing clients' scores on the TOA to the normative scores. Some therapists chose not to use the normative data at all; others continued to persevere with their use of the norms despite misgivings. Six therapists stated that they believed the norms for the TOA were not applicable to their client population. The small sample size of the normative group was a concern to two therapists interviewed. Another two therapists considered the use of norms for the TOA to be unimportant. Some therapists stated that they decided not to use the norms for the TOA after observing that other therapists were not using them. Others explained that they believed the use of the TOA norms would not be fair to the client. They were particularly concerned that the client might be labelled as a result of the performance scores. One therapist exemplified the hesitation expressed by many therapists about the use of the standardized scoring and norms in the following words:

> Respondent 6: *I think there must have been some reason why I didn't think it was fair for me to document those [scores in comparison to the norms]. I must have compared them to some psychology test and felt that it's not fair to write this judgment down, to be on someone's file forever. . . . I report everything as being my own impression, not absolute. Sometimes the things you put in the notes have a lot of power. They can make long-standing impressions on future people who are involved with the client.*

With regard to the third variation, 18 therapists (60%) reported that they modified the provision of the written and verbatim instructions for the TOA. Some therapists paraphrased the instructions; others used verbal prompting. They offered several reasons for choosing to adapt the provision of the verbatim or written instructions. Some stated that more information about clients' performance could be obtained if the verbatim instructions were modified. Others believed that presenting the TOA instructions in a standardized form was demeaning to clients. Several therapists emphasized that the method by which the assessment instructions are delivered should be individualized for each client. Four therapists reported that the provision of assessment instructions was altered to ensure that the client achieved success during the therapy session. One therapist explained as follows:

> Respondent 11: Occasionally, [I paraphrase the instructions] to meet the needs of an individual patient. It's difficult not to try and explain the instructions in another way and see if they can understand if you rephrase it. . . . The abstraction question, in the second edition, is poorly worded. I often need to rephrase it. "Skills" is a lingo word. Patients don't think of the specific things we do. I might reword [the question to say] "what do you need to be able to do in order to do this task?"

The information gleaned from the interviews with therapists who used the BaFPE-R indicated that there were perceived positive influences on the decision to use this assessment. Simultaneously, however, perceived needs and contingencies to alter its standardized administration appeared to exist. Some suggested interpretations of this paradox follow.

INTERPRETATIVE UNDERSTANDING

The results of this exploratory study support the assertions of other authors on the widespread practice of modifying standardized assessments in occupational therapy (Eakin, 1989; Fricke & Unsworth, 1992; Leonardelli Haertlein, 1992; Smith, 1992). The content of therapists' explanations provides some suggestions as to why assessment adaptation is occurring. Professional issues and values appeared to permeate the responses of most interviewees. The responses centered on the therapists' values and beliefs about clients' needs and the perceived obligations of occupational therapy practice.

Most therapists interviewed directly expressed or indirectly indicated an ambivalence toward standardized assessments. They expressed a need to use standardized assessments, such as the BaFPE-R, yet they were concerned about the incompatibility of the assessment with the therapeutic aims of their practice. Many stated that their decision to use the assessment was influenced by the professional image that their multidisciplinary team colleagues, especially psychiatrists and psychologists, associated with the use of standardized assessments. It appears that they used the reporting of the BaFPE-R results in team meetings as an indicator of professional status. These therapists described their use of the BaFPE-R as a means to developing a professional identity and improving the recognition and credibility afforded their profession. The BaFPE-R seemed to serve as an outward manifestation of the scientific base of occupational therapy.

This commitment to the use of a standardized assessment was often constrained by the perceived inability of the BaFPE-R to identify and address the specific needs of individual clients. Most therapists alluded to a desire to address the unique needs of each client rather than merely the manifestations or symptoms of the disease. Many reported that the guidelines of the standardized procedures inhibited their ability to attend to persons' needs. Although they did aspire to gain the acceptance and recognition of the multidisciplinary team, it appeared that following the administration protocol was incongruent with the therapists' inclination to treat clients as individuals.

Kielhofner (1992), Shannon (1977), and Yerxa (1983), among many others, have examined the relationship between the core values of occupational therapists and the influence of science, scientific methods, and the reductionistic approach to health and illness. These authors provide possible reasons for the ambivalence reported by the therapists interviewed in this study.

The education of occupational therapists includes instruction in the administration of standardized assessments and the necessity for the reliability and validity of such instruments. Additionally, through their education and socialization to practice, occupational therapists tend to adopt the core values and assumptions of the profession (Department of Health and Welfare Canada and Canadian Association of Occupational Therapists, 1983; Kielhofner, 1992; Yerxa, 1983). These values reflect a strong tendency "to focus on the assets of individuals and to emphasize the therapeutic process" (Kielhofner, 1992, p. 73). According to Kielhofner, "another deeply ingrained value of occupational therapy is the belief in capacity and the therapist's obligation to tease out that capacity" (1992, p. 73). The findings of this study illustrate the continuing commitment to those core values and beliefs that have underpinned the profession of occupational therapy since its inception. As Kielhofner stated, values "are very important guides to action" (1992, p. 73). Knowledge of the values expressed by the therapists in this study contributes to an understanding of the manner of using and modifying assessments such as the BaFPE-R.

The therapists modified the administration and scoring of the BaFPE-R to "tease out" their clients' capacities at the expense of the standardized protocol. It appears that the values of a humanistic, client-centered practice outweighed the values of a reductionistic, scientific approach to practice. Their desire to maintain and enhance client strengths rather than to focus on deficits appeared to guide the therapists' modified use of the standardized instrument.

IMPLICATIONS

The results of this study raise several questions in regard to occupational therapy research and practice. Most current research in the profession relies on the use of standardized assessments to measure the variables of concern. As this was an exploratory study, the findings described cannot be generalized to the use of other standardized assessments. Similar studies to the one reported here, examining the use of other standardized instruments are, therefore, required. Such research needs to address questions regarding the extent to which the nonstandardized administration of assessments influences the reliability and validity of research based on these assessment results.

The implications for clinical practice appear to be as salient as the implications for research. The results of this study were interpreted in terms of the strength of occupational therapists' commitment to approaches that emphasize each client's unique strengths. This interpretation challenges the profession to develop assessments that recognize the importance of that therapeutic goal, that is, to develop assessments that meet our clinical responsibilities, our values, and our clients' needs. Such instruments must demonstrate acceptable psychometric properties without diminishing our recognition of the capacities and holistic nature of our clients. The incongruity between professional values and the demands of standardization, as currently professed, require careful examination and, ultimately, resolution.

ACKNOWLEDGMENTS

We thank Samuel Noh, PhD. thesis co-advisor, and Helene Polatajko, PhD. of the thesis advisory committee. We are indebted to Carrie Clark for her critical evaluation, to Elizabeth Scott, MSc for her editorial assistance, and to Elizabeth Yerxa, EdD. for her encouragement and support. In addition, we thank all of the occupational therapists who participated in this study for their open and honest sharing of their clinical experiences.

This paper is based on research the first author conducted in partial fulfillment of the requirements for the degree of Master of Science at the University of Western Ontario, London, Ontario, Canada.

Appendix
Clinician Interview Guide: Revised

Demographic and Clinical information
1.1 When did you get your occupational therapy qualification?
1.2 At which university?
1.3 How long have you practiced here, at this facility?
1.4 And how long in psychiatry?
1.5 What clinical team are you affiliated with?
1.6 What is the average length of stay of patients on your unit?
1.7 What are your main duties?

Use of the Instrument
2.1 Are you using the first or second edition of the BaFPE? [Have you ever used the (other) edition?]
2.2 How often do you use it?
2.3 Which patients do you use the BaFPE with [describe age, diagnosis, acute or chronic]?

Purpose of the BaFPE
3.1 What do you think the purpose of the BaFPE is?
3.2 What do you think the developers of the BaFPE intended it for?

Administration of the BaFPE and Analysis of Results
4.1 Which of the subtests do you administer? [Why do you not use (___) subtest/component?]
4.2 Have you ever made any adaptations to the BaFPE?
4.3 How do you interpret patients' scores? [If norms not used, elaborate]
4.4 What do you use the results from the BaFPE for?
4.5 How much does the patient's performance on the BaFPE affect your planning?
4.6 Who do you discuss the evaluation results with?
4.7 Are other members of your multidisciplinary team familiar with the BaFPE?

Patient Reaction to the BaFPE
5.1 How do your patients react to the BaFPE?
5.2 How often are you unable to complete it in one session?
5.3 How often are you unable to complete it at all?
5.4 How long does it usually take for you to administer the BaFPE?
5.5 And to write up the results?
5.6 Do you think a shortened version of the BaFPE would be useful to you?

Knowledge of the BaFPE
6.1 How did you first learn about the BaFPE?
6.2 How were you trained to use it?
6.3 Are you familiar with the BaFPE manual?
6.4 Are you familiar with any studies that examine the BaFPE?

Evaluation of the Assessment
7.1 How much do you think the results on the BaFPE reflect the patients' actual functional status?
7.2 Do you think the BaFPE is reliable?
7.3 And valid?
7.4 What do you think are the strengths of the BaFPE?
7.5 And its weaknesses or shortcomings?
7.6 Do you think any of the items are inappropriate for cultural or other reasons?
7.7 Have you ever taught or trained another occupational therapist or occupational therapy student to use the BaFPE?
7.8 Have you ever recommended it to other occupational therapists or occupational therapy students?

Standardized Tests
8.1 How important do you think it is that we as occupational therapists in psychiatry use standardized tests?

Note. These questions guided the interview and were not asked verbatim. Probe questions, not shown here, were used to elucidate salient points raised by interviewees.

References

Bloomer, J. S., & Williams, S. L. (1978). *Bay Area Functional Performance Evaluation.* Palo Alto, CA: Consulting Psychologists Press.

Department of Health and Welfare Canada and Canadian Association of Occupational Therapists. (1983). *Guidelines for the client-centred practice of occupational therapy* (H39-33/1983E). Ottawa, ON: Department of National Health and Welfare.

Eakin, P. (1989). Assessments of activities of daily living: A critical review. *British Journal of Occupational Therapy, 52,* 11–15.

Fricke, J., & Unsworth, C. (1992). The status of activities of daily living: A Victorian perspective. *Australian Occupational Therapy Journal, 39,* 29–31.

Guba, E. G. (1981). Criteria for assessing the trustworthiness of naturalistic inquiries. *Educational Communication and Technology Journal, 29,* 75–91.

Hemphill, B. J. (1980). Mental health evaluations used in occupational therapy. *American Journal of Occupational Therapy, 34,* 721–725.

Houston, D., Williams, S., Bloomer, J., & Mann, W. (1989). The Bay Area Functional Performance Evaluation: Development and standardization. *American Journal of Occupational Therapy, 43,* 170–183.

Kielhofner, G. (1992). *Conceptual foundations of occupational therapy.* Philadelphia: F. A. Davis.

Krefting, L. (1990). Rigor in qualitative research: The assessment of trustworthiness. *American Journal of Occupational Therapy, 45,* 214–222.

Leonardelli Haertlein, C. A. (1992). Ethics in evaluation in occupational therapy. *American Journal of Occupational Therapy 46,* 950–953.

Lincoln, Y. S., & Guba, E. G. (1985). *Naturalistic inquiry.* Beverly Hills, CA: Sage.

Mann, W., Klyczek, J., & Fiedler, R. (1989). Bay Area Functional Performance Evaluation (BaFPE): Standard scores. *Occupational Therapy in Mental Health, 9,* 1–7.

Mann, W., & Klyczek, J. (1991) Standard scores for the Bay Area Functional Performance Evaluation Task Oriented Assessment. *Occupational Therapy in Mental Health, 11,* 13–24.

Marshall, C., & Rossman, G. B. (1989). *Designing qualitative research.* Newbury Park. CA: Sage.

Mover, E. A. (1984). A review of initial assessments used by occupational therapists in mental health settings. *Occupational Therapy in Health Care, 1,* 33–43.

Polgar, S., & Thomas, S. (1988). *Introduction to research in the health sciences.* New York: Churchill Livingstone.

Schatzman, L., & Strauss, A. L. (1973). *Field research.* Englewood Cliffs, NJ: Prentice-Hall.

Shannon, P. D. (1977). The derailment of occupational therapy. *American Journal of Occupational Therapy, 31,* 229–234.

Smith, R. O. (1992). The science of occupational therapy assessment. *Occupational Therapy Journal of Research, 12,* 3–15.

Spradley, T. S. (1979). *The ethnographic interview.* New York: Holt, Rinehart, & Winston.

Stein. F. (1988). Research analysis of occupational therapy assessments used in mental health. In B. J. Hemphill (Ed.), *Mental health assessment in occupational therapy: An integrative approach to the evaluative process.* Thorofare, NJ: Slack.

Thibeault, R., & Blackmer, E. (1987). Validating a test of functional performance with psychiatric patients. *American Journal of Occupational Therapy, 41,* 515–521.

Watts, J. H., Brollier, C., & Schmidt, W. (1988). Why use standardized patient evaluations? Commentary and suggestions. *Occupational Therapy in Mental Health, 8,* 89–95.

Williams, S. L., & Bloomer, J. S. (1987). *Bay Area Functional Performance Evaluation* (2nd ed.). Palo Alto, CA: Consulting Psychologists Press.

Yerxa, E. J. (1983). Audacious values: The energy source for occupational therapy practice. In G. Kielhofner (Ed.), *Health through occupation: Theory and practice in occupational therapy* (pp. 149–162). Philadelphia: Davis.

Chapter 17

Innovation and Leadership in a Mental Health Facility

The American Journal of Occupational Therapy

1995, 49(7): 595–606

Joanne Valiant Cook

Joanne Valiant Cook, PhD. OT(C), is Assistant
Professor, Department of Occupational Therapy,
Faculty of Applied Health Sciences, Elborn
College, The University of Western Ontario
London, Ontario, Canada N6G 1H1.Canada.

KEY WORDS

- philosophy
- sociology

ABSTRACT

*For 3½ years an occupational therapist perse-
vered in efforts to introduce an innovative
outpatient service of multidisciplinary team
case management within a general community hospital. The service was intended to meet
the needs of discharged clients with severe
mental illnesses who were attempting to live
successfully and satisfactorily in the community. The reality of attempting to initiate change
in medical bureaucracies involves ongoing
negotiation and persuasion, issues of power
and politics, differing cultural visions, and
strongly committed leadership. This case study
describes the developmental process of innovation and the contribution of occupational
therapy philosophy and practice to the therapist's emergent leadership in promoting cultural change. Some of the lessons to he learned
from this case study by others who would
attempt institutional innovation include
articulating a clear vision that uses new language, building coalitions, and being flexible
and persistent.*

This article presents a case study description
and analysis of the long negotiation process of
implementing change in services and service
delivery for clients with severe mental illness
who were outpatients of an acute care psychiatric unit of a general hospital. The change—
the formation of a multidisciplinary team to
provide ongoing, coordinated care—was proposed and negotiated for by an occupational
therapist.

The purpose of this article is to reveal and
interpret the developmental process involved in
seeking to make organizational, program, or
service changes in medical bureaucracies. At a
time when health services are in a state of
change or flux in terms of demands from the
public and funders, it seems useful for providers
of mental health services to be aware of and
prepared for the delays and roadblocks they
may encounter as they attempt change. Such
understanding may support the change-makers
in maintaining the perseverance that is often
required to achieve successful innovations.

This case study is one component of an
extended ethnographic research study, conducted by the author between 1983 and 1989 in a
medium-sized Canadian city, of the evolution
of an outpatient clinic for clients with schizophrenia. Although the events described in this

article took place more than a decade ago, a current ongoing research study of an attempt at introducing a new rehabilitation service in a large provincial psychiatric hospital (analogous to state psychiatric hospitals in the United States) reveals that similar processes of development are occurring. That is, although the context of events in terms of time and place are different and thus one cannot generalize the results of the 1980s study, it does appear that the processes themselves and the analysis of those processes meet the criterion of "transferability" (Lincoln & Guba, 1985, pp. 297, 316) to situations where health care professionals are attempting to introduce new services. Case study analysis of organizational change may offer lessons that can assist those who wish to be leaders of innovations in programs and interventions in health care.

The process of innovation that is described here occurred before participant observation at the site began. The history was obtained from an analysis of all available documentation of the process and in-depth, tape-recorded and transcribed interviews with key participants including the occupational therapist; the directors of the departments of psychiatric services, social work, psychology, and day care therapy; and all the members of what became known as the Schizophrenia Clinic Team. The history of the process is, therefore, a reconstructed account based on the participants' memories as well as written reports and minutes of meetings. The sequence and description of events were consistently reported by the above named informants and supported by the written sources. The criterion of credibility for qualitative studies (Krefting, 1991; Lincoln & Guba, 1985) would thus appear to be partially met by the triangulation of sources and the later prolonged engagement and my observations at the site. In addition, this reconstruction was read and supported by three of the participants in the study, thus providing the "member checks" that Lincoln and Guba (1985, p. 314) recommended as another technique to enhance the credibility of findings.

This article is organized in two parts. Part I provides a chronological description of the process of initiating change in mental health services and an analytic understanding of the difficulties in implementing new programs of care. Part II examines the role of leadership in fostering change and the contribution of professional ideology to the commitment to effecting change.

PART I: THE DEVELOPMENTAL PROCESS OF INNOVATION

The Context for Change

By the late 1970s, the neglect and seeming abandonment to the streets of deinstitutionalized persons with chronic mental illness was being described in professional journals, exposed in the popular press, and examined by commissions of inquiry (Bachrach, 1983; Cook, 1988). Some of the professional staff members in the Psychiatric Services Unit of the hospital described in this case study were increasingly concerned about the lack of programs, coordination of services, and even the availability of access to the resources that did exist, for an ever-growing population of clients requiring on-going care. The occupational therapist described the situation in her place of employment at that time as follows:

At that point the treatment of schizophrenia was done on an individual basis. Therapists and psychiatrists were working independently. There were no formal mechanisms for coordinating treatment. Individuals who were really ill could quite easily have as many as four therapists. So you had multiple therapists but no mechanism for coordinating. If you had a concern or problem or you wanted to clarify something, you tried catching the psychiatrist in the breezeway or coffee lounge or in the hall. It was a very loosey-goosey system. It has a rather humorous sound to it, but in actual fact, with the nature of schizophrenia and the kinds of multiple problems that our clients[1] had, for myself and for other people it was very ineffective and at times dangerous. Crisis intervention was almost impossible because there was no unified approach as to how the case was going to be handled. You really didn't have the opportunity to discuss the outpatient approach with the psychiatrist or other staff, so it was really challenging.

On a more global level, Psychiatric Services had no unified concept of how we were going to treat schizophrenia. Some people used a medical approach, some people used a psychological approach, some people used a supportive centered approach, some humanistic, and there were even people who had a more layman approach. So we had a lot of problems. People were coming from different angles and there was no opportunity for collaboration. Clients were not being informed or educated about their illness. They often had very poor compliance with treatment as a result. There was a revolving door that was incredible. People would be bopping in and out—I'm talking about the more seriously ill. We had what we called the "lounge crowd" of young schizophrenics that would hang around the hospital and smoke and drink coffee. They had no sense of direction, but it was more symptomatic of the problem that they had.

Families were blamed for the illness. A lot of families became very distressed. I received numerous calls and letters from parents wanting help. At that time people were actually being referred to Social Work to be assessed to see if family pathology was causing the illness.

The starting point, really, for us were the patients, their families, and their needs. And the needs were multiple. Several clinicians and representatives from all disciplines were really concerned about the situation and really wanted to improve our aftercare for, at that point, what we called "the chronic population." And the result of that was informal meetings.

By 1980, the environmental pressures for improved and more available services to deinstitutionalized clients were increasing. The members of the newly formed local chapter of the Friends of Schizophrenics (an organization similar to the National Alliance for the Mentally Ill [NAMI] in the United States) were requesting professional help for their ill relatives and for themselves. The physicians, both general practitioners and psychiatrists, at the hospital were also finding the increasing numbers of persons who were chronically ill a demanding responsibility due to the multiple social and functional problems with which these clients presented. The revolving door problem, crisis episodes, and the "lounge crowd" worried the hospital administrators.

The First Initiatives: 1979–1980

In the late months of 1979, one of the psychiatrists began to feel overwhelmed by the pressure of the large caseload of patients with schizophrenia that he was carrying:

> *I had reached the stage where I couldn't go any further. . . . I couldn't handle it . . . there wasn't sufficient back up . . . there was a steady increase year by year. . . . So at that time I presented a seminar, at one of Friday morning inservices [in-house education series] on the problem of schizophrenia. I became convinced that we had to do something about it.*

A small group of clinicians, including the occupational therapist, a social worker, and a nurse who were also concerned about the lack of coordination and follow-up of outpatients, began to meet once a week for short periods with this psychiatrist to discuss these issues in regard to his patients. In late May 1980, the occupational therapist wrote a memo to her department manager outlining in considerable detail the need for and benefits of a formally designated, multidisciplinary, outpatient team for the coordination of services for the chronically ill who required continuing care (see Appendix A). The combination of the psychiatrist's inservice, the occupational therapist's memo, and the visit of a British psychiatrist who pointed out the inadequacies of care for this specific population led the Director of the Psychiatric Services to bring the issue before the Professional Advisory Committee for Psychiatric Services (PAC). This body met monthly to plan, approve, and evaluate services and programs. It was composed of department chiefs or managers from the various disciplines and hospital administration. Three months later, a Task Force on Continuing Care, chaired by the Chief of Social Work, was convened to define the current needs of the chronic population, to establish their future needs for programs, and to submit a report by the end of the year.

The Initial Negotiations: August 1980–March 1982

The task force included the clinicians who had been meeting weekly with one psychiatrist and other department chiefs and representatives. The task force met regularly for 8 months and then held a 2-day workshop in an attempt to reach consensus on how to proceed with its mandate. The divisive issue was whether a program should be established to provide care for a small number of the most obviously disabled, clearly defined, chronic, users of resources (the position of the Chairperson of the task force) or whether a service only for patients with schizophrenia, both newly diagnosed and chronic, should be undertaken (the psychiatrist's position).

In the minutes of the PAC meeting of May 11, 1981, the Chairperson of the task force is reported as stating that "after nine months of work the Task Force was grinding to a halt." One month later he reported that, although some short-term goals, such as establishing a list of needy patients, had been met, the problem of defining the population to be served was at an "impasse situation" and would probably require resolution by PAC. On October 26, 1981, PAC requested recommendations from the task force for review. In December 1981, the Chairperson of the task force submitted to PAC a "majority proposal for a continuing care program for chronic psychiatric patients" which was to begin with a modest caseload of 32 patients who would be provided with the services of a multidisciplinary team. The report was tabled for several months until the psychiatrist's minority report favoring the establishment of a program for patients diagnosed as having schizophrenia was presented to PAC on March 8, 1982.

The minority report contained indications of the problems and conditions encountered by those who had such high hopes for the policy of deinstitutionalization and to which the occupational therapist was responding in recommending a team-coordinated service. As Cameron (1978) had written, "the severely mentally ill, on the other hand, are more professionally frustrating; treating them has been largely eschewed with the reorganization of the health system" (p. 323). The minority report outlined the reality of practice, which had resulted in many persons with chronic mental illness suffering from neglect in the community:

> *If we are drawing up a program covering all types of chronic mental illness, then I would see no special role for a psychiatrist in the program apart from what is happening now. We would be dealing with very much the same patients we have around the unit now and each of them are [sic] under the care of a psychiatrist. I am unclear as to how we could develop a meaningful program for these patients because most of them are really just being carried and there is not too much hope for therapeutic improvement. I feel it will be difficult to find a psychiatrist who would devote himself to the chronic care program as envisioned by our committee, because it would soon become a dumping ground for patients who are really untreatable. On the other hand it might be possible to find a psychiatrist for an active and interesting schizophrenia program, which I think is much more important for this area.*

After much discussion, a compromise motion was offered to PAC: "that the various individuals from departments involved meet to establish a team to begin dealing with chronic patients—specifically schizophrenic patients—in a formalized fashion."

Planning the Schizophrenia Clinic: April 1982–December 1982

The members of what was designated as the Continuing Care Team first met in April 1982. The membership included the original members of the group who had been meeting regularly with the psychiatrist and representatives from the Day Therapy and Nursing Departments. The director of the Psychiatric Services Department asked the occupational therapist to be the chairperson of the team meetings. In June 1982, after three meetings, the chairperson submitted a report on the team's progress, which included issues of patient identification, the development of a registry system, and a preliminary model of team functioning in regard to coordination of treatment and review of patients' progress. The team continued to meet once a week for 1 hr. In a transcribed interview the therapist—chairperson described the process that led to the proposal for a Schizophrenia Clinic:

> We looked at the schizophrenic clients we were working with that had problems and we studied them all in depth and we made lists of patients and worked out what themes were emerging. The whole process was really unsatisfactory because all we were doing was studying, but in the meantime our clients were still having problems and nothing was happening. So, finally the team got frustrated and decided what we really needed was a team approach for starters and we needed good case management. That was what was emerging from the discussions. So we decided that the best approach would be to develop a schizophrenia clinic and [the psychiatrist] actually called it The Schizophrenia Clinic. That's where the beginning for that concept came from.

In December 1982, a formal proposal written by the occupational therapist—chairperson was submitted to PAC (see Appendix B). The proposal reflected all the concerns expressed in her May 1980 memo, but now they were more specifically detailed in terms of establishing a schizophrenia clinic that would meet the "combined needs of psychiatrists, other professional staff, the patient, his family and community agencies." The proposed clinic format retained the private relationship of psychiatrists to their clients but gave them each a block of time to meet with the multidisciplinary team to discuss their roster of clients and plan for the coordinated delivery of services.

Resistance to and Acceptance of the Plan: January 1983

At the January 1983 meeting of PAC, the Chief of Social Work (and former Chairperson of the task force) in a written memo and in person at the meeting, criticized the schizophrenia clinic proposal in terms of its scope, staffing, and program design. He argued persuasively for the development of "a quality service for a smaller number of chronic patients [rather than] diffusing our efforts by attempting a limited service for all schizophrenic patients." He further argued that there were insufficient staff resources to mount the clinic as proposed and that more specific programs needed to be developed. The Chairperson of the Continuing Care Team had recently been appointed Senior Occupational Therapist for Psychiatric Services and in that capacity now attended PAC meetings. As she listened to the arguments against the proposal she told me that she began to "feel desperate." She was sure PAC would turn down the proposal and ask for the development of a program or programs for a population (rather than establishing a clinic format with team input to meet the needs of individuals); then the whole process would go back to the beginning and it would take another 2 years or more to reach any decision. She said, "as an [occupational therapist] I have started a lot of new programs here and I know that approach doesn't work." Her feeling of desperation was also influenced by the recent suicide of one of her clients. She believed that the death might have been prevented had the clinic concept been realized, so she argued "that if we could just start with good case management even though we didn't have a lot of resources, then at least we would be making some inroads and giving it a start." After much discussion, PAC agreed—with the proviso that the Clinic Team develop a program proposal to be submitted to the District Health Council for independent funding. The departments of social work, day therapy, and occupational therapy each agreed to give 6 hr of staff member time per week to the clinic.

The occupational therapist and the social worker on the Continuing Care Team were asked to write the proposal for additional funding, within some severe limits imposed by PAC members and particularly by the Director of Psychiatric Services. They were told to keep the proposal modest and to only request funding for a half-time social worker and half-time nurse. (The original plan from the Continuing Care Team included additional day therapy and occupational therapy staff.) PAC believed that the existing services with their 6-hr per week commitment were adequate. In addition, the Director believed that there was a greater chance of securing funding if the proposal was small.[2]

The occupational therapist reported that she

> fought and advocated for increased occupational therapy involvement as the department's resources were stretched to the limit. Moreover, we deal with this population of clients more than any other department. It was an uphill fight and it's typical of the problems of recognition for the contribution of occupational therapy as a professional service.

The application for funding had to be submitted only 2 weeks after PAC approved the clinic proposal. Many unpaid, overtime hours were spent in completing the forms required by the Ministry of Health guidelines. At the last moment, the Director of Psychiatric Services agreed to include a request for additional occupational therapy time but not for day therapy time. With the exception of the staffing requests, the proposal submitted (see Appendix C) was, in essence, the same program proposed in the submission to PAC, which itself was very similar to the multidisciplinary team concept proposed in the original memo sent by the therapist to her department manager (see Appendices A and B).

The Implementation of the Clinic— March 1983

The psychiatrist from the Continuing Care Team was appointed as the Director of the Schizophrenia Clinic, and the occupational therapist was given the *informal* title of Team Coordinator (i.e., responsibility for day-to-day administration of the clinic but without administrative authority).

The first formal case conference clinic was held in March 1983 before funding was approved. By September 1983 the occupational therapist in her role as Team Coordinator had, by persuasion, letters, and memos, convinced all the psychiatrists who had a roster of clients with schizophrenia to schedule regular clinics with the team. In October 1983, the provincial Ministry of Health granted the program funding for a trial period of 2 years, with permanent funding dependent upon two annual Ministry evaluations. It was the first schizophrenia clinic in Canada. There were various service programs (such as vocational assessment and training, social skills groups, and activities of daily living groups) throughout the country at that time but no multidisciplinary clinics offering individualized, client-centered, case management to a population with a specific condition.

This process of innovation took more than 3 years to reach fruition. In the late 1960s, when deinstitutionalization was well under way, a critical account of the problems faced by workers in mental health facilities reported that "innovative talking has been encouraged, while innovative action has been resisted" (Graziano, 1969, p. 10). Similarly, almost 20 years later Kinston pointed out that "getting new ideas into the health system and properly used is a long term effort" (1983, p. 1163). As the narrative above illustrates, the idea for a multidisciplinary team service for the persons with severe mental illness took several years and a great deal of effort to reach implementation. An understanding of the obstacles and barriers to innovation in mental health care requires an exploration of the realities of bureaucratic organization, of cultural differences in the health professions and practices, and of differences in power between interested stakeholders.

Understanding Obstacles and Barriers to Innovations in Health Care

A useful framework for summarizing the process of initiating this innovation is Tichy's (1981, 1983) conceptual scheme of *problem cycles.* He stated that there are three systems in mutually influencing relationships in any organization: the technical, the political, and the cultural. Any organization has

> *three basic dilemmas . . . the technical design problem . . . social and technical resources must be arranged so that the organization produces some desired result . . . the political allocation problem . . . allocating power and resources . . . who will reap benefits . . . [and] the ideological and cultural mix problem . . . to determine what values need to be held (Tichy, 1981, p. 165).*

In very simplified terms, what occurred during the developmental process described here can be conceptualized as follows: There was a technical problem—the provision of services to a new clientele, the deinstitutionalized client with chronic illness; the proposed solution to this technical problem involved cultural change in values, practices, and organizational structure; the cultural change proposal became the focus of political negotiation, challenge, and opposition. Each of these waves of activity took place within a medical bureaucracy in a time of changing social and political approaches to persons who were mentally ill. These varying cycles, contexts, and historical circumstances were intertwined in the long process that eventually led to the adoption of the innovative change.

The Reality of Barriers to Innovation Within a Bureaucracy

Many of the propositions developed by Downs (1967) on the problems of change in bureaucracies were borne out during the ongoing negotiations for the initiation of the Schizophrenia Clinic. For example, Downs stated that in large bureaucracies "nearly every major structural or behavioral change is preceded by study of the need for such a change carried out by one or more committees" (1967, p. 275). The 3 years required to implement the original idea proposed by the occupational therapist can be partially explained by the barriers posed to innovation in bureaucracies. The

appointing of committees, then a task force, then a workshop, then a feasibility team, and so on, each needing approval from yet another layer of the hierarchy, bogged down the decision-making process in terms of both time and competing alternative approaches. An additional problem was that this change was initiated from the bottom up in an organization accustomed to directives issued from the top down. Those with the authority to make decisions— the members of PAC—were department and administrative chiefs who were not involved in day-to-day interaction with these clients. Most of those working toward the implementation of a multidisciplinary outpatient service were lower-level staff employees in terms of the hierarchical arrangement of decision making, until the occupational therapist became a member of PAC. The problems of change initiated from the bottom up in a bureaucracy that "can mire staff in a morass of detail and conflict" (Weissman, 1982, p. 44) were evident in this attempt to develop a new service. That is, organizations that are arranged in hierarchical form, with clearly defined departments and professional role definitions, are more likely to require longer time frames for negotiation toward decision making because of the multiplicity of interests, professional practices, and authoritative channels.

The Reality of Cultural Differences in Delaying Consensus

Morgan (1986) identified another important factor in understanding the process of change in organizations. "Traditionally the change process has been conceptualized as a problem of changing technologies, structures and [people] . . . [but] . . . effective change also depends on changes in images and values that are to guide action . . . organizational change implies cultural change" (pp. 135–138). Some of the delays encountered in developing the Schizophrenia Clinic resulted from a dispute over values and behavioral solutions. The opposing proposals from the Chairperson of the task force and the Continuing Care Team chaired by the occupational therapist illustrate the cultural diversity. One proposed defining the problem as a question of use of services and the need to establish *group* programs for the chronic users of such services. The other proposed an *individualized,* psychiatrist-team—directed, direct service delivery to a more clearly identified population in need of specialized services. These were different philosophies of intervention, evidenced different values as to the neediest population, and proposed different professional responses as a solution.

The emergent solution for a case management service took many months of cultural defining work by the Continuing Care Team. This process was not just one of innovation but one of fundamental cultural change. The focus of practice was to be on the community and the clients who lived there, rather than on inpatient care. The approach was to be individualized, coordinated services to the client and family, not the provision of group programs. The services were to be integrated, comprehensive, and coordinated by a collaborative and overlapping team, rather than fragmented, technical expertise provided by several departments. The primary goal was rehabilitation (maintaining and enhancing function), not treatment to effect cure. The new service was designed to provide continuing after-care, not short-term, acute care.

Although the cultural solution among the members of the Continuing Care Team evolved through consensus, its eventual adoption depended on the ability to mobilize support for the proposal within the hospital. Both the delayed nature of this innovation process and the eventual adoption were influenced by political activity and differential access to power.

The Reality of Power and Politics in Negotiating for Change

In their classic work on psychiatric institutions, Strauss, Schatzman, Bucher, Ehrlich, and Sabshin (1964) conceived of the institution as an arena of negotiation and the eventual working structure and practices as a negotiated order. Several illustrations of the negotiating process culminating in the Schizophrenia Clinic have been provided. However, the process of negotiation was not between equals in each context. The adoption of the proposal depended on the ability to mobilize the power resources within the hospital.

As Kanter (1983) pointed out, there is a "political side to innovation . . . it requires campaigning, lobbying, bargaining, negotiating, caucusing, collaborating and winning votes. That is, an idea must be sold . . . and [there is a need] for power to turn ideas into action" (p. 216). Or as Graziano (1969) so cogently put it, "the *conception* of innovative ideas in mental health depends upon creative, humanitarian, and scientific forces, while their *implementation* depends, not on science or humanitarianism, but on a broad spectrum of professional and social politics" (p. 10).

Traditionally, in mental health facilities, decision-making power is vested in the medical profession, department heads, and top administrators. In this hospital, the decision-making body was the PAC composed of such persons. Initially, neither of the two prime movers for the innovation (the psychiatrist and the occupational therapist) was a member of this body. It was only at the end of the process, by virtue of a promotion, that the occupational therapist was able to attend the meetings and lobby for the adoption of the clinic proposal. Occupational therapists as a group have traditionally held less powerful positions among medical professionals. Maxwell and Maxwell (1977) attributed this lack of power to the history of medical sponsorship and hence control of occupational therapy, to the diffuse and not-well-understood expertise of its practitioners, to its association with chronicity and rehabilitation rather than the more dramatic acute-care medical practice, and to its being a predominantly female profession. This lack of power has led to a pattern of adaptation to the health care hierarchy that was characterized as "diffidence" by Maxwell and Maxwell (1977, p. 83).

Perhaps, in this case, the occupational therapist's "diffident" pattern of lobbying for support by writing memos and being part of the task forces and committees, but being unable to directly participate in the decision-making level of the hierarchy, partially accounts for the length of time it took to finally implement the original idea. In spite of being able to secure the support of the Director of Psychiatric Services, the innovation was almost lost due to the skillful, persistent, and, as later events proved, prophetic opposition of the Chief of Social Work who served as the Chairperson of the initial task force.[3] As Downs (1967) pointed out, opposition to change is more likely to occur when the change will reduce the resources one has to control and decrease the importance of the functions currently fulfilled. The proposed clinic format would be under the control of the medical profession. The opposing proposal for group programs would have provided opportunities for an expansion of Social Work jurisdiction and, hence, control. The detailed critique of the clinic proposal in terms of its inadequacies in design, goals, and resources almost blocked the innovation. In the end, the proposal was approved because it met the interests of those who had control over the decision—the psychiatrists and the hospital administrators. The former would get the support services they needed and the latter could be seen to be providing further community service (which, in their interest, also resolved the lounge crowd nuisance and the revolving door problem) but at a low cost because the program was to be funded by an external grant from the Ministry of Health. The power brokers had to be convinced that it was in their interests to approve the program. The length of time required for the lobbying, persuading, and stating the case that the occupational therapist pursued was prolonged by political opposition from those who had something to lose or nothing to gain if her innovative idea was adopted.

Persistence and Innovation: Professional Values and Cultural Leadership

This chronology of the process of effecting an innovation in the delivery of mental health services illustrates the lengthy negotiations, persuasion, meetings, and discouragements faced by those who would initiate change in medical bureaucracies. This chronology makes understandable those situations in which service providers give up their attempts to improve service delivery. Why, in this situation, did an occupational therapist persevere to institute this innovation? What enabled her to persevere in spite of setbacks, delays, and opposition? In part II of this case study, some possible answers to those questions are explored. The thesis to be argued is that the philosophy (values and beliefs or professional ideology) adhered to and the professional practice experience of the primary change agent were important personal resources and stimuli for leadership activities.

PART II: THE ROLE OF PROFESSIONAL IDEOLOGY IN LEADERSHIP AND CULTURAL CHANGE

Kanter (1983) described those who effect change or innovation as entrepreneurs. She wrote "entrepreneurs are above all visionaries. They are willing to continue single-minded pursuit of a clearly articulated vision, even when the line of least effort or resistance would make it easy to give up" (p. 239). What enabled the occupational therapist in this case study to continue pushing for change while others gave up the fight when consensus could not be reached? What can account for the eventual acceptance of her original proposal for an outpatient multidisciplinary team? Why did she emerge as the informal leader of a cultural change and its eventual implementation? One possible interpretation is that her professional affiliation and experience as an occupational therapist provided her with the beliefs and values (professional ideology) that were used as personal resources for initiating change.

The Nature and Function of Professional Ideologies

Wilson defined ideology as

> a set of beliefs about the social world and how it operates, containing statements about the rightness of certain social arrangements and what actions would be undertaken in the light of those statements. An ideology is both a cognitive map of sets of expectations and a scale of values in which standards and imperatives are proclaimed. Ideology thus serves both as a clue to understanding and as a guide to action, developing in the mind of its adherents an image of the process by which desired changes can best be achieved (1973, pp. 91–92).

Similarly, Marx characterized the ideology of a profession as a "morally charged mandate for action" (1969, p. 81). The literature on organizational life cycles and organizational culture examines the importance of ideology as a resource in creating new meaning in innovative activity, to legitimate those activities and to develop an identity or ethos that provides direction and purpose (Abravanel, 1983; Lohdahl & Mitchell, 1981; Smircich, 1983). Thus, the primary function of ideology is prescriptive.

If ideology provides the stimulus to action, one can presume that when innovative activities are proposed within an organization, there is a different ideology underpinning those proposals. Ideology

> becomes a central feature of the innovative organization. The ideology summarizes the values and ideals that the founders intended the new organization to epitomize . . . by using the ideology as a resource, the founders . . . may be able to generate commitment . . . and value consensus. (Lohdahl & Mitchell, 1981, pp. 186–187)

The adherence to ideological values can serve to attach meaning to situations and the actions required within them. Those meanings and prescriptions for action are the resources of those who lead cultural change.

The Role of Leadership and Shared Meaning in Innovation: The Cultural Connection

In an analysis of leadership, Smircich and Morgan (1982) stated:

> Leadership [is] The Management of Meaning . . . Leadership is realized in the process whereby one or more individuals succeeds in attempting to frame and define the reality of others . . . they emerge as leaders because of their role in framing experience in a way that provides a viable basis for action. (pp. 257–258)

Schein (1985), in an analysis of cultural change in organizations, declared that

> as I began to think through the issues of how culture changes, I again realized the centrality of leadership—the ability to see a need for change and the ability to make it happen. Much of what is mysterious about leadership becomes clearer . . . if we link leadership specifically to creating and changing culture. (pp. x–xi)

Hall (1982) defined leadership as being "what a person does above and beyond the basic requirements of his [sic] position. It is the persuasion of individuals and innovativeness in ideas and decision making that differentiates leadership from the sheer possession of power" (p. 161). Bennis (1979) expanded this definition by stating that "leadership involves more than managing, more than just being an idea man [sic], it involves questioning the routine" (p. 42). There are three requisite characteristics for determining leadership or change agent implied in the foregoing quotations: (a) the ability to recognize the need for change; (b) the ability to define, create, or develop meaningful realities or bases for action to meet the need; and (c) the capacity to mobilize resources to implement the change.

The occupational therapist in this case study went beyond the mere requirements of her job, questioned the routine modes of therapeutic practices with persons with chronic mental illness, and proposed an alternative reality of service. In proposing a new service, she was introducing a different ideological system of beliefs, that is, a different cultural frame for practice. Both the psychiatrist and the occupational therapist on the Continuing Care Team saw a need for change in the after-care services for clients with chronic mental illness. The psychiatrist defined it in terms of requiring support services from others:

> [T]o treat patients with schizophrenia is a lifetime job . . . the social problems are so great. It seemed to me that the psychiatrists would be willing to treat schizophrenics if they got support. Just as I was prepared to treat them if I got support.

On the other hand, the occupational therapist had defined the need in terms of ongoing, individualized client care that required the coordination and integration of services and workers by enhancing communication through a formally structured team mechanism. Both professionals worked toward defining the situation, but from different perspectives. With the exception of his minority report to PAC, the psychiatrist did not participate as actively in the various task forces and meetings as did the occupational therapist, nor did he outline in writing the kind of detailed proposals supported by treatment principles that the therapist continuously circulated (see Appendices A and B). These various written memos and proposals documented the therapists' vision of service (Bennis, 1979) and they began to establish a meaning structure as the basis of action.

It is the third requisite that most distinguished the occupational therapist rather than the psychiatrist as the primary change agent and emergent leader. Kanter (1983) stressed "the link between individual entrepreneurs and their coalitions or teams. Individuals initiate . . . and then work through teams to bring ideas to innovation. Prime movers push—by getting more and more people involved in action vehicles that express the change being promoted" (p. 35). Because of her participation in the various task forces and committees and her appointment to PAC and chairmanship of the

Continuing Care Team, the therapist slowly gathered support from others who came to share her definitions and they, through interaction, began to develop shared understandings of the need for and type of change required.

It is "shared meanings that permit organized activity to emerge and assume coherence . . . for unless meanings are in some sense shared, there can be no alignment and co-ordination of action" (Morgan, 1984, p. 315). The occupational therapist described the final consensus on meaning in terms that confirm Louis's (1983, p. 50) statement that: "A key premise of a cultural view is that meaning is emergent and intersubjectively negotiated."

> We decided what we needed was a team approach, for starters, and we needed good case management. That was what was emerging from the discussions. With the problems we had, we had to start with the clinic, the team, and case management. That was the only logical place to start, but interestingly enough that took a long time to evolve—that concept. It seems so obvious when you look at it, but it wasn't obvious when we were groping with the start. At one point people were looking at starting a program here in the hospital—a social program, a work program, etc.—and that would have been putting the cart before the horse. You can't rehabilitate on that basis.

The ongoing consultations in weekly meetings and the written proposals on goals, objectives, and rationales prepared by the occupational therapist were instrumental in bringing the clinic to being, for, as Kanter (1983) stated, "prime movers push in part by repetition" (p. 296). In the midst of the ambiguity and ad hoc nature of the 3-year process of initiating the multidisciplinary clinic idea, the therapist's written proposals provided some structured meaning even as they were being negotiated.

However, as Schein (1985) contended, "cultures do not start from scratch. Founders and group members always have prior experience to start with" (p. 221). This insight on prior experience leads to questions about the content of the ideology underpinning the innovation known as the Schizophrenia Clinic.

Professional Ideology as a Resource in Promoting Innovation: The Values of Occupational Therapy

In 1986, 3 years after the clinic was established, the occupational therapist provided for some new members of the team what she termed a historical review of the clinic development in the following words:

> [My] purpose is to provide some information about the clinic's development, to help us regain, or for the new people, to gain an understanding of our philosophy, central concepts and organization . . . What I'm wanting to highlight through this review is that there are certain central concepts that are important to the clinic. Number one is that we are client centered. We are looking at the client first and administration second. Now that is why the program was established. Secondly, that we wanted to look at the development of a holistic, coordinated approach. As we all know, individuals with schizophrenia have a multiplicity of problems and really require a team effort. When you look at the clinic, each member of the team has a very specific role. There is some overlap, but there are so many things to look at, that a team effort is required. Along with the team approach is the understanding that the clients are going to relate to a team, not just one individual. So if someone leaves or is sick, or on holiday, that client doesn't feel like he has no one to relate to—they have got a team. The third concept is that schizophrenia is a mental illness and that informing clients and their families about the diagnosis is important and that education is really going to facilitate community adjustment. Along with that concept is our feeling that client participation in their treatment and taking responsibility is important. The fourth is case management and the importance of good linkage between the community and the hospital resources and really helping the client to make the links and have access to that. A final point that is essential to clinic functioning is that it is a point of contact for clients, community, and staff.

Most occupational therapists reading the above quotation will recognize the description of the Schizophrenia Clinic as an embodiment of many of the fundamental beliefs, values, and principles of practice of the profession. The writings of many of those honored by their profession with the Eleanor Clarke Slagle lectureship in the United States (American Occupational Therapy Association, 1985) or the Muriel Driver Lectureship in Canada (Baptiste, 1988; Carswell-Opzoomer, 1990; Judd, 1982; Law, 1991; Polatajko, 1992) and the Canadian publication on *Guidelines for the Client Centered Practice of Occupational Therapy* (Canadian Association of Occupational Therapists, 1991), among others, espouse those central values and beliefs of occupational therapy that Yerxa has stated "speak to vital human needs and ensure that people with chronic conditions will be able to lead satisfying, productive lives instead of being throw away people in tomorrow's world" (Yerxa, 1991, p. 2).

Smith (1984) has advised that those who would attempt organizational change must provide a new language, as the old language maintains the old ways. In contrast to the traditional language of psychiatric practice, there are different conceptions for services illustrated in this therapist's historical review and in the documents and proposal for the establishment of the multidisciplinary team clinic (see Appendices A, B, and C): *holistic,* not specific psychotherapeutic care; *clients,* not patients; *quality aftercare* for clients and families, not acute care for the ill patient; *case management* and *education* to promote *function,* not just medical treatment to effect cure; *participation* of clients and families in treatment planning, not passive reception of service; and *coordination* of services, not brokerage or fragmentation of expertise.

In focusing her efforts on developing comprehensive services for persons with chronic mental illness, the therapist in this case study also reflected the commitment to those persons often devalued by other professional and lay groups. Yerxa has commented on this essential value of occupational therapy practice:

> Otherwise devalued, mental patients were perceived humanistically by the pioneers in

occupational therapy as people worthy of dignity . . . the valuing of a person's essential humanity in spite of severe and sometimes chronic disease, was central to the practice of the original therapists . . . The historical values of the profession have been transmitted to modern occupational therapists, as may be seen in current patient advocacy efforts as well as in occupational therapists' traditional provision of services to the most severely and chronically disabled patients. Such patients are often seen as "beyond help" by many other professionals because of extensive and irreversible pathologies. (1983, p. 151)

Perspectives differ on the need for innovation in services for the deinstitutionalized clients in this study, as enunciated by the psychiatrist and the therapist. With the institution of the Schizophrenia Clinic, the psychiatrists gained the back up, supportive services to deal with non-medical needs of these clients, which were often responsible for their previous neglect by many professionals (Baxter & Hopper, 1982; Cameron, 1978; Cook, 1988; Grob, 1980, 1983; Morrissey & Tessler, 1982). Although one of the premises of deinstitutionalization policy was to provide access to psychiatric care in the community, the resistance to working with this clientele by psychiatrists and some other professionals was unpredicted (Cameron, 1978). The basic needs of persons with schizophrenia are for functional, educational, and supportive services, not the talking therapies that many professionals prefer to offer. Further, the difficulty of working with persons with severe mental illness must not be discounted in understanding the reluctance of many professionals to accept them as clients. Often any progress they make may be small and may take place at a very slow pace. There may be setbacks and relapses and the clients themselves can sometimes be demanding, belligerent, frustrating, and uncooperative (Estroff, 1981; Pranger & Brown, 1992; Price, 1993). In this case the occupational therapist's commitment to serving the chronically ill was crucial in instigating the long process of improving the services available to them.

Professional Values, Leadership, and Change

The Schizophrenia Clinic as envisioned and, in most respects, as embodied reflected the fundamental values and practice beliefs of occupational therapy to which the therapist in this case study was clearly committed. This commitment appeared to serve as an important driving force in her consistent efforts to realize a vision of improved service. But it has also been noted that leadership requires more than vision and ideas. Successful change masters also require "a longer time horizon, conviction in an idea, no need for immediate results or measure and a willingness to convey a vision of something that might come out a little different when finished" (Kanter, 1983, p. 239).

This process to effect organizational change began with the initiative of a professional in the middle ranks of a hierarchically structured medical bureaucracy. By most accounts such efforts from "the grass roots" (Kanter, 1983, p. 180), the "muddling" middle manager (Feldman, 1980, p. 3) or the "lower level staff change agent" (Weissman, 1982, p. 4) are doomed to failure or as Kanter puts it, "withering" (1983, p. 102). Generally, this lack of success is due to the inability to mobilize resources, particularly political power and support (Graziano, 1969) and due to the general inertia and resistance to change in service bureaucracies (Downs, 1967; Golembiewski, 1985; Kanter, 1983; Kinston, 1983; Mechanic, 1980). In such contexts and circumstances, said Mechanic,

[u]nusual leadership is often necessary. . . . A change in direction requires a leader who can communicate to others the sense of excitement in a new venture and who has the organizational skills to bring the necessary people and organizations together. In the absence of a strong incentive—such as available funding—it is extraordinarily difficult to build the necessary momentum. (1980, p. 179, emphasis added)

In spite of the barriers and obstacles to innovation, a leader did emerge who was able to maintain the momentum to eventually put a multidisciplinary team and the clinic together. Her leadership position came about as much by default as by appointment. It appears that by always maintaining the idea of a holistic, multidisciplinary, coordinated, education and case management service she kept the cultural vision in the foreground. The role of defining the reality, of imparting a sense of mission, of creating a new cultural form led to her emergent leadership. As others came to share those understandings and see that it gave purpose and shape to their hopes and working life, her position as unofficial team coordinator solidified. The Schizophrenia Clinic as implemented was a somewhat altered creation but was based nevertheless upon the occupational therapist's original vision of a multidisciplinary team designed to coordinate services for persons with chronic mental illness.

Much of what we read in professional journals and the popular press documents the powerlessness of so-called lower-level participants to effect change in organizations. In this case, one person did make a difference. A new delivery of services was established that reflected the occupational therapist's values and beliefs about the importance of client participation, the individual worth of those with chronic illness, the necessity of continuous and ongoing support, the client's potential for growth, and the recognition of the holistic nature of humans, which requires coordination and integration of services to meet their varied needs. Yerxa (1983) discussed the difficulties and challenges faced by therapists who strive to maintain those values in medically dominated settings:

> Owing to [the value differences between medicine and occupational therapy], occupational therapists have sometimes had difficulty implementing their values in the traditional medical setting. . . . Occupational therapy has been sufficiently audacious to create and sustain its own unique model of practice while surviving within, and contributing to, health in the medical milieu. In many respects this persistence of professional values and a singular philosophy, in the midst of conflicting ideals and philosophies, has been intrepidly daring (p. 157).

When the therapist in this case was asked why she kept trying for so long to effect change when so many others might have given up, her explanation was somewhat less sophisticated than Yerxa's, but value-laden nevertheless. She said "the bottom line was improved patient care and that's what sees you through all this muck." The profession and its clients need more change making therapists who are so committed to professional values that they "intrepidly" see their way through "all the muck."

CONCLUSION: LESSONS TO BE LEARNED

Nothing changes quickly. Those who wish to initiate new programs or services within bureaucratic organizations must be prepared to be persistent and persuasive over a long time period.

Have a clear and consistent vision. Change agents are often required to clearly articulate the components of change to many participants in a variety of meetings.

Maintain the vision with new language. In order to change a culture (both the values and the practices) new meaning must be developed through the use of new terminology used consistently when explaining or negotiating for change.

Put it in writing. In this case study, the therapist was the one person who kept the mission in front of others by writing memos and proposals for the change. In turn, those written proposals maintained the vision by reiterating new language.

Build coalitions. Change is much more likely to occur if it is supported by other professionals and administrators. This factor also adds to the time line but is necessary for success in both the initiation phase and the maintenance of the innovation once implemented.

Recognize stakeholders' interests. This follows from building coalitions. Everyone involved in institutional change has "turf" or professional concerns that can hinder or help the process of change. Being aware of such interests means that adjustments and compromises can be made to change proposals to encourage support.

Be flexible. This follows from the previous lesson. It does not mean compromising the vision for change but allows for the adjustments necessary to build strong coalitions.

Don't give up or give in. As shown in this case study, initiating change often requires a long term commitment of energy. One's values can be resources in maintaining enthusiasm. Hold on to them.

Notes:
1. The terms *client* and *patient* were used interchangeably by the Clinic staff members, although *client* had become the preferred term by the conclusion of this study.

2. Ironically, the Director explained to me in an interview that he had been mistaken. In fact, the Ministry of Health totally funded as requested all proposals ranked number 1 and 2 by the District Health councils. The Schizophrenia Clinic proposal was ranked number 1 and thus could have received much larger funding. The lack of adequate funding was a source of many subsequent problems in the clinic's development.

3. The Chief of Social Work's criticism of the scope and ambition of the clinic proposal proved over the years to be valid as the team struggled with inadequate human and material resources to meet the needs of an ever-increasing clientele.

Appendix A
Outpatient Multidisciplinary Team Memo (May 26, 1980), Abridged

A team approach would provide a mechanism for:
1. Identifying patient needs, establishing treatment goals, developing and implementing treatment programs
2. Coordinating and integrating treatment programs
3. Providing a systematic review of patient progress
4. Improving quality of care
5. Improving communication among staff and facilitating consistent patient treatment
6. Promoting development of treatment programs based on clearly identified patient needs
7. Maintaining staff morale and impetus in treating this challenging group of patients

Appendix B
Proposal for Schizophrenia Clinic (December 13, 1982), Abridged: Objective and Goals for Clinic

The overall objective of the clinic is to promote the development of good quality treatment services for schizophrenic patients and their families in the community. More specific goals include the following:
1. Provide a formal system for organizing the delivery of treatment care to schizophrenia patients including psychiatric and psychosocial aspects
2. Develop a multidisciplinary team approach to the outpatient treatment of schizophrenic patients
3. Provide a system of mutual staff support and peer consultation
4. Provide a point of contact for the patients, their families and community agencies
5. Promote research, education and program development in the area of schizophrenia

Appendix C
Summary Outline Of Program (Ministry Application: January 1983)

It is proposed to establish an aftercare clinic for schizophrenic patients and their families that will comprise several components. A system of case management involving the assignment of a prime therapist and the contribution of a multidisciplinary team will be put in place with a designated psychiatrist in charge. Members of the team will act both as direct service providers and as consultants in their particular area of expertise.

The clinic will perform a coordinating function in relation to existing programs that serve the schizophrenic patient, e.g., outpatient, day therapy and social/recreation programs.

The clinic will provide a point of contact for staff, patients, their families, and community agencies. Patient and family crisis situations will receive quick and thorough response with the aim of preventing relapse and/or admission to hospital.

The clinic program will offer patient and family education about the medical and psychosocial aspects of schizophrenia in the form of teaching and support groups.

Finally, the program, through focusing on one particular patient population, will develop an intimate knowledge of gaps in service for the schizophrenia patient and consequently will produce comprehensive recommendations for further program development.

ACKNOWLEDGMENTS

I acknowledge the valuable feedback received from Betty Yerxa, EdD. LHD (Hon), OTR, FAOTA. and Helene Polatajko, PhD, OT(C), as well as the reviewers for the *American Journal of Occupational Therapy*.

This research was supported by the Social Sciences and Humanities Research Council of Canada Doctoral Fellowship program.

References

Abravanel, H. (1983). Mediatory myths in the service of organizational ideology. In L. Pondy, P. I. Frost, G. Morgan, & T. C. Dandridge (Eds.), *Organizational symbolism* (pp. 273–293). Greenwich, CT: JAI Press.

American Occupational Therapy Association (1985). *A professional legacy. The Eleanor Clarke Slagle lectures in occupational therapy, 1955–1984*. Rockville, MD: Author.

Anthony, W., Cohen, M., & Farkas, M. (1990). *Psychiatric rehabilitation*. Boston: Center for Psychiatric Rehabilitation.

Bachrach, L. (Ed.) (1963). *Deinstitutionalization. New directions for mental health services series*. San Francisco: Jossey-Bass.

Baptiste, S. (1988). Chronic pain, activity and culture. *Canadian Journal of Occupational Therapy, 55,* 179-185.

Baxter, E., & Hopper, K. (1982). The new mendicancy: Homeless in New York City. *American Journal of Orthopsychiatry, 52*(3), 393–408.

Bennis, W. (1979). Why leaders can't lead. In R. Kanter & B. Stein (Eds.), *Life in organizations* (pp. 36–48). New York: Basic.

Cameron, J. (1978). Ideology and policy termination. Restructuring California's mental health system. In J. May & A. Wildavsky (Eds.), *The policy cycle* (pp. 301–328). Beverly Hills, CA: Sage.

Canadian Association of Occupational Therapists (1991). *Occupational therapy guidelines for client-centered practice*. Toronto, ON: CAOT Publications.

Carswell-Opzoomer, A. (1990). Occupational therapy: Our time has come. *Canadian Journal of Occupational Therapy, 57*(4), 197–204.

Cook, J. V. (1988). Golfman's legacy: The elimination of the chronic mental patient's community. *Research in the Sociology of Health Care, 7,* 249–281.

Downs, A. (1967). *Inside bureaucracy*. Boston: Little, Brown.

Estroff, S. E. (1981). *Making it crazy: An ethnography of psychiatric clients in an American community*. Berkeley, CA: University of California Press.

Feldman, S. (1980, Fall). The middle management muddle. *Administration in Mental Health,* pp. 3–11.

Golembiewski, R. T. (1985). *Humanizing public organizations*. Mt. Airy, MD: Lomond.

Graziano, A. M. (1969). Clinical innovation and mental health power structure: A social case history. *American Psychologist, 24* (1), 10–18.

Grob, G. N. (1980). Abuse in American mental hospitals in historical perspective: Myth and reality. *International Journal of Law and Psychiatry, 3,* 295–310.

Grob, G. N. (1983). Historical origins of deinstitutionalization. In L. L. Bachrach (Ed), *Deinstitutionalization* (pp. 15–30). San Francisco: Jossey-Bass.

Hall, R. H. (1982). *Organizations. Structures and process*. Englewood Cliffs, NJ: Prentice-Hall.

Judd, M. (1982). The challenge of change. *Canadian Journal of Occupational Therapy, 48*(4), 117–124.

Kanter, R. M. (1983). *The change masters*. New York: Simon & Schuster.

Kinston, W. (1983). Hospital organization and structure and its effect on inter-professional behaviour and the delivery of care. *Social Science and Medicine, 17*(16), 1159–1170.

Krefting, L. (1991). Rigor in qualitative research: The assessment of trustworthiness. *American Journal of Occupational Therapy 45*(3), 214–222.

Law, M. (1991). The environment: A focus for occupational therapy. *Canadian Journal of Occupational Therapy, 58*(4), 171–180.

Lincoln, L., & Guba, E. (1985). *Naturalistic inquiry*. Newbury Park, CA: Sage.

Lodahl, T. M., & Mitchell, S. M. (1981). Drift in the development of innovative organizations. In J. R. Kimberly, R. H. Miles, & Associates (Eds.), *The organizational life cycle* (pp. 184–207). San Francisco: Jossey-Bass.

Louis, M. R. (1983). Organizations as culture-bearing milieux. In L. Pondy, P. J. Frost, G. Morgan, & T. C. Dandridge (Eds.), *Organizational symbolism* (pp. 39–53). Greenwich, CT: JAI.

Marx, J. H. (1969). A multidimensional conception of ideologies in professional arenas: The case of the mental health field. *Pacific Sociological Review, 12*(2), 75–85.

Maxwell, J. D., & Maxwell, M. P. (1977). *Occupational therapy. The diffident profession*. Kingston, ON: Queen's University.

Mechanic, D. (1980). *Mental health and social policy*. Englewood Cliffs, NJ: Prentice-Hall.

Morgan, G. (1984). Opportunities arising from paradigm diversity. *Administrative Science Quarterly, 16*(3), 306–327.

Morgan, G. (1986). *Images of organization.* Beverly Hills: Sage.

Morrissey, J. P., & Tessler, R. C. (1982). Selection processes in state mental hospitalization: Policy issues and research directions. *Research in Social Problems and Public Policy, 2,* 35–79.

Polatajko, H. (1992). Naming and framing occupational therapy: A lecture dedicated to the life of Nancy B. *Canadian Journal of Occupational Therapy, 59,* 189–200.

Pranger, T., & Brown, G. (1992). Burnout: An issue for psychiatric occupational therapy personnel? *Occupational Therapy in Mental Health, 12*(1), 77–92.

Price, S. (1993). New pathways for psychosocial occupational therapists. *American Journal of Occupational Therapy, 47,* 557–559.

Schein, E. (1985). *Organizational culture and leadership.* San Francisco: Jossey-Bass.

Smircich, L. (1983). Organizations as shared meanings. In L. Pondy, P. I. Frost, G. Morgan, & T. C. Dandridge (Eds), *Organizational symbolism* (pp. 55–56). Greenwich, CT: JAI.

Smircich, L., & Morgan, G. (1982). Leadership: The management of meaning. *The Journal of Applied Behavioural Science, 18*(3), 257–273.

Smith, K. (1984). Philosophical problems in thinking about organizational change. In P. S. Goodman & Associates (Eds.), *Change in organizations* (pp. 3 16–374). San Francisco: Jossey-Bass.

Strauss, A., Schatzman, L., Bucher, R., Ehrlich, D., & Sabshin, M. (1964). *Psychiatric ideologies and institutions.* New York: Free Press of Glencoe.

Tichy, N. (1981). Problem cycles in organizations and the management of change. In J. R. Kimberly, R. H. Miles, & Associates (Eds.), *The organizational life cycle* (pp. 163–183). San Francisco: Jossey-Bass.

Tichy, N. (1983). *Managing strategic change. Technical, political and cultural dynamics.* New York: Wiley.

Weissman, H. H. (1982). Fantasy and reality of staff involvement in organizational change. *Administration in Social Work, 6*(1), 37–45.

Wilson, J. (1973). *Introduction to social movements.* New York: Basic.

Yerxa, E. J. (1983). Audacious values: The energy source for occupational therapy practice. In G. Kielhofner (Ed.), *Health through occupation. Theory and practice in occupational therapy* (pp. 149–162). Philadelphia: F. A. Davis.

Yerxa, E. J. (1991). Occupational therapy and medicine: A comparison of values. *The Link, 7,* 1–2.

Chapter 18

"Doing" in Mental Health Practice: Therapists' Beliefs About Why It Works

The American Journal of Occupational Therapy

1997, 51(8): 662–670

Sandra Moll, Joanne Valiant Cook

Sandra Moll, MSc, OT(C), is Case Manager/Living Skills Coordinator, Hamilton Program for Schizophrenia, 350 King Street E., Suite 102, Hamilton, Ontario L8N 3Y3, Canada.
Joanne Valiant Cook, PhD, OT(C), is Assistant Professor, Department of Occupational Therapy, Faculty of Applied Health Sciences, Elborn College, The University of Western Ontario, London, Ontario, Canada.

KEY WORDS

- planning process
- occupational therapy
- therapeutic activities

ABSTRACT

Objective. *The purpose of this study was to explore the beliefs of occupational therapists working in mental health regarding the therapeutic value of "doing" as a treatment modality. Doing was defined as any activity or action-oriented approach that was identified and used by the participating therapists.*

Method. *Eleven occupational therapists working in a variety of mental health areas were observed as they conducted 3 to 6 regularly scheduled therapy sessions. They were then interviewed about their activity-related beliefs. Audiotapes of the 44 treatment sessions and 11 interviews were transcribed and then coded to identify emergent themes and categories of beliefs about activity.*

Results. *Participants used a variety of activities in both task-based and verbally based treatment sessions. Multiple reasons for activity use were cited, particularly in relation to the task-based sessions. Two main themes related to the value of activity were (a) benefits of activity for the client and (b) benefits in facilitating the process of therapy. Categories of client-related benefits included skill development; impairment reduction; self-awareness; positive self-concept; interaction or connection with others; healthy, balanced routines; pleasure; and enhancement of occupational role performance. Perceived effects on the therapeutic process included creating a therapeutic context, enhancing client readiness, facilitating communication, and providing an organizing framework.*

Conclusion. *Occupational therapists working in mental health hold diverse beliefs about the value of doing in treatment. Basing practice on clearly identified and evidence-based beliefs will assist in ensuring a viable and valued future for the profession in this important domain of health services.*

Occupational therapists in the mental health system face increasing competition from professionals and paraprofessionals in the delivery of rehabilitation services (Foto, 1996; Paul, 1996). Validation of our role in this area of practice demands clear articulation of our unique contributions and evidence-based rationales for our intervention.

Occupation, activity, or "doing" have traditionally been identified as the hallmark and essential uniqueness of occupational therapy practice (American Occupational Therapy Association [AOTA], 1995; Canadian Association of Occupational Therapists [CAOT], 1991). The profession was founded on a belief in the therapeutic value of activity or occupation (Meyer, 1922; Reilly, 1962). However, reasons for using action-oriented treatment modalities have changed considerably over time. They have gone from beliefs in the value of doing as an essential part of daily life to beliefs about doing as a means to reaching other therapeutic goals and, again, back to beliefs about the value of doing in daily life and, therefore, the ultimate goal of the therapy process (Bing, 1981; Kielhofner, 1992; Kielhofner & Burke, 1983). Although changes in beliefs about the value of doing have been reported, there has been little systematic study of the clinical reasoning process of therapists working in mental health, particularly with respect to their selection and use of treatment modalities.

The current study was designed to explore the beliefs of this population regarding the therapeutic value of doing as a treatment modality. Doing was defined as any activity or action-oriented approach that was identified and used by the therapists. The terms *doing* and *activity* were used interchangeably. Although there has been considerable controversy in the occupational therapy literature about distinctions among the terms *activity, task,* and *occupation* (Christiansen, 1990; Kielhofner, 1982, Nelson, 1988; Polatajko, 1992), *activity* continues to be commonly used to refer to the broad range of treatment modalities that therapists use (Allen, 1987; AOTA, 1995; CAOT, 1991).

LITERATURE REVIEW

Beliefs about and the use of activity in mental health practice have changed considerably over time. When the profession was initially founded, mental health practice was based on principles of the Moral Treatment era (Bing, 1981; Kielhofner & Burke, 1983). Programs of daily living activities were designed to normalize the disorganized behavior of persons with mental illness (Bockoven, 1971). A wide variety of activities were used, such as fishing, gardening, games, dancing, reading, and sewing circles (Bockoven, 1971). One of the early occupational therapy approaches to treatment, which was based on the Moral Treatment philosophy, was termed *habit training* (Slagle, 1922). This approach involved a carefully designed schedule of activities in order "to give the patient a well-balanced day as nearly approaching the normal as possible in an institutional set-up" (LeVesconte, 1935, p. 11).

The influence of the medical model in the late 1940s led to a shift in therapists' beliefs about and use of activity. In mental health, a psychodynamic approach was advocated, and the focus was on clients' impairments and reduction of pathology (Azima & Azima, 1959; Fidler, 1958). Projective media, such as drama, dance, drawing, and clay, were often used (Wittkower & Johnston, 1958). Knowledge of group dynamics was also advanced during this era (Howe & Schwartzberg, 1986). The emphasis of therapy was on verbally based approaches; tasks or activities were used primarily to facilitate group process (Bissell & Mailloux, 1981; Kielhofner & Burke, 1983).

Increasing dissatisfaction with occupational therapy roles and restricted identity in the 1960s and 1970s (Diaso, 1971; Mosey, 1971) led to further changes in therapists' use of activity in the 1980s and 1990s. There has been a shift from using activity as a treatment modality to enabling occupational performance as an end goal (Kielhofner, 1992). Provision of *task opportunities* is still considered a valued approach to treatment. However, environmental modification and counseling interventions are considered to be equally valid (Kielhofner, 1992). Concerns have been expressed about this trend by some authors who maintained that because of the profession's strong belief in the therapeutic value of activity or occupation, action-oriented treatment modalities should continue to be an integral part of occupational therapy practice (Allen, 1987; Fidler, 1991; Hettinger, 1996).

Studies of psychiatric occupational therapy in the 1980s revealed that a variety of treatment activities were used, ranging from macrame and woodworking to cooking, games, and field trips (Barris, Cordero, & Christiaansen, 1986; Dickerson & Kaplan, 1991; Duncombe & Howe, 1985; Javetz & Katz, 1989; Stein & Tallant, 1988; Taylor & Manguno, 1991). However, the use of craft-oriented treatment modalities decreased over time, whereas treatment modalities related to communication skills and activities of daily living (ADL) became the most frequently used (Barris et al., 1986; Duncombe & Howe, 1985; Gohl-Giese & Eliason, 1986; Javetz & Katz, 1989; Stein & Tallant, 1988; Taylor & Manguno, 1991).

Of all these studies that described the overall trends in activity use, only two examined the association between therapists' treatment goals and specific treatment modalities (Barris et al., 1986; Duncombe & Howe, 1985). Both studies had therapists rate the frequency with which treatment goals (from a list developed by the researchers) were associated with particular treatment approaches. The studies revealed that therapists used a wide range of goals and that activities were often used to meet multiple goals. The treatment goal most commonly cited was skill development (e.g., communication, cognitive, task skills). Studies of occupational therapists' clinical reasoning also indicate that therapists tend to cite multiple reasons for using a particular treatment approach and that these reasons may vary, depending on the perceived needs of a particular client (Fleming, 1994).

Overall, studies of activity use in mental health practice reflect that therapists use a variety of treatment modalities and that changes have occurred in their use of these modalities over time (e.g., decreased use of crafts, increased use of skill-training approaches). Verbally oriented modalities that focus on skill development seem to be among the most common approaches, although there is much variation both within and between therapists. In general, research examining therapists' beliefs about the value of activity has been limited. Most of the studies were conducted more than a decade ago, and their use of predetermined lists of treatment goals did not capture the potential richness, complexity, and variety of reasons therapists use in selecting interventions. To obtain an in-depth understanding of therapists' beliefs, they need to be examined within the context of day-to-day practice, considering the impact of individual clients and types of treatment modalities.

METHOD

Design

A qualitative, naturalistic research design was adopted. Schatzman and Strauss (1973) stated that communicating with participants in their natural situation reveals "the nuances of meaning from which their perspectives and definitions are continually forged" (p. 6).

Participants

Eleven therapists from five facilities in southwestern Ontario participated in the study. Facilities were selected to ensure variation in both location and type of practice. Two psychiatric hospitals and three general hospitals were represented. These facilities were located in four different urban centers. Participants ranged in clinical experience from 5 months to 9 years and came from a variety of educational backgrounds, including five universities and two foreign colleges. Nine worked in an inpatient mental health setting, and seven worked in acute care. Eight had a mixed caseload, and the other three worked in specialty areas (i.e., psychogeriatrics, a community-based schizophrenia program, a program for survivors of childhood sexual abuse).

Data Collection

Data were collected over approximately 2 to 3 weeks at each facility. Each participant was observed conducting 3 to 6 regularly scheduled therapy sessions that they identified as typical of their daily practice. During the sessions, the investigator recorded notes, as unobtrusively as possible, about the content of the dialogue and the observed behavior of the therapist and client(s). Most therapy sessions were audiotaped as well. Forty-four sessions were observed: 15 individual and 29 group.

After the observation period, participants were interviewed about their activity-related beliefs and practices. The audiotaped, semistructured interviews were approximately 1.5 hr in length. General as well as session-specific reasons for activity use were explored.

Data Analysis

Transcribed data from the observations and interviews were reviewed, coded, and recoded in an iterative process of organizing the data and generating categories, themes, and patterns. Several classification schema were explored before selecting the one that best represented the participants' responses and enabled description of their beliefs and practices.

Trustworthiness was established through triangulation of data sources and methods. The combination of interview and observation methods plus the use of a variety of data sources (i.e., participants from different facilities, repeated observations with each participant) meant that information from one source or method could be cross-checked for confirmation from another (Krefting, 1991; Lincoln & Guba, 1985). Member checking was also conducted with 10 of the 11 participants. The 10 participants reviewed the final themes and patterns, which they believed accurately captured their perceptions and beliefs about activity use. In addition, the investigator maintained a reflexive journal so that the research process and product could be audited.

RESULTS

Types of Therapy Sessions

Upon observing overall patterns of activity use in both individual and group sessions, it became evident that there were two main types of sessions: task based and verbally based. Task-based sessions were classified as such if the primary focus for the client was observed to be on performance of a particular task(s). In some sessions, clients worked on individual projects (e.g., crafts, baking, computer work), and in others, clients worked together on a group project (e.g., newsletter committee, group meal). In a few task-based sessions, clients participated in action-oriented exercises (e.g., playing catch, passing around objects). Regardless of the treatment modalities used, the focus in each treatment session was on performance of the activity. Although there was some conversation, it was usually social in nature. Problems related to the client's illness were not discussed. Approximately 30% of the observed sessions were classified as task based.

Verbally based sessions, on the other hand, were observed to be organized around a particular issue or topic rather than on a task. Activities were used to varying degrees and at different stages in the sessions but appeared to be auxiliary to the focal point or topic(s) being addressed. The names of the groups reflected their focus on a particular topic or issue. For example, several groups were called communication or coping skills groups. The names of the other groups included predischarge, social action, and assertiveness training. More than half of these sessions were classified as "teaching–learning" sessions because they seemed to have an educational focus, with lesson plans, information written on the board or on handouts, and homework assignments. Activities identified by the therapists in these groups included role playing, written work sheets, and experiential exercises to facilitate "here-and-now" learning. The other verbally based sessions were classified as "support-and-planning" sessions because their focus seemed to involve discussing how the client was doing in his or her therapy and daily life and then planning how to proceed from there. Although talking was usually the main focus, written exercises were sometimes used (e.g., reading material, journals, goal setting work sheets). One other type of verbally based session, although not observed, was described by several therapists. This was classified as "intrapsychic exploration" because its focus seemed to be on exploring feelings and thoughts and development of insight. Projective techniques and experiential exercises were often the identified activities used in these sessions. Approximately 70% of the observed sessions were classified as verbally based.

Overall, in the task-based sessions, the doing seemed to be of central importance. In verbally based sessions, the main doing was verbal in nature, and the identified treatment modalities seemed to be used to supplement the verbal discussion regarding a particular topic. It was important to know the overall goals of the verbally based sessions because the activity often served a specific function in achieving the overall goal(s). The type of session, therefore, provided important contextual information for understanding the reasons for using activity within the session.

Participants' Reasons for Activity Use

Several general features were evident in the participants' responses regarding their reasons for using activity. Some participants found it difficult to articulate their rationale, explaining that they did not consciously consider specific reasons before using the activity. Their intuitive approach to using activity is illustrated as follows:

Therapist D2: I think sometimes I am not 100% sure of all the different ways I'm using an activity and, therefore, I don't feel competent in describing it. Like, I have an idea, I have a goal in using this, or an idea [that] perhaps I haven't even formulated . . . into a goal. I just think, "Ok, this seems appropriate; this might work; I'm going to try it."

However, one of the most striking features of the responses was the diversity in the identified benefits of using activity. Participants usually gave long lists of reasons for why they used an activity. This was particularly evident in reference to the task-based sessions in which activity was a central feature. One participant described the multiple benefits of using activity in a craft group:

Therapist B2: We use a variety of leisure-type craft activities, but also you can do work—activities like typing and using a computer in that group—and we use those activities to look at sort of more the mental components of things like concentration, organization, things like that and looking at self-esteem and leisure interests within that. So that's how we'd use the activity—also as an observation.

In general, participants spoke with more animation and at greater length about the value of activity for a specific client than about the value of activity in general practice. For example, group protocols listed standard benefits of using activities (e.g., increasing task skills, self-esteem, motivation, social skills), yet when talking about individual clients within the group, participants provided rich narratives about the value of activity for the client. The variety and complexity of the perceived benefits are illustrated in the following description of the benefits of woodworking for one client:

Therapist B1: Unfortunately, J. was in a very, very major depression, and a lot of his self-confidence and feelings about himself were really low, and he was feeling that he wasn't the breadwinner in the house; he wasn't able to provide for his family. The farm that he had worked on all his life wasn't doing well financially. He had to sell off large chunks of it, and so on. And so, productivity was a real concern for him. One, because of his psychovegetative symptoms as well as from his self-esteem standpoint. I felt it very important to be able to have him working on something. One that he could accomplish and say, "OK, I'm doing stuff, I'm able to get things done," especially for his self-esteem, but also just to get him up and out of bed and doing something so that he could generate more energy and so on within himself.

Additionally, as alluded to earlier, reasons for using activity varied, depending on the type of session and the activities themselves. The term *activity* was used to refer not only to treatment modalities related to self-care, productivity, and leisure, but also to pencil-and-paper tasks that were used to supplement verbal discussion. Descriptions of the participants' reasons for using activity will further highlight differences between these two approaches to activity use.

Specific Reasons for Activity Use

Despite the diversity in descriptions of the benefits of activity, two main themes emerged repeatedly: (a) the benefits of activity for the client and (b) the effects of the activity on the therapeutic process. Within each theme, several categories were identified on the basis of narratives from at least two to three participants.

Client-related benefits. Client-related benefits cited by the participants were classified into eight main categories: skill development; impairment reduction; increased self-awareness; positive self-concept; interaction or connection with others; healthy, balanced routines; pleasure; and connection to valued occupational roles.

Most participants described the value of activity in promoting *skill development*. In the task-based sessions, activity was identified as a means to promote development of cognitive skills (e.g., concentration, organization, problem solving) as well as a means to promote occupational performance skills (e.g., cooking, budgeting, work skills). In the verbally based sessions, the main focus of the session was often on a particular skill (e.g., problem solving, assertiveness, nonverbal communication), and

tasks (e.g., self-assessment questionnaires, role plays) were used to facilitate knowledge acquisition and skill practice. Many participants commented generally on the value of doing to facilitate learning. For example:

> *Therapist A2: It helps them get the information in a manner that's consistent with my philosophy, which is that doing is better than just observing.*

Participants identified *impairment reduction* activities as beneficial in remediating a variety of symptoms. Walking, for example, was described as part of a desensitization program for a client with agoraphobia, and cooking was described as a way of helping clients with anorexia confront their phobias about food. Experiential activities (e.g., imagery exercises, striking a tackle dummy) were identified as useful in overcoming defenses and facilitating the healing process in survivors of childhood abuse.

Increasing self-awareness through written exercises used in the verbally based sessions (e.g., self-assessment questionnaires, journals, writing out goals) was frequently cited as useful in facilitating reflection and awareness of personal attributes and abilities. Projective activities (e.g., collages, drawing) and experiential exercises were also identified as a means of facilitating self-awareness. For example:

> *Therapist E3: [In reference to experiential activities] So it's those kinds of things where you can see that it can really help people to figure out what they're trying to contend with. Rather than it all just being talked about, actually doing activities . . . will help them cope with it and deal with it. They can actually visualize what's going on. Also, to get people in touch with their feelings.*

Many participants stated that the role of activity in promoting a *positive self-concept* was beneficial. They maintained that the client's self-concept improved as a result of completing projects in the task-based sessions. Completing the project reportedly produced a sense of accomplishment and increased self-esteem. In addition, several participants emphasized the value of the actual end-product, explaining that positive feedback from others improved the client's self-confidence. Repeatedly performing a task, or even performing a task that the client was already good at, was described as a way of enhancing a sense of self-efficacy or self-esteem. Several verbally based sessions specifically focused on self-esteem, and tasks (e.g., reading text, playing a game) were used to facilitate learning and reflection on the identified topic.

Comments related to the value of activity in promoting *interaction or connection with others* indicated that participants believed in the importance of social interaction, not as simply a means to develop social skills, but as a basic human need and, therefore, an end goal in itself. For example, the participant who worked in the psychogeriatric ward identified social interaction as a fundamental need for her clients:

Therapist A1: Our original reason [for developing the task-based group] was because the patients on the ward have no human contact other than hands-on care. And we just thought, "Wouldn't it be nice if they had somebody touch them, or hold them, or move them, or talk to them, or stimulate them in some way so that they're getting something other than sitting in their chair and having the TV turned on in front of them all day long?"

Activity in both individual and group sessions reportedly provided the context within which social interaction could occur. For example:

Therapist B2: [Rationale for baking group with clients who were fairly high functioning] . . . getting group cohesion . . . making it more social for people to work on an activity together, and the social interaction that happens after the thing's made, and getting feedback on that, and that sort of thing.

Participants indicated that for some clients, activity in the task-based sessions fulfilled a basic need to participate in meaningful activity and promoted *healthy, balanced routines*. For example:

Therapist D1: [In reference to value of newsletter committee for a male outpatient client] He is looking at that as being a productive use of his

time—the social part of it as well as an opportunity to do something structured. And I really think that's important for him. . . . So for him individually, that's his goal. He likes to be involved in doing something.

Several participants also talked about the structure provided by activity as a way for clients to normalize their daily routines. They hypothesized that if clients were able to engage in regular, healthy activities in the hospital, they might learn to do this at home as well. For example:

Therapist D2: We try to have one [session a week] that's sort of a recreational–leisure activity, like a game, inside–outside, go for a walk, do some exercise, something like that. . . . And [a word game] and games like that. And we hope that by doing that on a regular basis, they will also indirectly pick up on the fact that it's good to incorporate these types of activities into your daily schedule or into a routine. So, we're hoping that will pick up on a lot of things in an indirect way.

According to participants, activities that provided *pleasure* were valuable. Pleasurable activities included those that were soothing, relaxing, and enjoyable or ones that produced a sense of personal satisfaction. Many participants talked about the importance of incorporating activities that were fun for the clients. For example:

Therapist E3: I guess my feeling, being here in the hospital, is that a lot of the people . . . come in here under a lot of pressure, and they are very stressed out, and fun hasn't been something that's been a part of their life for a while because they've [gotten] very entrenched in all of their problems. And so in the group, we do try and focus on the sort of lighter side of things too. Just so that it gets them back in touch with the feeling of having fun.

It is interesting to note that not all participants were comfortable identifying pleasure as a primary reason for using activity. One participant commented that she felt guilty when using games that the clients perceived as fun or enjoyable:

Therapist D2: [Asked about why she sounded apologetic when describing an activity that the clients enjoy] Because I'm using games. I don't want to be confused with a recreationist. I think, "I'm using games." I have to go home and tell my husband that I played a game with patients and then explain how that is therapeutic.

In general, ensuring that the activity was enjoyable for the client was described as important, but pleasure was not usually identified as the sole reason for using an activity.

There were three sessions conducted by the participants that appeared qualitatively different from the rest. Descriptions of the impact of activity within these sessions seemed to relate to its function in connecting the client to valued past, present, or future *occupational roles.* Activities were described as having particular, idiosyncratic meaning to the clients in relation to their occupational roles. For example, the participant who worked on a psychogeriatric ward described the meaning of passing familiar objects to clients with severe cognitive impairments. She explained that holding a simple object like a teddy bear or doll might "spark awareness" of the client's past role as a parent of small children. Clients who were previously unresponsive would become animated, cuddling or talking to the doll in their arms. A second participant talked about the occupational role that was created for one of his clients who participated on a newsletter committee. For this client, the committee was viewed as volunteer work—a way of helping others and "giving back" to the program. The impact of activity on present and future occupational roles was also described by a third participant who was working on budgeting with an outpatient client. This participant described the impact of the sessions on the client's relationship with her spouse, who was an accountant. As the client learned and applied budgeting skills, her role within the marriage reportedly changed. In all of these sessions, the activity seemed to relate to some aspect of the client's past, present, or future occupational roles.

Effects on the therapeutic process. The other main rationale for using activity relates to the participants' perceived value of activity in facil-itating the process of therapy. This rationale was particularly evident in comments about activity in the verbally based sessions. Effects on the therapeutic process were classified into four main categories: establishing a therapeutic context; enhancing client readiness or receptiveness, facilitating communication, and providing an organizing framework.

Several participants explained that activity may assist in *establishing a therapeutic context* or nonthreatening milieu. They explained that it redirects the focus of attention, thereby increasing clients' comfort level. Furthermore, activity may act as a unifying factor, establishing a common ground between clients. For example:

Therapist E3: You know, depending on the activity too, it can take away from people being sort of put on the spotlight, which is very uncomfortable for some people. . . . I feel that by doing that [activity] too, that people do feel a part of being in a group—everyone's doing the same thing.

Participants identified several ways in which activity could be used to *enhance client readiness or receptiveness.* One participant talked about playing chess with a client as a way of engaging him in the therapy process and, therefore, establishing rapport. She explained that "he was so paranoid that I wasn't able to do a lot, so he took control of the sessions, and he wanted to play chess." Activities were also described as being useful in focusing the attention of clients on the topic being discussed. Interesting or fun activities were described as a means of generating interest and readiness to receive information. For example, one participant believed that "if you can get people laughing, then the moment right after is a teachable moment."

Activity also contributed to *facilitating communication.* Many participants talked about using activities such as games, questionnaires, and role playing as catalysts for generating thoughts and feelings for subsequent discussion. Activity was also described as an alternative medium through which clients could express their thoughts and feelings. For example, drawing or collages were described as agents for nonverbal communication. Several participants also talked about using activity to regulate or control discussions, particularly with talkative clients. Writing tasks and relaxation exercises were identified as ways of ensuring that the participant would get some "air time" with the client.

Participants further described activity as *providing an organizing framework* for the session. Written activities, such as journals or work sheets, were identified as particularly useful in structuring the session, organizing information delivery, or summarizing information that was covered.

DISCUSSION

This study was designed to explore occupational therapists' beliefs about activity use within the context of their practice in mental health settings. One of the most striking findings was the considerable diversity and complexity in the participants' beliefs about the effectiveness of various treatment modalities. Treatment activities were used in many different ways, for many different reasons. Participants often identified layers of meaning that the "doing process" entailed not only for the client, but also for the overall process of therapy.

Diversity of Beliefs

Fleming (1994) noted that choosing activities that serve several purposes simultaneously is typical of occupational therapy practice. In her discussion of the clinical reasoning process of therapists, she stated that "therapists never do only one thing at a time" and "never do anything for just one reason" (p. 34). The technique of activity analysis supports identification of multiple goals for any one activity (Lamport, Coffey, & Hersch, 1989). The diversity may be further attributed to the therapists' attempts to reconcile established principles of treatment with the unique needs and abilities of each client (Fleming, 1994). Therapists in our study

repeatedly emphasized the importance of individualizing treatment. Their narratives about interventions with individual clients were often lengthy and multifaceted. In addition, they discussed the importance of engaging the client in the process of therapy, which seemed to add another layer to the perceived value of the activity. Treatment planning, therefore, seemed to involve consideration of a combination of factors that involved the activity, the client, and the process of therapy.

The range of benefits associated with activity also reflected the diversity of and shifts in activity use described in the literature on successive eras in the profession's development (Kielhofner, 1992; Kielhofner & Burke, 1983). For example, the value of activity in promoting healthy habits and routines reflected the principles of habit training characteristic of early occupational therapy practice. On the other hand, benefits related to impairment reduction and facilitation of verbal communication were consistent with principles of activity use in the 1950s and 1960s. Finally, benefits related to skill training and occupational performance seemed to be consistent with principles of activity use in the 1980s and 1990s. Identified benefits, therefore, were not restricted to one particular era within the profession's development.

It is important to note that comments about the multipurpose nature of activity primarily referred to treatment modalities used in the task-based sessions. Activities in these treatment sessions involved "traditional" modalities such as crafts, ADL, and vocational activities. The majority of sessions conducted by the participants, however, were classified as verbally based. Unlike the task-based sessions, treatment activities in the verbally based sessions were often used for a specific purpose (e.g., to facilitate discussion, to organize information delivery).

Different Types of Doing

Our finding that "learning modalities" used in the verbally based sessions predominated over traditional craft and ADL-oriented modalities is consistent with patterns of activity use reported in the literature (Gohl-Giese & Eliason, 1986; Javetz & Katz, 1989; Taylor & Manguno, 1991). Both Fidler (1981, 1991) and Huss (1981) expressed concern about the use of verbally based approaches in psychosocial occupational therapy. They argued that the depth of meaning of occupational therapy activities may be lost and that therapists who stressed verbally based approaches were devaluing traditional occupational therapy media in an effort to gain credibility with other disciplines. The therapists in our study spoke with more animation about nontraditional media characteristic of verbally based sessions (e.g., projective collages, group exercises, questionnaires) than about the more traditional media used in the task-based sessions (e.g., crafts, ADL tasks). They usually emphasized the verbally based rather than the ADL-oriented or task-based sessions, and one of the participants talked about being embarrassed about using games or crafts in therapy.

Although it appears that therapists might be abandoning their central focus on the value of doing, another perspective is possible. It may be that the doing focus has shifted from the modality used in therapy to the end goal of the therapeutic process. Kielhofner's (1992) description of the emerging paradigm of the 1980s and 1990s emphasizes a return to the fundamental values of meaningful occupation, but the focus is on the outcome rather than on the process of therapy. He emphasized that provision of task opportunities may be one approach to treatment, but other approaches such as verbal counselling may be equally valid. For example, in verbally based sessions that focus on assertiveness, the "meaningful doing" may not be completing a written questionnaire but rather being able to assertively ask one's boss for a raise. The occupational performance outcome may have many layers of meaning and benefits for the client. The increased focus on doing that occurs outside of the therapeutic session makes sense in this era of shortened hospital stays and increased focus on community intervention.

Directions for Future Research

This study was exploratory in nature, examining one aspect of clinical practice—beliefs about the therapeutic value of doing as a treatment modality. Analysis was conducted with a relatively small group of mental health occupational therapists. It would be interesting to investigate whether similar beliefs are held by therapists working in other geographical regions or other practice areas and to compare the beliefs held by therapists with those held by consumers of occupational therapy services.

The study findings provide a glimpse into the complex clinical reasoning process as it relates to beliefs about the therapeutic value of activity. More in-depth research could be conducted to investigate how beliefs about activity affect the process of treatment planning. For example: How do therapists balance the needs of individuals versus groups in selecting treatment modalities? Are there other important factors that influence the process of activity selection and treatment? What types of clinical reasoning are evident as therapists apply their beliefs about activity to the process of treatment planning?

Other studies could examine and empirically test occupational therapy practitioners' beliefs about the value of doing. This empirical research would not only provide evidence to support practitioners' beliefs, but also contribute to validating our services. Such research will require development of outcome measures that operationalize our beliefs about the multiple benefits of the doing process.

CONCLUSION

Doing has historically been a fundamental component of occupational therapy practice in mental health. Many of the beliefs held by therapists about the value of the doing process are not evident to the uninformed observer. According to Fleming (1994), "Although what they do looks simple, what they know is often quite complex" (p. 24). Basing mental health occupational therapy practice on clearly identified and evidence-based principles of activity, doing, or occupation will assist in ensuring a viable and valued future for the profession in this important domain of health services.

ACKNOWLEDGMENTS

This study was funded by a grant from the Canadian Occupational Therapy Foundation. It is based on the first author's thesis work in partial fulfillment of the requirements for the master of science in occupational therapy degree at The University of Western Ontario.

References

Allen, C. K. (1987). Activity: Occupational therapy's treatment method, 1987 Eleanor Clarke Slagle lecture. *American Journal of Occupational Therapy, 41,* 563–575.

American Occupational Therapy Association. (1995). The philosophical base of occupational therapy. *American Journal of Occupational Therapy, 49,* 1026.

Azima, H., & Azima, F. J. (1959). Outline of a dynamic theory of occupational therapy. *American Journal of Occupational Therapy, 13,* 215–221.

Barris, R., Cordero, J., & Christiaansen, R. (1986). Occupational therapists' use of media. *American Journal of Occupational Therapy, 40,* 679–684.

Bing, R. K. (1981). Occupational therapy revisited: A paraphrastic journey, 1981 Eleanor Clarke Slagle lecture. *American Journal of Occupational Therapy, 35,* 499–518.

Bissell, J. C., & Mailloux, Z. (1981). The use of crafts in occupational therapy for the physically disabled. *American Journal of Occupational Therapy, 35,* 369–374.

Bockoven, J. S. (1971). Occupational Therapy—A Historical Perspective: Legacy of moral treatment—1800s to 1910. *American Journal of Occupational Therapy, 25,* 223–225.

Canadian Association of Occupational Therapists. (1991). *Occupational therapy guidelines for client-centred practice.* Toronto, Ontario: Author.

Christiansen, C. (1990). The perils of plurality. *Occupational Therapy Journal of Research, 10,* 259–265.

Diaso, K. (1971). Occupational Therapy—A Historical Perspective: The modern era—1960 to 1970. *American Journal of Occupational Therapy, 25,* 237–242.

Dickerson, A., & Kaplan, S. H. (1991). A comparison of craft use and academic preparation in craft modalities. *American Journal of Occupational Therapy, 45,* 11–17.

Duncombe, L., & Howe, M. C. (1985). Group work in occupational therapy: A survey of practice. *American Journal of Occupational Therapy, 39,* 163–170.

Fidler, G. S. (1958). Some unique contributions of occupational therapy in treatment of the schizophrenic. *American Journal of Occupational Therapy, 12,* 9–12, 36.

Fidler, G. S. (1981). From crafts to competence. *American Journal of Occupational Therapy, 35,* 567–573.

Fidler, G. S. (1991). The challenge of change to occupational therapy practice. *Occupational Therapy in Mental Health, 11*(1), 1–11.

Fleming, M. H. (1994). The search for tacit knowledge. In C. Mattingly & M. H. Fleming (Eds.), *Clinical reasoning: Forms of inquiry in a therapeutic practice* (pp. 22–34). Philadelphia: F. A. Davis.

Foto, M. (1996). Nationally Speaking—Multiskilling: Who, how, when, and why? *American Journal of Occupational Therapy, 50,* 7–9.

Gohl-Giese, A., & Eliason, M. L. (1986). Changes in the frequency of use of occupational therapy treatment modalities from 1978 to 1985: Educational implications. In *Occupational therapy education: Target 2000 proceedings* (p. 149). Rockville, MD: American Occupational Therapy Association.

Hettinger, J. (1996, May 30). Why OT will continue to flourish. *OT Week, 10*(22), 14–15.

Howe, M. C., & Schwartzberg, S. L. (1986). *A functional approach to group work in occupational therapy.* Philadelphia: Lippincott.

Huss, A. J. (1981). From kinesiology to adaptation. *American Journal of Occupational Therapy, 35,* 574–580.

Javetz, R., & Katz, N. (1989). Knowledgeability of theories of occupational therapy practitioners in Israel. *American Journal of Occupational Therapy, 43,* 664–675.

Kielhofner, G. (1982). A heritage of activity: Development of theory. *American Journal of Occupational Therapy, 36,* 723–730.

Kielhofner, G. (1992). *Conceptual foundation of occupational therapy.* Philadelphia: F. A. Davis.

Kielhofner, G., & Burke, J. P. (1983). The evolution of knowledge and practice in occupational therapy: Past, present and future. In G. Kielhofner (Ed.). *Health through occupation: Theory and practice in occupational therapy* (pp. 3–54). Philadelphia: F. A. Davis.

Krefting, L. (1991). Rigor in qualitative research: The assessment of trustworthiness. *American Journal of Occupational Therapy, 45,* 214–222.

Lamport, N. K., Coffey, M. S., & Hersch. G. I. (1989). *Activity analysis handbook.* Thorofare. NJ: Slack.

LeVesconte, H. P. (1935). Expanding fields of occupational therapy. *Canadian Journal of Occupational Therapy, 53*(11), 9–15.

Lincoln, Y. S., & Guba, E. G. (1985). Naturalistic inquiry. Newbury Park, CA: Sage.

Meyer, A. (1922). The philosophy of occupation therapy. *Archives of Occupational Therapy, 1,* 1–10.

Mosey, A. C. (1971). Occupational Therapy—A Historical Perspective: Involvement in the rehabilitation movement—1942 to 1960. *American Journal of Occupational Therapy, 25,* 234–236.

Nelson, D. L. (1988). Occupation: Form and performance. *American Journal of Occupational Therapy, 42,* 633–641.

Paul, S. (1996). The Issue Is—Mental health: An endangered occupational therapy specialty? *American Journal of Occupational Therapy, 50,* 65–68.

Polatajko, H. J. (1992). Naming and framing occupational therapy: A lecture dedicated to the life of Nancy B. *Canadian Journal of Occupational Therapy, 59,* 189–199.

Reilly, M. (1962). Occupational therapy can be one of the great ideas of 20th century medicine, Eleanor Clarke Slagle lecture. *American Journal of Occupational Therapy, 16,* 1–9.

Schatzman, L., & Strauss, A. L. (1973). *Field research: Strategies for a natural sociology.* Englewood Cliffs, NJ: Prentice-Hall.

Slagle, E. C. (1922). Training aides for mental patients. *Archives of Occupational Therapy, 1,* 11–17.

Stein, G., & Tallant, B. K. (1988). Applying the group process to psychiatric occupational therapy part 1: Historical and current use. *Occupational Therapy in Mental Health, 8*(3), 9–27.

Taylor, E., & Manguno, J. (1991). Use of treatment activities in occupational therapy. *American Journal of Occupational Therapy, 45,* 317–322.

Wittkower, E. D., & Johnston, A. M. (1958). New developments in and perspectives of psychiatric occupational therapy. *Canadian Journal of Occupational Therapy, 25*(1), 5–11.

Chapter 19

Enjoyment Experiences as Described by Persons with Schizophrenia: A Qualitative Study

Canadian Journal of Occupational Therapy

1998, 65(4): 183–192

Heather Emerson, Joanne Cook, Helene Polatajko, Ruth Segal

Heather A. Emerson, M. Sc., O.T. (C) is an Occupational Therapist at London Psychiatric Hospital, 850 Highbury Avenue, P.O. Box 2532, Station A, London, Ontario, N6A 4H1
Joanne Valiant Cook. Ph.D., O.T. (C) Associate Professor
Helene Polatajko, Ph.D., O.T. (C) Department Chair
Ruth Segal, Ph.D., O.T. (C) Assistant Professor, all in the School of Occupational Therapy, Faculty of Health Sciences, Elborn College. The University of Western Ontario, London, Ontario, N6G 1H1

KEY WORDS

- human activities and occupation
- mental health
- personal satisfaction

ABSTRACT

Csikszentmihalyi's (1990) assertion that persons with schizophrenia do not experience "flow" states provided the impetus for a study exploring the enjoyment experiences of nine persons with schizophrenia. Data were gathered using an audio taped semi-structured interview and analyzed using qualitative methods. Five themes emerged regarding the informants' subjective experiences: excitement, accomplishment, relaxation, social connectedness, and being interested. The first two themes parallel flow states, disputing Csikszentmihalyi's assumption that individuals with schizophrenia are unable to experience flow. The third theme may be a precursor to flow. The remaining two themes are distinct from flow, suggesting that for the informants in this study, enjoyment was a broader construct than flow.

The purpose of this study was to explore enjoyment as experienced by persons with schizophrenia. The study was motivated by the wish to examine assertions found in the literature on schizophrenia (Grinker & Holzman, 1973; Spaulding & Sullivan, 1992), and the literature on flow (Csikszentmihalyi, 1990), that people who have this illness do not derive enjoyment from involvement in activities.

Occupational therapists believe that enjoyment and intrinsic motivation occur when individuals engage in occupations that are challenging, but not overwhelming (Arnsten, 1990; Doble, 1988; Florey, 1969; Kielhofner, 1992). The experience of becoming absorbed in a "just-right challenge" is considered to be therapeutic and crucial to one's sense of well-being (Yerxa et al., 1989). In recent years occupational therapists have cited literature on flow by Csikszentmihalyi (1988, 1990) which stresses the importance of a balance between skills and challenges (Law, 1991; Primeau, Clark, & Pierce, 1989; Yerxa et al., 1989).

Csikszentmihalyi (1990) has used the terms *enjoyment* and *flow* interchangeably to describe an intrinsically-rewarding experience that occurs when people are involved in activities that they perceive as offering manageable challenges. Flow is a subjective state characterized by a positive affective state, high motivation, high cognitive efficiency, and high activation (Csikszentmihalyi, & Mei-Ha Wong, 1991). According to Csikszentmihalyi (1993), flow states involve concentration on an activity, a sense of control over one's actions, and a clear sense of purpose. During flow there is a temporary reprieve from one's worries, a loss of self-consciousness, and a distorted sense of time (Csikszentmihalyi, 1990, 1993). The experience of flow involves a merging of awareness with action, immediate clear feedback, and a sense that the activity is rewarding and meaningful (Csikszentmihalyi, 1990).

Flow states are thought to relate to self-esteem, life satisfaction, productivity (Carlson & Clark, 1991; Csikszentmihalyi, 1993; Massimini, Csikszentmihalyi, & Carli, 1987) and to the ability to cope with stress (Graef, 1975; Logan, 1988). The potential for flow is felt to be both universal and individualized. The literature on flow suggests that it exists across a variety of cultures, ages, and social classes (Carlson & Clark, 1991; Massimini, Csikszentmihalyi, & Delle Fave, 1988). The characteristics of flow appear to be the same in all cultures, although the contexts differ (Csikszentmihalyi, 1990). While there seem to be differences from person to person in the tendency to experience flow (Csikszentmihalyi, 1990; Csikszentmihalyi & Mei-Ha Wong, 1991; Kimiecik & Stein, 1992; Massimini et al., 1988), it is assumed that, with the exception of people with schizophrenia, just about everyone has the potential to experience flow (Csikszentmihalyi, 1990).

Csikszentmihalyi (1990) suggested that persons with schizophrenia may lack the ability to experience flow states. He writes:

Some individuals may be constitutionally incapable of experiencing flow. Psychiatrists describe schizophrenics [sic] as suffering from anhedonia, which literally means "lack of pleasure." This symptom appears to be related to "stimulus over inclusion," which refers to the fact that schizophrenics are condemned to notice irrelevant stimuli, to process information whether they like it or not. . . . Unable to concentrate, attending indiscriminately to everything, patients who suffer from this disease not surprisingly end up unable to enjoy themselves (p. 85).

Schizophrenia is an illness characterized by symptoms which include psychosis, environmental hypersensitivity, distractibility, and reduced ability to feel pleasure (American Psychiatric Association, 1994; Braff, 1993). Effects of these symptoms may include withdrawal, anxiety, and reduced ability to initiate and sustain involvement in activities (Anthony & Liberman, 1992; deVries & Delespaul, 1989; Gross, 1986; Spaulding & Sullivan, 1992). Much of the psychiatric literature on schizophrenia suggests that persons with this illness have reductions in their ability to enjoy activity involvement. For example, following an analysis of interviews with young persons with schizophrenia, Grinker and Holzman (1973) wrote:

A second feature of all schizophrenics [sic] in our groups of patients is their pleasureless demeanor. Although some schizophrenic [sic] patients reported having had fun during childhood, for the most part these young patients reported a pervasive inability to derive much joy from life. Even when moderately successful in their accomplishments during their hospitalization, they showed a kind of dampening in their joy and an absence of pleasure . . . Further, the view of their own future described by the schizophrenic [sic] patients held little prospect of amelioration (p. 174).

Occupational therapy practitioners have traditionally worked to develop opportunities for persons with schizophrenia to engage in purposeful activity, or occupation (Hayes, 1989; Krupa & Thornton, 1986; Meyer, 1921/1986). They believe that, for these clients, occupation has a role in promoting enjoyment (Shoichet &

Oakley, 1978), minimizing disorganization and skill loss (Kielhofner, 1992; Krupa & Thornton, 1986), developing a temporal perspective (Suto & Frank, 1994), influencing affect (Boyer, Colman, Levy, & Manoly, 1989), and reducing positive symptoms (MacRae, 1991). Since occupational therapy practitioners use occupation as a therapeutic tool it is important that they understand its effects on their clients. Yerxa et al. (1989) wrote, "To fully understand occupation, it is necessary to comprehend the experience of engagement in it" (p. 9).

The effects of activity, or occupation, on persons with schizophrenia are not well understood. Some authors have suggested that externally-imposed challenges may be overwhelming and harmful for individuals with schizophrenia (Goldberg, Schooler, Hogarty, & Roper, 1977; Gross, 1986; Schooler & Spohn, 1982). Other authors report beneficial effects of activities that are matched to abilities, but do not supply empirical evidence to support this claim (Shoichet & Oakley, 1978), or do not distinguish the characteristics of activities that are helpful (Linn, Caffey, Klett, Hogarty, & Lamb, 1979; Scott & Griffith, 1982). Still others suggest that although persons with schizophrenia may not be harmed by involvement in manageable activities, they will not derive feelings of accomplishment or pleasure from them, due to irreversible damage to the noradrenergic reward system (Grinker & Holzman, 1973; Meehl, 1962; Rado, 1956; Stein & Wise, 1971).

While the medical literature, including DSM IV (American Psychiatric Association, 1994), presents a discouraging picture of the ability of activities to enable persons with schizophrenia to experience enjoyment, more recent work from the field of psychosocial rehabilitation suggests involvement in meaningful activities can help such persons overcome the effects of the illness (Spaniol, Gagne, & Koehler, 1997; International Association of Psychosocial Rehabilitation, 1994). Supportive rehabilitation programmes in education, employment, and social activities have success in enabling more satisfying community lives for persons with severe and persistent mental illness (Anthony, Cohen, & Farkas, 1990). Although measurement of the construct of enjoyment is not reported in these studies, one might infer that a component of satisfaction is enjoyable or pleasurable experiences. Anthony (1993) discusses how mental health systems which are re-oriented to a vision of recovery can enable persons with mental illness to change "the frequency and duration of symptoms. . . . That is, symptoms interfere with functioning less often, and for briefer periods of time" (p. 19). Thus, the negative symptoms of dulled affect, anhedonia, and lack of interest or pleasure may diminish when persons are engaged in occupations of choice.

In addition, first person accounts by persons with this illness reflect some evidence of activity enjoyment (Hamara, Pallikkathayil, Bauer, & Burton, 1994; Leete, 1989; MacDonald, 1964). For instance, MacDonald (1964) wrote:

Just as instinct often guided me in matters of eating, and working, and playing, so it seems to guide me in matters of hobbies. Without this reliance on natural cycles of creative drive, critical periods, and periods of test, none of the creative activities which have made my life meaningful would be possible (p. 183).

Leete (1989) described a sense of motivation and confidence associated with work:

It (work) gives me something to look forward to everyday and a skill to learn and to improve. It is my motivation for getting up each morning. In addition, my hours are passed therapeutically as well as productively. As I work, I become increasingly self-confident, and my self-image is bolstered. I feel important and grown up, which replaces my usual sense of vulnerability, weakness, and incompetence (p. 197).

While such descriptions do not directly address flow, they do reflect some evidence of activity enjoyment, thus suggesting the need for further investigation of assumptions in the literature about the lack of the potential of activity to promote enjoyment among persons with schizophrenia. Insufficient evidence is available to dismiss or confirm the potential for flow, and the potential of occupation to promote flow, among individuals with this disorder. Information on the experience of enjoyable activities among persons with this illness is needed to better identify factors that might characterize, lead to, and enhance these experiences. Such information would be relevant to occupational therapy practitioners who are concerned with motivating their clients to engage in occupation.

Massimini et al. (1987) have suggested that monitoring the experience of flow in everyday contexts could provide information applicable to psychiatric rehabilitation. They noted emotional atrophy among people with psychiatric illnesses. They hypothesized that if flow models apply to this population, then the prescription for psychiatric patients would include involvement in activities that are challenging, but do not overwhelm the individual's skills. If individuals with schizophrenia were able to experience flow, and flow was able to mitigate against some of the symptoms of schizophrenia, it would be important to gather information about the conditions that influence its occurrence. With this additional knowledge, occupational therapy practitioners could gain a better understanding of the potential of activity and could be more helpful in enabling their clients to discover occupations that promote a sense of well-being and enjoyment.

The study reported here examines accounts of enjoyment as described by persons with schizophrenia, and lends support to the suggestion in the psychosocial rehabilitation literature that persons with schizophrenia derive satisfaction from engagement in occupation. Qualitative methods were used to explore descriptions of enjoyment provided by individuals with schizophrenia to gain a better understanding of whether they experience enjoyment, and, if so, what factors characterize their enjoyment experiences.

METHODS

The qualitative paradigm was selected to allow for the exploration of perspectives held by individuals (Lincoln & Guba, 1985; Merrill, 1985). Yerxa (1991) wrote that the flexibility of qualitative research is suited to complex interactions such as those that influence occupational experience.

Subjective reports have been found to improve scientific understanding of schizophrenia (Bernheim & Lewine, 1979; Brekke, Levin, Wolkon, Sobel, & Slade, 1993; Hamara et al., 1994; Shulman, 1968). The value of such reports is influenced by a number of factors including the mental state of the contributor (Hurlburt, 1990) and the skill, flexibility and persistence of the researcher (Marshall & Rossman, 1989; Spradley, 1979). Hurlburt (1990) and Delespaul and deVries, (1987) studied subjective experiences of persons diagnosed with schizophrenia and reported that, when not in an acute phase of their illness, the informants provided clear descriptions of their emotional experiences.

The interview format is important in determining the quality of data gathered. In a study of wellness and schizophrenia Hamara et al. (1994) noted that a focused interview protocol was needed to elicit clear descriptions of the thoughts and feelings of participants. While relevant information about the subjective experience of activity can be gathered from persons with schizophrenia, a degree of structure and persistent probing are needed to gain an in-depth understanding of important concepts (Liberman, 1989; Strauss, 1989).

A semi-structured, focused interview method was chosen for this study. Open-ended questions were used with probes to explore concepts in more depth. Attempts were made to verify, but not interpret, descriptions during the interview.

SAMPLE

Lincoln and Guba (1985) stated that the sample size should be large enough to permit an adequate amount and range of information, and that saturation occurs when interviews no longer bring in new information that alters the hypotheses. According to McCracken (1988), in many cases saturation can be achieved with eight participants.

A provincial psychiatric hospital was selected as the point of entry because of its accessibility, the diversity in its population, and the availability of data for triangulation. Members of two out-patient clinical teams provided potential research participants with information about the study and asked whether they were willing to be contacted by the researcher. If the client agreed, the team member relayed this information and the researcher telephoned to discuss the study. If the person indicated an interest in participating, the researcher established a time for the interview.

The final sample consisted of nine adults who met the following four inclusion criteria: ability to speak English, diagnosis of schizophrenia or schizoaffective disorder applied by a licenced psychiatrist, ability to give informed consent to participate, and not currently in an acute phase of the schizophrenic illness. (Some participants had at one time been diagnosed as having a schizoaffective disorder, and other times as having schizophrenia. The diagnosis at the time of the study is listed on Table 1). All informants were followed regularly by a treatment team member and considered by the team to be stabilized by psychotropic medication. A demographic description of the participants is provided in Table 1.

DATA GATHERING

The interviewer was introduced as a researcher and interviews were held in a variety of places including coffee shops, restaurants, an informant's apartment, and the hospital grounds. To increase comfort, the interviewer and informant spent a few minutes getting to know each other before starting the interview. Attempts were made to keep the relationships informal.

During the interview informants were asked to describe something that they enjoyed doing.

Table 1
Demographic Data for the Nine Informants

Variable	Category	(n) Informants
Age	20–29	3
	30–39	3
	40–49	1
	50–59	2
Gender	Male	6
	Female	3
Diagnosis		
	schizophrenia unspecified	2
	paranoid schizophrenia	2
	schizoaffective disorder	3
	schizophrenia & personality disorder	1
	schizophrenia & substance abuse	1
Age of Onset		
	childhood	1
	adolescence	4
	20–30	4
Marital Status		
	single	6
	married/common-law	1
	separated/divorced	2
Living Situation		
	independent alone	3
	with family of origin	3
	with common-law spouse	1
	supervised setting with others	2
Number of Children		
	0	5
	1	4
Highest Formal Education		
	partial elementary school	1
	partial secondary school	3
	high school diploma	3
	post secondary diploma/degree	2
Employment Status		
	unemployed	6
	casual/part-time employment	3
Main Income Source		
	Family Benefits (Disability)	5
	Welfare	1
	Family	1
	Earnings/Grants	2
Medications		
	Antipsychotic medications	9

They were asked whether they had ever become so involved in doing something that they lost track of time, and if so, to describe these experiences. In addition, they were prompted to describe different time periods in their lives in terms of the ways they liked to spend their time. All informants were given an opportunity to add additional information that might help the researcher to understand how it felt for them to do the things they liked to do.

Interviews were audio taped and transcribed verbatim by the researcher. Each data collection session took approximately two hours including time for consent forms and initial conversation. The in-depth interview itself ranged between forty minutes and one hour.

A methods log was maintained to document interactions with participants, and operational notes about the interview process and context. Ongoing observations were recorded in a field notebook. Members of the university thesis advisory committee were consulted to discuss expectations and responses during data collection and analysis.

DATA ANALYSIS

The initial analysis involved open coding so that codes emerged from what was in the data, rather than from a predetermined set of categories. Data were coded several different times. Methods were based on techniques designed for constant comparison (Glaser & Strauss, 1967), utilizing and categorizing (Lincoln & Guba, 1985), and domain analysis (Spradley, 1979). The analysis process included open review of the transcripts, categorization of information, memo writing, review of the transcripts, and recategorizing as themes and relationships emerged. The thesis committee members blind coded portions of the data to check for agreement in analysis. While this study yielded several interesting findings, those reported here will be confined to the themes of the enjoyment experiences described by informants.

RESULTS

Each of the informants described several experiences that he or she had enjoyed. These descriptions were categorized by grouping similar expressed feelings. Five main themes, related to the way enjoyment was experienced by informants, emerged. On the basis of the words informants used in their descriptions, these themes were designated: Excitement, Accomplishment, Relaxation, Social Connectedness, and Being Interested.

For each theme, sample quotes from informants are provided. Repetitive or unnecessary material has been omitted from the quote as indicated by three ellipsis points (. . .). To ensure anonymity, identifying data have been replaced by a blank line.

EXCITEMENT

Several informants identified experiences that were exciting for them. During excitement informants experienced "high" feeling or sense of exhilaration:

Like you get these natural highs, like from skiing or white water; that's a really good experience . . . Skiing.[. . .] I was in Ellicottville in New York State and I did the wall [. . .] it's a hill with a slope about like that (gestures) and that was pretty exhilarating. . . . You're concentrating on keeping your weight forward. And shifting your weight from ski to ski.

Along with the feeling of exhilaration, there was a heightened sense of arousal and energy:

I like to do aerobics, and lifting the weights, and sit-ups. And I like to get the adrenaline going. . . . I like the adrenaline feeling, the working of all that adrenaline. [. . .] . . . you feel like you're all pumped up . . . It just feels good.

Informants described the role concentration and challenge played in the experience of excitement.

Chess is like a war game. . . . It's kinda like war. Exciting. . . . Sometimes I concentrate and sometimes I don't . . . then I get serious, because I see him coming the way he's coming . . . then I get involved because I know it's too dangerous for me now for the game. I might lose it. So then I start to try hard and sometimes I win, and sometimes

I lose, but it's a challenge, you know. . . . You don't get nothing from it . . . but good feelings, good ideas . . . different moves . . . it's a challenge, like.

Karate is a great outlet to get high because when you do a kata. A kata is like a series of movements. I think it has to do with your breathing . . . And the way you kiai, because . . . when you're done you are just standing there and you feel really high. . . . Your arteries are pumping, and you feel . . . a little light-headed. . . . And you're focusing on where you are going to punch, and where you put your feet, and where to look. Your focus is the point where you look.

For the informants in this study, excitement seemed to occur during a variety of challenging activities including recreation, sport activities, and competitive games.

ACCOMPLISHMENT

A second theme of enjoyment that emerged from informants' descriptions was the experience of accomplishment. Expressed feelings connected with this type of experience included pride, self-efficacy, and satisfaction:

You are accomplishing things and you are having a good time at the same time. And you feel good about what you are doing . . . I thought my work was good, so I was feeling proud of my work . . . I enjoyed it because it occupied my time and it was an accomplishment.

One of the things I've enjoyed is writing the book that I'm writing. It's a science fiction murder mystery. . . . You are writing to an audience which is the world and probably future history. People after you're dead will be reading it . . . When I get an hour done I feel as if I've accomplished something during the day. I feel that I'm not going to go to my grave not having accomplished something in my life.

For some informants there was a feeling of power associated with accomplishment:

If you win a fight you feel like you have accomplished. You feel like "wow. I'm power tripping. I got power now. I'm where it's at . . . I wanted to be

someone. . . . Not just a wimp or something . . . that you could push away . . . [. . .] And you really control your fists. You do really good. . . . I always felt like nothing if I wasn't fighting you know.

In addition to this sense of self-satisfaction, informants talked about becoming focused on an activity or challenge and ceasing to worry about other factors. One informant described his frame of mind during model building:

I really don't think a whole lot. I don't think too much about it other than I want to get it finished. [. . .] You have to have everything in the right place and you have to get it even . . . right in the middle . . . like that looks as close as I'm likely to get it.

Other informants talked about becoming focused during creative and intellectual activities:

If I'm at home by myself and I'm drawing something, or working on my art work, I just get so involved with it that uh, I forget about everything.

You get enthused. You may come in with other thoughts in your head. For example, What will I eat for supper tonight? . . . Then all of a sudden you start reading and your thoughts start coming back to the research and the individual you are studying, and then you forget about the other things. And they go to the back of your mind. . . . People can be coming and going and I may not notice them so well to the extent that my mind is focused.

A few informants described a loss of awareness of their actions, and a sense that their behaviours were occurring automatically without having to think about them:

And then, all of a sudden just as you go the next paragraph, it comes right to you. You might have to think for, you know 15 seconds, and then all of a sudden the action seems to follow and so on. . . [. . .] You sit down and all of a sudden your thoughts, and the plot just form in your mind and right on the screen.

I'd do my art work and I'd be watching T.V. and before I knew it was like two o'clock in the morning. Like what happened to—like I don't remember the shows I watched. All I cared about was

doing this motion (Gestures drawing motion).
[. . .] And then . . . I'd get up, take a look at it,
and I'd think "Wow! How did I do that?"

Activities that were connected with the informants' experiences of accomplishment included helping others, creative arts, and some antisocial activities (i.e. fighting).

RELAXATION

Informants also described enjoyment feelings involving the experience of relaxation. Feelings of peace, or calmness were associated with this type of experience:

I'd just take a nice drive out to _____ Creek.
It's quiet. It's not overly crowded like some of the
beaches are, and other . . . fishing spots around.
I can just . . . kind of be at one with nature and
myself. It's calming. It's relaxing.

Peaceful. Like for instance that one right there
(points to drawing) . . . when I was working on
the female, like. . . . I felt very peaceful. But, the
figures that are her shadow are more emotional
than the female figure itself.

Some informants discussed a sense of relief or release of tension associated with the relaxation experience. When asked to describe the feelings he had when doing art work, one informant responded:

Oh, uh, relieving . . . [. . .] I think I said earlier,
'Relieving.' . . . Feeling that it is okay to feel good.

Another informant had experienced comparable feelings after physical activity:

I'd feel good. Coming out of the gym I'd feel all
. . . relaxed and that. . . . It was . . . kind of feeling like . . . a relief feeling.

The informants' descriptions of relaxation reflected the absence of worries:

There's no anxiety involved with camping you
know . . . if it's going to rain it's going to rain, and
that's the only thing you have to worry about . . .
and that's not even the biggest problem.

As the activities linked with relaxation were less demanding, informants' total attention was not required to deal with challenges inherent in the task. Some energy was available to reflect on one's situation or appreciate the surroundings:

I think about lots of things. Just how beautiful
the place is right where I'm at. How fortunate I
am to be there. . . . I can even sometimes take a
book with me when I am getting sort of, reeling
in and out. Casting out my line . . . I just start
reading a bit. . . . Because it's peaceful. . . . [. . .]
Well, fishing. I don't need to take a twelve pack
fishing with me. I don't necessarily have to when
I am practicing my guitar.

SOCIAL CONNECTEDNESS

A fourth category of enjoyment experience described by informants was that of being socially connected. This experience was characterized by feelings of belonging, communication with others, security, and trust:

When I feel like I am loved, I feel a great enjoyment because . . . I get to feel towards a person,
I get to care about a person . . . I trust this man
fully. And it's love. Like . . . enjoyment is such a
word—love—it's enjoyment.

Pleasure dominates . . . it gives you a sense that
you are worth something. A sense of worth. That
you are part of a community that . . . is going
some place.

The experience of social connectedness involved a focus on others, or on oneself in relation to others. Sometimes there is a component of feeling in sync with others:

It felt good. It was good. [. . .] . . . like thinking
what other people are thinking. Like uh, they'd
laugh, so I'd laugh too, eh?

Activities through which informants had experienced social connectedness included social, recreational, educational, and intimate activities. Relationships with animals, memories, and mystical beliefs had also provided these feelings for some informants.

BEING INTERESTED

A final category of enjoyment described by some informants was the experience of being interested. This experience included a sense of curiosity, fascination, or discovery:

It's kind of a mental feeling of . . . having mental pleasure. It's sort of an intellectual pleasure in acquiring knowledge and experience of watching a play, or finding out a new fact in science, or writing a book and that. . . . Anticipation is one of the feelings. I'm interested in finding out how my characters are going to talk to one another and what they are going to do next and so on. I like chemistry . . . I like . . . collecting coins . . . and collecting stamps. That kind of thing I liked to do in school. I've got a bunch of old coins still. . . . Interesting would be a word for collecting coins. It's like an interest. [. . .] . . . Sometimes to observe. [. . .] I would imagine you are exercising your powers of observation . . . maybe curiosity.

The experience of being interested entailed mental arousal and alertness:

I watched a Shakespearean play. . . . It was How you like it. And I really loved the play. . . . I was thrilled with the way the actors would never forget their lines. Their behaviour was perfect. . . . I saw a play called Checkmate . . . and it was very realistic the way they interacted with each other. . . they could do everything so perfect night after night. . . . That's something remarkable to me. That kind of feeling. . . . That they can do that. That their skills are so good. It's like trapeze artists. They never fall.

If I get really involved in a book and I can't set it down . . . I get lost in time, there. Kind of get lost in the book.

The experience of being interested differed from accomplishment, in terms of the performance demands it placed on the informant. With interest, the informant was taking information in and processing it, without necessarily having to act on it. Informants did not seem to have such a strong awareness of action goals, or a sense that their own performance would make a difference. Attention was focused on the incoming stimulation, rather than on one's self, one's output, or one's worries:

It's kind of fun meeting people. [. . .] . . . they have something interesting to say. . . . (re. Strawberry social) . . . There was a lot of people there all getting some strawberries. [. . .] I was watching them dance.

You sit there and watch the world go by. Watch everything go by.

Activities through which informants had experienced being interested included education, spectator events, hobbies, entertainment, and hallucinations for one informant. As he described:

I used to like it when I would look in the back of people's heads and look through their eyes, and see what they were looking at . . . And I'd see all the colours. [. . .] I was like a little boy . . . enjoying like. Looking around. That's all I wanted to do was look at everything. That gave me good feelings. Good satisfaction.

DISCUSSION OF FINDINGS

An initial incentive for this exploration was to determine whether individuals with schizophrenia experience enjoyment. The literature about the effects of schizophrenia (Grinker & Holzman, 1973; Meehl, 1962, Stein & Wise, 1971) and the literature about flow (Csikszentmihalyi, 1990) painted a picture of persons with schizophrenia as not being able to experience enjoyment. These assumptions are disturbing as they raise questions about the belief held by occupational therapists that activities matched to an individual's needs and abilities are intrinsically motivating (Arnsten, 1990; Florey, 1969; Yerxa, 1993).

The findings of this study suggest that, contrary to much of the literature on schizophrenia, individuals with this illness do experience enjoyment. There are indications in these findings that may account for the inconsistencies between the findings reported here and in the literature on schizophrenia. The timing of the study may be important. Some of the studies on schizophrenia were conducted on persons while they were in an acute phase of their illness (Grinker & Holzman, 1973), whereas the informants in this study were not considered to be in an acute phase of their illness. Support for the relevance of this timing comes from the fact that in a study comparing anhedonia scores of long-term out-patients with schizophrenia to those of controls, the differences were not great enough to support the use of anhedonia scales for diagnostic purposes (Cook & Simukonda, 1981).

Another consideration that may account for discrepancies between the findings reported here and those in the literature on schizophrenia relates to the availability of activity. To find out whether individuals with schizophrenia enjoy activities, there must be opportunities available to engage in activities with the right conditions for their enjoyment. In literature describing reduced enjoyment among persons with schizophrenia, the opportunities to engage in activity were restricted (Kearns & Taylor, 1989; Suto & Frank, 1994), not discussed (Grinker & Holzman, 1973) or not matched to subjectively-perceived needs and abilities of participants (Goldberg et al., 1977; Schooler & Spohn, 1982).

An additional consideration that may explain some of the differences between the findings reported here and the literature on schizophrenia is that the other studies did not use an emic approach. An emic perspective focuses on the insider's way of understanding experiences (DePoy & Gitlin, 1994). Schooler and Spohn (1982) based their findings on a battery of objective measures while Grinker and Holzman (1973) based their remarks about their clients' enjoyment on observations and psychiatric interviews. The use of an emic approach may have provided new insights into the perspectives and subjective experiences of persons with schizophrenia in this study. Hence, this approach needs to be given more attention in the literature on persons with this illness.

The descriptions provided by the informants in this study enabled the researcher to gain an understanding of the properties of their experiences of enjoyment. The way in which informants experienced enjoyment was consistent with literature on the way most people experience enjoyment (Allen, 1985; Csikszentmihalyi, 1988; Laliberte, 1993; Stephens & Craig, 1990; Wankel, 1993).

Flow experiences involve concentration, automatic actions, and a sense of control over outcomes (Csikszentmihalyi, 1990). During flow people focus away from their worries; lose track of time, and experience high energy, interest, and arousal (Csikszentmihalyi, 1993). These feelings are experienced during activities that offer manageable challenges with meaningful outcomes as determined by participants' perceptions of their abilities, and environmental demands (Csikszentmihalyi, 1988).

In this study, concentration or focus occurred during experiences of excitement and accomplishment. Automatic actions, feelings of losing track of time and worries were also described as part of the accomplishment experience. Energy, interest, and arousal were high in both excitement and accomplishment. The essential components of flow are reflected in the informants' descriptions of excitement and accomplishment experiences.

The experience of being interested shares properties with flow. Csikszentmihalyi (1990) considered interest an essential ingredient of flow. Being interested does not seem to involve the same demands for performance, nor sense of control over outcomes, as flow. In addition to being enjoyable in itself, the experience of being interested may be a precursor, or essential condition, for flow.

The experiences of social connectedness and relaxation were described as enjoyable by informants, but are not discussed in the flow literature. Although these themes are not discussed in the literature on flow, they are identified as sources of enjoyment in the literature on occupation, and leisure. A benefit of activity involvement is its role in maintaining connectedness with friends and family (Laliberte, 1993; MacGregor, 1995; Stephens & Craig, 1990;

Wankel, 1993). Common reasons documented for participating in enjoyable activities are to relax (Stephens & Craig, 1990) and escape pressures (Allen, 1985).

There are implications of the findings with respect to the understanding of enjoyment and flow. The fact that informants identified experiences as enjoyable that fall outside the realm of flow suggests that enjoyment is a broader construct that is not limited to flow experiences. Hence, these two terms do not appear synonymous. Csikszentmihalyi's use of the words enjoyment and flow interchangeably may be misleading, and cause his readers to overlook potential sources of enjoyment beyond flow. Since flow is a specific type of enjoyment, it can best be understood if authors specify it as flow and keep working to develop knowledge about its properties. In addition, other forms of enjoyment need to be explored for their unique properties.

This study pointed to interesting and fruitful lines of investigation for future research. Due to the limitations of this study, the research needs to be replicated using the emic approach with a larger population. In this study the sample size was small and it is unlikely that saturation (Lincoln & Guba, 1985) occurred. As with other qualitative studies, generalization is not possible. The lack of prolonged involvement (Lincoln & Guba, 1985) with the informants, and the researcher's biases as an occupational therapist may also have influenced the study. While as a researcher the aim was to ensure that the findings depicted the views of informants, as a therapist the hope was to validate assumptions about the potential of activity to promote enjoyment for clients.

Despite these limitations, the study had several strengths. The use of the emic perspective allowed the researcher to explore the perspectives of informants and to question assumptions about enjoyment among persons with schizophrenia. The research committee provided feedback to ensure that findings were grounded in the data. There were indicators to suggest that informants were not simply saying what they thought the interviewer would want to hear. For example, informants spoke of activities that would be discouraged by health professionals (such as car theft, making explosives, and drug use) and other data sources supported their disclosures. Member checks were carried out with seven informants to confirm the researcher's impressions of what they had said. These factors offer support for the credibility of the study.

This study pointed to the need for additional research in several areas. More research is needed on enjoyment and persons with schizophrenia to determine if, and how, enjoyment is experienced by others with schizophrenia. The construct of flow should be re-examined and explored for its relevance not only to persons with schizophrenia, but to persons with other disabling conditions as well. More information is needed about the conditions, benefits, barriers and strategies involved in enabling enjoyment of occupation for persons with disabilities. With a better understanding of these factors occupational therapy practitioners may be able to more effectively use occupation to promote enjoyment, and use enjoyment to promote occupational engagement among persons with disabilities.

ACKNOWLEDGEMENTS

The authors wish to thank the informants for sharing their experiences and giving us a better understanding of their views.

References

Allen, L. (1985). An analysis of the social unit of participation and the perceived psychological outcomes associated with most enjoyable recreation activities. *Leisure Sciences, 7,* 421–439.

American Psychiatric Association. (1994). *Diagnostic and statistical manual of mental disorders* (4th ed.). Washington, DC: Author.

Anthony, W. (1993). Recovery from mental illness: The guiding vision of the mental health service system in the 1990s. *Psychosocial Rehabilitation Journal, 16,* 11–23.

Anthony, W., Cohen, M., & Farkas, M. (1990). *Handbook of psychiatric rehabilitation.* Needham Heights, MA: Allyn and Bacon.

Anthony, W., & Liberman, R. (1992). Principles of practice of psychiatric rehabilitation. In R. Liberman (Ed.), *Handbook of psychiatric rehabilitation* (pp. 1–29). Needham Heights, MA: Allyn and Bacon.

Arnsten, S. (1990). Intrinsic motivation. *American Journal of Occupational Therapy, 44,* 462–463.

Bernheim, K., & Lewine, R. (1979). *Schizophrenia: Symptoms, causes & treatments.* New York: W. W. Norton.

Boyer, J., Colman, W., Levy, L., & Manoly, B. (1989). Affective responses to activities: A comparative study. *American Journal of Occupational Therapy, 43,* 81–88.

Braff, D. (1993). Information processing and attention dysfunctions in schizophrenia. *Schizophrenia Bulletin, 19,* 233–239.

Brekke, J., Levin, S., Wolkon, G., Sobel, E., & Slade, E. (1993). Psychosocial functioning and subjective experience in schizophrenia. *Schizophrenia Bulletin, 19,* 599–608.

Carlson, M., & Clark, F. (1991). The search for useful methodologies in occupational science. *The American Journal of Occupational Therapy, 45,* 235–241.

Cook, M., & Simukonda, F. (1981). Anhedonia and schizophrenia. *British Journal of Psychiatry, 139,* 523–525.

Csikszentmihalyi, M. (1988). Introduction. In M. Csikszentmihalyi & I. Csikszentmihalyi (Eds.), *Optimal experience: Psychological studies of flow in consciousness* (pp. 3–14). Cambridge, UK: Cambridge University Press.

Csikszentmihalyi, M. (1990). *Flow: The psychology of optimal experience.* New York: Harper & Row.

Csikszentmihalyi, M. (1993). Activity and happiness: Towards a science of occupation. *Occupational Science: Australia, 1,* 38–42.

Csikszentmihalyi, M., & Mei-Ha Wong, M. (1991). The situational and personal correlates of happiness: A cross-national comparison. In F. Strack, M. Argyle, & N. Schwartz (Eds.), *Subjective well-being* (pp. 193–212), Toronto, ON: Pergammon Press.

Delespaul, P., & deVries, M. (1987). The daily life of ambulatory chronic mental patients. *Journal of Nervous and Mental Disease, 175,* 537–544.

DePoy, E., & Gitlin, L. (1994). *Introduction to research: Multiple strategies for health and human services.* St. Louis, MO: Mosby.

deVries, M., & Delespaul, P. (1989). Time, context and subjective experience in schizophrenia. *Schizophrenia Bulletin, 15,* 233–245.

Doble, S. (1988). Intrinsic motivation and clinical practice: The key to understanding the unmotivated client. *Canadian Journal of Occupational Therapy, 55,* 75–81.

Florey, L. (1969). Intrinsic motivation: The dynamics of occupational therapy theory. *American Journal of Occupational Therapy, 23,* 319–322.

Glaser, B., & Strauss, A. (1967). *The discovery of grounded theory: Strategies for qualitative research.* Chicago, IL: Aldine Publishing.

Goldberg, S., Schooler, N., Hogarty, G., & Roper, M. (1977). Prediction of relapse in schizophrenic outpatients treated by drug and sociotherapy. *Archives of General Psychiatry, 34,* 171–184.

Graef, R. (1975). Flow patterns in everyday life. In M. Csikszentmihalyi (Ed.), *Beyond boredom and anxiety: The experience of play in work and games.* (pp. 140–160). San Francisco, CA: Jossey-Bass.

Grinker, R., & Holzman, P. (1973). Schizophrenic pathology in young adults. *Archives of General Psychiatry, 28,* 168–175.

Gross, G. (1986). Basic symptoms and coping behavior in schizophrenia. In J. Strauss, W. Boker, & H. Brenner (Eds.), *Psychosocial treatment of schizophrenia* (pp. 126–135). Toronto, ON: Hans Huber.

Hamara, E., Pallikkathayil, L., Bauer, S., & Burton, M. (1994). Descriptors of wellness by individuals with schizophrenia. *Western Journal of Nursing Research, 16,* 288–300.

Hayes, R. (1989). Occupational therapy in the treatment of schizophrenia. *Occupational Therapy in Mental Health, 9,* 51–68.

Hurlburt, R. (1990). *Sampling normal and schizophrenic inner experience.* New York: Plenum.

International Association of Psychosocial Rehabilitation Services: Publications Committee. (Eds.). (1994). *An introduction to psychiatric rehabilitation.* Boston, MA: Centre for Psychiatric Rehabilitation.

Kearns, R., & Taylor, S. (1989). Daily life experience of people with chronic mental disabilities in Hamilton, Ontario. *Canada's Mental Health, December,* 1–4.

Kielhofner, G. (1992). *Conceptual foundations of occupational therapy.* Philadelphia. PA: F.A. Davis.

Kimiecik, J., & Stein, G. (1992). Examining flow experiences in sports context: Conceptual issues and methodological concerns. *Journal of Applied Sport Psychology, 4,* 141–160.

Krupa, T., & Thornton, J. (1986). The pleasure deficit in schizophrenia. *Occupational Therapy in Mental Health, 6,* 65–78.

Laliberte, D. (1993). *An exploration of the meaning seniors attach to activity.* Unpublished master's thesis, London, ON: University of Western Ontario.

Law, M. (1991). Muriel Driver Lecture—The environment: A focus for occupational therapy.

Canadian Journal of Occupational Therapy, 58, 171–179.

Leete, E. (1989). How I perceive and manage my illness. *Schizophrenia Bulletin, 15,* 197–200.

Liberman, P. (1989). "Objective" methods and "subjective"experiences. *Schizophrenia Bulletin, 15,* 267–275.

Lincoln, Y., & Guba, E. (1985). *Naturalistic inquiry.* Beverly Hills, CA: Sage Publications.

Linn, M., Caffey E., Klett, C., Hogarty, G., & Lamb, H. (1979). Day treatment and psychotropic drugs in the aftercare of schizophrenic patients. *Archives of General Psychiatry, 36,* 1055–1066.

Logan, P. (1988). Flow in solitary ordeals. In M. Csikszentmihalyi & I. Csikszentmihalyi. (Eds.), *Optimal experience: Psychological studies of flow in consciousness.* (pp. 172–180). Cambridge: Cambridge University Press.

MacDonald, N. (1964). Living with schizophrenia. In B. Kaplan, (Ed.). *The inner world of mental illness.* (pp. 173–184). New York: Harper and Row.

MacGregor, L. (1995). *An exploratory study of the personal experience of occupational deprivation.* Unpublished master's thesis, London, ON: University of Western Ontario.

MacRae, A. (1991). An overview of theory and research on hallucinations: Implications for occupational therapy intervention. *Occupational Therapy in Mental Health, 11,* 41–60.

Marshall, C., & Rossman, G. (1989). *Designing qualitative research.* Newbury Park, CA: Sage Publications.

Massimini, F., Csikszentmihalyi, M., & Carli, M. (1987). The monitoring of optimal experience. *Journal of Nervous and Mental Disease, 175,* 545–549.

Massimini, R., Csikszentmihalyi, M., & Delle Fave, A. (1988). Flow and biocultural evolution. In M. Csikszentmihalyi, & I. Csikszentmihalyi (Eds.), *Optimal experience: Psychological studies of flow in consciousness.* (pp. 60–81). Cambridge, UK: Cambridge University Press.

McCracken, G. (1988). *The long interview.* Newbury Park, CA: Sage Publications.

Meehl, P. (1962). Schizotaxia, schizotypy, schizophrenia. *American Psychologist, 17,* 827–838.

Merrill, S. (1985). Qualitative methods in occupational therapy research: An application. *Occupational Therapy Journal of Research, 5,* 213–222.

Meyer, A. (1921/1982). Worth repeating: The philosophy of occupational therapy. *Occupational Therapy in Mental Health, 2,* 79–86.

Primeau, L., Clark, F., & Pierce, D. (1989). Occupational therapy alone has looked upon occupation: Future applications of occupational science to pediatric occupational therapy. *Occupational Therapy in Health Care, 6,* 19–32.

Rado, S. (1956). *Psychoanalysis of behavior: Collected Papers.* New York: Grune & Stratton.

Schooler, C., & Spohn, H. (1982). Social dysfunction and treatment failure in schizophrenia. *Schizophrenia Bulletin, 8,* 85–98.

Scott, D., & Griffith, M. (1982). The treatment of schizophrenia. *Small Group Behavior, 13,* 415–422.

Shoichet, R., & Oakley, A. (1978). Notes on the treatment of anhedonia. *Canadian Psychiatric Association Journal, 23,* 487–491.

Schulman, B. (1968). *Essays in schizophrenia.* Baltimore, MD: Williams and Wilkins.

Spaniol, L., Gagne, C., & Keohler, M. (Eds.). (1997). *Psychological and social aspects of psychiatric disability.* Boston, MA: Centre for Psychiatric Rehabilitation.

Spaulding, W., & Sullivan, M. (1992). From laboratory to clinic: Psychological methods and principles in psychiatric rehabilitation. In R. Liberman (Ed.). *Handbook of psychiatric rehabilitation.* (pp. 30–55). Needham Heights, MA: Allyn and Bacon.

Spradley, J. (1979). *The ethnographic interview.* New York: Holt, Reinhardt, & Winston.

Stein, L., & Wise, C. (1971). Possible etiology of schizophrenia: Progressive damage to the noradrenergic reward system by 6-hydroxydopamine. *Science, 171,* 1032–1036.

Strauss, J. (1989). Subjective experiences of schizophrenia: Toward a new dynamic psychiatry. *Schizophrenia Bulletin, 15,* 179–187.

Stephens, T., & Craig, C. (1990). *The well-being of Canadians: Highlights of the 1988 Campbell's Survey.* Ottawa, ON: Canadian Fitness and Lifestyle Research Institute.

Suto, M. & Frank, G. (1994). Future time perspective and daily occupations of persons with chronic schizophrenia in a board and care home. *The American Journal of Occupational Therapy, 48,* 7–18.

Wankel, L. (1993). The importance of enjoyment of adherence and psychological benefits from physical activity. *International Journal of Sports Psychology, 24,* 151–169.

Yerxa, E. (1991). Nationally speaking: Seeking a relevant, ethical, and realistic way of knowing for occupational therapy. *The American Journal of Occupational Therapy, 45,* 199–204.

Yerxa, E. (1993). Occupational science: A new source of power for participants in occupational therapy. *Occupational Science: Australia, 1,* 3–10.

Yerxa, E., Clark, F., Frank, G., Jackson, J., Parham, D., Pierce, D., Stein, C., & Zemke, R. (1989). An introduction to occupational science: A foundation for occupational therapy in the 21st century. *Occupational Therapy in Health Care, 6,* 1–17.

Chapter 20

Client-centred Care Means That I Am a Valued Human Being

Canadian Journal of Occupational Therapy

1999, 66(2): 71–82

Deborah Corring, Joanne Cook

Deborah J. Corring, M.Sc. O.T., O.T. (C) is Programme Co-leader, at London/St. Thomas Psychiatric Hospital, St. Thomas, Ontario. She also operates an independent business—Client Perspectives, 126 Chalet Crescent, London, Ontario N6K 3C6 E-mail: dcorrin2@julian.uwo.ca
Joanne V. Cook, Ph.D., O.T. (C) is an Associate Professor, School of Occupational Therapy, Elborn College, University of Western Ontario, London, Ontario N6G 1H1
E-mail: jvcook@julian.uwo.ca

KEY WORDS

- client-centred practice
- consumer attitudes
- mental health services

ABSTRACT

Canadian occupational therapists have increasingly adopted a client-centred approach to practice. Interpretation of what "client-centred" means has been diverse and varied. Professionals have written about the characteristics of this approach to care but no reported studies could be found that examined the client's perspective. The omission of the client perspective is puzzling when partnership, client involvement in decision making, and client empowerment are thought to be fundamental elements of this approach to practice.

A qualitative research approach, using focus groups was employed to explore the opinions and perspectives of individuals with experience of mental illness and the mental health service delivery system. Seventeen individuals participated in three focus groups to discuss the meaning of a client-centred approach to practice. Participants assessed the inadequacies of past and present practices and recommended needed changes. Their central message was the need for individuals with mental illness to be viewed as valuable human beings by service providers and by society.

THE RESEARCH ISSUE

Canadian occupational therapists have increasingly adopted a client-centred approach to practice (Blain & Townsend, 1993; Gage & Polatajko, 1995; Hobson, 1996). Interpretation of what being client-centred means, as well as its impact on the profession and its clinical practices, has been diverse and varied (Gage & Polatajko, 1995). An extensive review of occupational therapy and related health and social sciences literature provided a listing of the characteristics of this approach to care from a professional perspective but no reported studies could be found that specifically examined the client's perspective. In particular, the purpose was to examine with individuals who were experienced with mental illness and the mental health service delivery system, their definition of the characteristics of a client-centred care service delivery system in order to compare them with the characteristics as described by the professionals. Since our study, there has been one published study by Rebeiro and Allen (1998), which explores the meaning of client-centred care from the clients' perspective.

LITERATURE REVIEW

The term "client-centered" was first used by Carl Rogers (1939). In *Client-Centered Therapy,* Rogers (1951) outlines the propositions of his theory of client-centred care. He describes and emphasizes the importance of individuality, holism, sense of self, the influence of the environment, values development, actualization, and goal-directed behaviour both for an individual's overall development and as part of the client-therapist relationship.

Discussion of the term "client-centred" began for many Canadian occupational therapists after the release of the *Guidelines for the Client-Centred Practice of Occupational Therapy* in 1983 by the Canadian Association of Occupational Therapists (hereafter identified as CAOT) and continued as further documents were released in 1986, 1991, and 1993. The CAOT guidelines are used consistently as a reference point for discussions of client-centred care in the occupational therapy literature (since this study was conducted a new conceptual model of practice has been published by CAOT in 1997, *Enabling Occupation: An Occupational Therapy Perspective*).

Sumsion (1993) observed that after ten years of exposure in the literature and at conferences, there were very few Canadian therapists who had not heard of the model. She wondered if occupational therapists had really "integrated" the client-centred concept into daily practice in the way that was intended, She questioned whether occupational therapists involved the client as the primary decision maker so that the client was the one directing the treatment. "Does the therapist really give up some control, or do some therapists use this model as an exercise for less involvement with the client?" (p. 7). Sumsion asserts that this approach to practice requires that therapists are willing to accept the greater challenge of engaging the client in the process of problem solving.

The CAOT Guidelines impact study (Blain & Townsend, 1993) concluded that the most frequent or constant use of the guidelines was by those involved in administering occupational therapy services. They concluded that their results indicated that the Guidelines had not produced a fundamental, paradigm shift from traditional practice to a client-centred practice although they had fostered considerable growth by occupational therapists towards such a shift.

Articles have been written to address application of the guidelines in various areas of occupational therapy practice (Hobson, 1996; Madill, Tirull-Jones, & Magill-Evans, 1990; Stewart & Harvey, 1990; Waters, 1995). The "guidelines model" has also been evaluated both as a model for practice and as a conceptual model (McColl & Pranger, 1994). McCall and Pranger concluded that its use as a conceptual model was acceptable, but it was considered problematic as a model of practice due to structural, conceptual and technical variances and the lack of explanation of several important relationships.

Occupational therapists have also discussed client-centred care's fit with another service delivery model. Krupa and Clark (1995), after an extensive discussion of case management services design and principles, point out that the guidelines' emphasis on collaborative partnerships with the client is consistent with the principles of case management service delivery for the seriously mentally ill.

In 1995, Law, Baptiste, and Mills provided a detailed definition of client-centred care from a professionals' perspective as an approach to care "which embraces a philosophy of respect for, and a partnership with, people receiving services" (p. 253). They outline seven key concepts of client-centredness including: autonomy/choice, partnership, responsibility, enablement, contextual congruence, accessibility, and respect for diversity.

Barriers to implementing client-centred practice were identified by Law et al. (1995) and verified by other authors (CAOT, 1993; Gage & Polatajko, 1995; Sumsion, 1993; Townsend, 1992; Woodside, 1991). The barriers include therapists who are confused about how client-centred practice translates into their everyday work, therapists who are uncomfortable with the shift in power in the therapeutic relationship, the client's willingness and ability to make decisions and exercise power, and, a working environment that continues to value a traditional biomedical approach to delivering services.

Related concepts, such as that of holistic practice (McColl, 1994), the helping relationship (Lloyd & Maas, 1993), occupational therapy's social vision (Townsend, 1993) and the active roles that clients can play in health care issues (Woodside, 1991) and in programme evaluation and research (Clark, Scott & Krupa, 1993) can also be found in the occupational therapy literature. Two models that share many of the same principles as client-centred care are the Planetree model (Jenna, 1986; Jirsh, 1993; MacStravic, 1988; Martin, 1990; Sherer, 1993) and psychosocial rehabilitation (Beard, Propst, & Malemud, 1982; Cnaan, Blankertz, & Saunders, 1992; Estroff, 1983; Freund, 1993). In the Planetree model, patients choose to participate in decisions about their care; are responsible for themselves; are listened to by staff; are given personal choices regarding meal, shower and bed times; have ready access to educational resources concerning their illness; have free access to clinical charts; and can expect services to come to them rather than the reverse (Martin, 1990). Similarly, central to the practice of psychosocial rehabilitation (PSR), are the values of client empowerment, client choice, equipping people with skills, hope, self-determination, contextual relevance, individualization of services, environmental modification, early intervention, advocacy and staff commitment to the philosophy (Cnaan et al., 1992). These two models are very similar to the principles of client-centred care as described by Law et al. (1995). However, PSR was the only model found in the literature search that had consistently involved its clients in the development of its principles and practices. The omission of a client perspective in the discussion of a client-centred approach to practice is puzzling when partnership, client involvement in decision making and client empowerment are thought to be fundamental elements of this approach to practice (Law et al., 1995).

There has been increasing evidence in the literature of the benefits of client involvement in service evaluation and planning (Clark et al., 1993; Dubin, Goering, Wasylenki & Roth, 1995; Greenfield, Kaplan, & Ware, 1985; Hart & Bassett, 1975; Lazare, Eisenthal, & Wasserman, 1975; Pulice, McCormick, & Dewees, 1995; Woodside, 1991). Many of the evaluation instruments have been developed by service providers or by professional evaluation agencies (for example, the tool kit for measuring psychosocial outcomes prepared by the research committee of the International Association of Psychosocial Rehabilitation Services, 1995). However, there was also evidence in the literature that discrepancies existed between clients' and professionals' opinion and perspectives concerning fundamental elements of practice (Dellario, Anthony, & Rogers, 1983; Mayer & Rosenblatt, 1974; Prager & Tanaka, 1980; Sullivan & Yudelowitz, 1996). Health care clients have become increasingly vocal about their desire to be part of the planning for service delivery systems that are more responsive to their needs (Chamberlin, Rogers, & Sneed, 1989; Church, 1994; 1993; 1992; Church & Capponi, 1991; Ridgeway, 1988). Other models of care that share similar principles with client-centred care have demonstrated that client involvement in the development of philosophy and principles and their application to practice has been of considerable benefit (Cnaan et al., 1992; Jenna, 1986).

In summary, the literature reviewed indicated that soliciting a client perspective of client-centred care will be a useful addition to the knowledge base in occupational therapy's conception of client-centred care.

METHODS

A qualitative research approach using focus groups was used in order to understand the emic perspective (DePoy & Gitlin, 1994; Morgan, 1988, 1993). A modified participatory action strategy was also employed (Kaufman, 1993; Rogers & Palmer-Erbs, 1994). Two mental health clients were involved as members of the research team in all phases of the project. These persons had been active in patient councils, peer support and self-help iniatives with other mental health clients. They participated in project design, data collection, data analysis, and as facilitators in the focus groups.

Participants

Participants in this study were adults who have a history of mental illness and contact with the mental health services delivery system. They resided in two cities located in Southwestern Ontario and were recruited from local consumer/survivor agencies. Recruitment strategies included letters of information concerning the project; an advertisement placed in the agency newsletter; and person-to-person recruitment by the executive director of the agency. Table 1 summarizes the demographic characteristics of the participants.

A preliminary set of focus group questions was developed. Very broad topic questions were chosen to emphasize the participants' perceptions of what client-centred care would look like, and to describe how their own experiences with mental health care had led them to their conclusions. The four preliminary questions were: 1) What does client centred care mean to you?; 2) If mental health services revolved around you and your needs, what would they look like?; 3) What sorts of things in a hospital or community agency help or hinder a person with your kind of needs to achieve their goals in life?; 4) If you were asked by the people who decide what and how mental health services are provided to you as a mental health client, what would you suggest is the number one priority?

Table 1
Participant Demographics

Caracteristics		N
Gender	Male	7
	Female	10
Marital Status	Married	6
	Single	5
	Separated/Divorced	5
	Widowed	1
Age Range	18–35	2
	36–50	11
	51–65	4
	Over 65	0
Type of Living Arrangement	Own home/apartment	15
	Boarding home	2
Employment Status	Paid Work	2
	Volunteering	5
	Not working	10
Year of first experience with mental health system	1950–1959	1
	1960–1969	5
	1970–1979	4
	1980–1989	4
	1990–1996	3
Date of most recent hospitalization	1980–1989	3
	1990–1996	8
	Not applicable	5
	Not answered	1
***Types of experience with mental health system**	**G.H. in-patient	6
	**G.H. out-patient	7
	Community Agency	14
	Consumer Agency	14
	**P.P.H. in-patient	6
	P.P.H. out-patient	9
	Family Physician	8
	Crisis/Help Line	6
	***Other	6
***Current experience with mental health system**	G.H. in-patient	0
	G.H. out-patient	2
	Community Agency	3
	Consumer Agency	12
	P.P.H. in-patient	0
	P.P.H. out-patient	6
	Family Physician	7
	Crisis/Help Line	2
	****Other	4

*   Participants chose as many items as were appropriate for them
**   G.H. = General Hospital, P.P.H. = Provincial Psychiatric Hospital
***   Responses included such things as volunteer at Canadian Mental Health Association, seeing a private psychologist or psychiatrist, trust in God, family services, sexual assault centre and nerve specialist
****   Responses included such things as applying for disability pensions, help from friends, Homes for Special Care, and incest support worker

Each of the focus groups, which lasted from two to three hours, was audio taped and transcribed verbatim. The transcripts of the focus group audiotapes, along with field notes contained in the field journal, were reviewed several times by the researcher and assigned preliminary category codes. Categories were expanded or condensed in order to respond to themes noted within the data. Quotes illustrating the categories were identified, sorted according to category, and evaluated for clarity of message and ability to relay the themes expressed by clients. The data were organized under two main themes, three categories under each theme, and several elements under each category.

Member checks were done in person with focus group members in both cities. A copy of the draft analytic categories and sub-categories as well as a verbal explanation by the researcher of interpretations and preliminary conclusions were presented to those able to attend. There was agreement that all of the items were reflective of the groups' discussions. Some important suggestions were made for changes in descriptors of themes and categories and some elements were added. Specifically, participants preferred the term *service provider* to *professional*. They preferred that service providers rather than the system be named as not accountable and insensitive/inflexible. They preferred the term *disillusionment* to *apathy* and then added the elements of the negative effect on the healing process to the category of the effect on the client in the client/service provider relationship. They also added the element "had to meet their own needs" to the category of the effect on the client in the social and mental health system and, the element "laws" to the category of what's needed.

The criteria of credibility, transferability, dependability and confirmability (Lincoln & Guba, 1985) were met through the use of several strategies. The data were triangulated in this study through the use of field notes, transcripts, the involvement of many participants in focus groups, and the use of two facilitators and

one observer (the researcher) in each of the focus groups. Both the member checking groups and debriefing with an academic advisor ensured credibility (Lincoln & Guba, 1985). The results section provides sufficient detail of participants' verbatim quotations to permit the reader to assess transferability. Dependability and confirmability were met through an audit of all data sources and data reconstruction by an academic advisor.

RESULTS

The term *client* was used in this paper as opposed to the terms patient or consumer because this study was exploring the concept of client-centred care, and because the term *client* is reported to be the preferred term for mental health clients (Mueser, Glynn, Corrigan & Baber, 1996).

It should be noted that after raising the general question concerning the client perception of client-centred care, participants in each of the focus groups found it necessary to first describe their past experiences with their illness and the mental health service delivery system, before they were able to return to the question of client-centred care. Results of this study are presented through the use of descriptive statements, illustrated by selected verbatim quotations from the transcripts of the focus groups. Quotations were chosen for two reasons: to present the reader with the most succinct, articulate expression of client opinion and/or to convey the dramatic effect that events and practices have had on these individuals.

The quotations are categorized under three main themes: 1) the client in the client/service provider relationship; 2) the client in the social and mental health system; and 3) client-centred care means I am a valued human being. Within the first two themes there are three categories which reflect the participants' need to discuss prior experiences as well as look at client-centred care. These are titled *what's wrong, the effect on the client* and *what's needed*. Within each of the categories there are several elements which are listed in the order they appeared in the transcripts; they are not ranked in order of importance or frequency. Most of the elements appeared several times in the transcripts. The final theme is the concluding analytic theme, client-centred care means I am a valued human being.

THE CLIENT IN THE CLIENT/SERVICE PROVIDER RELATIONSHIP

What's Wrong

Within the focus groups the clients provided descriptions of what has been wrong, and what is currently wrong, with relationships these individuals have with service providers. These examples were provided frequently by all 17 focus group participants. In regard to **negative attitudes,** there were several examples given of derogatory attitudes, sarcasm, harsh words, and "put downs" that clients considered unnecessary and harmful.

> Participant A: . . . this whole, this client run or client care for thing is their attitude and the attitude is one that is derogatory towards the client. They're considered to be less than human, that they did something wrong in the first place to get mentally ill. Treatment is often accompanied in punitive style where the patient is made to feel it's their fault if they're upset, their fault if they're crying, . . . I know restraints are sometimes necessary but the whole attitude and the way it's done and the harsh words that come to you, the voice level, the sarcasm is not necessary . . .

Participants stated that service providers seemed **indifferent to them as human beings.** They talked about service providers being too busy to deal with their concerns. They often felt unimportant and insignificant in the overall process of service delivery.

> Participant D: I made the comment one time that my psychiatrist doesn't care whether I live or die. I believe that. If I do believe that how on earth am I going to relate to him? Then why would I tell him anything about me or put any faith in him? Like when I walk in I want some

kind of response - an emotional response, that I exist as a human being, that it matters that I'm there, that I'm doing as well as possible, because if it doesn't matter, if it doesn't make a difference then I don't see the point in being there.

Service providers' **superficial knowledge of clients** was discussed as a source of frustration. The participants queried how service providers could make choices for them, make decisions concerning appropriate treatments, and diagnose so quickly when they had gained so little insight into the complexities of their clients as individuals and the life experiences that had shaped them.

> Participant A: Oh, oh I was diagnosed as having a personality disorder like within a week of being there. Personality disorder, that's an easy pigeon slot, for you know, a lot of things . . .

Clients were very conscious of the **status difference** between themselves and professionals. They talked of the professionals who had learned all that they know through books, professionals who discounted their life experiences as valuable sources of knowledge, and professionals who thought that their credentials somehow made them better than their clients.

> Participant F: What I would like to see is a sort of advocate that would be between the psychiatrist at the top and the client at the bottom. There would be a mediator or somebody in between in serious situations, and . . . you would move away from that when the person got a little stronger. So that is sort of going, . . . just one to one in bad situations, it's just not, I guess it's just that authority figure . . . being able to cope with that.

Participants talked extensively of their experiences with service providers who had used **techniques that did not meet client needs.** In their opinion, this lack of success was often due to so little time being spent in developing a relationship with the client.

> Participant E: One of the things I was looking for were answers and I'm still looking for those same damn answers today. How to deal with

yourself financially, how to manage money, how to manage your time, just ordinary simple damn living and so you're . . . you feel that reject of not belonging here.

Descriptions of the **lack of trust** in relationships with service providers were pervasive. Clients had lost faith in service providers because of promises made and not kept, confidences broken, not being believed, and an unwritten but clear understanding that clients complaining about poor staff practices was not acceptable.

Participant H: No we don't [get believed]. People don't believe us. It's very true. They question everything we do, professionals are put up here on pedestals and we're the rug on the floor.

Stigma is experienced by clients at all levels of society and the mental health system but the perception that **service providers stigmatize the mentally ill** client was also pervasive.

Participant A: and everyone goes oh, oh you have cancer, but if it's a mental illness stay away. Labels are for jars, not for people and still to this day . . . oh, they don't give you credit for changing. Twelve years, it's been twelve years and I still hear the whispers [from staff] . . . and . . . there was never any closure for the treatment that I go to, do you know what I mean by that?

Effect on the Client

The effect on the client of these past difficulties in the client/service provider relationship was described in a variety of ways. **Fear** of hospitalization, **fear** of the wrath of service providers if they complained, and **fear** of their own illness are common experiences for mental health clients.

Participant I: The people would complain but that is the only time they would complain, because they are so afraid of that person at that home. They will say don't let them find out we said this, you know.

The deep sense of **disillusionment with service providers** that clients have come to accept was expressed.

Participant E: Okay, so what's the use of me putting the effort into going out there [the hospital] if you have the Mexican stand-off, where you sort of stare at each other and you don't say anything to each other because there's nothing to say.

An **impaired self-esteem** resulting from their previous experience with the system has left these clients with the belief that they cannot play a valued role in their own health care. Some clients had considerable difficulty in conceptualizing their role in client-centred care.

Participant A: I don't think I'd have a role [referring to decisions about her own care]. Whatever they say goes. I, I don't have any. I don't have any input into it whatsoever.

The **negative effect on the healing process** of a poor client/service provider relationship was added during the member checking phase. One participant in the member check group had expressed it as follows:

Participant E: But part of the thing is you're looking for answers and if you're not finding answers what do you do? You quite often give up looking for answers or you stay still.

What's Needed

One suggestion of what's needed in the client/service provider relationship is the need for service providers wishing to practice in a client-centred fashion **to value and appreciate the life experience of their clients** and **recognize their expert knowledge of themselves.** They need to believe in their clients' potential, respect them as human beings, treat them like the adults they are, and not add to the stigma that already exists in their lives.

Participant L: She [the service provider] seems to think that she's the only expert on this in the field. Well I live it, I should know just as much or more than her because I'm the actual person surviving it.

The need for service providers to **change the way they deliver services, get close, and be**

welcoming to the client were referred to in several quotations.

Participant H: A pat on the back once in awhile instead of a kick in the back of the knees or a hug like (participant's name) says—the love. We don't get the love from professionals like and a lot of people when you say love think sex, that's not what I'm talking about. Love as in you've done good for yourself. Give us credit instead of stamping us out for things we didn't do . . .

Participant J: . . . it's all those little things, consideration, sensitivity, respect—it all is shown in the way you treat people. Little things like even the HS [an abbreviation from the Latin term referring to an evening snack] lunch ya know. If HS lunch is made at five o'clock and the toast is left to sit there until seven o'clock and it's ice cold, well who cares what they eat, they can have anything, they're only mental patients you know.
I would want more one on one . . . sincere care because that is what health care is all about, sincere caring. Like I want to become a nurse because I care about people and I like to help people and this is what it is all about, but that's not what it's all about out there [the hospital].

A great deal of discussion in the focus groups centred around the need for clients to talk things through with others and that **talking takes time.** They want service providers to listen, to get to know them before they can expect trust, and to consider them as people and as more important than paperwork.

Participant M: Take time for each one, you don't put a time limit like a fifteen minutes per patient cause some can't open up that fast.

Participants talked about the need for a common understanding between clients and service providers, a common respect, and the creation of an atmosphere that would promote healing. They want a shared philosophy that encourages all players to work together in partnership, on a **common ground,** so that issues of power and control are not hindering the process of change.

Participant G: Maybe if they had the time, a smaller caseload, whatever if it was possible, take the time to get to know them and actually talk to them just maybe not just sit there and listen

completely but talk with them, not like doctor/patient more like two people, two humans talking back and forth and that way one isn't higher than the other, you're both just sitting there talking.

Participants felt they could play an important role in the **education of professionals.** They spoke of providing opportunities for professionals to understand what it is like to live with mental illness and to live on their very limited incomes.

Participant N: . . . we have to educate the professionals ourselves, us with the mental illness because we have the illness and we have the experience of the illness. They see it from the outside, they can help us but we have to help them.

THE CLIENT IN THE SOCIAL AND MENTAL HEALTH SYSTEM

What's Wrong

As focus group participants discussed the concept of client-centred care, several comments were made concerning the negative consequences of the social and mental health system and the stigma they encounter. The system included institutional care as well as community and public resources, such as boarding homes, the public trustee and the municipal and provincial income supplement programmes. It became clear that, to practice in a client-centred way, the service provider would also have to advocate for change in the larger system. As will be seen, clients are interested in working with service providers to effect change in the system and to promote public education.

Service providers whom these people encounter, in institutions, in boarding homes, in welfare offices, and in virtually every part of the system are perceived as **not being held accountable.** Clients are often not informed how their money is being managed, are often exploited, and are actively discouraged from complaining. When they do complain the system does not repair the problem or damage and the clients are left to suffer the consequences.

Participant K: . . . I find out from (participant's name) that I don't know if it's the Public Trustee or who does it but I'm paying a $1000 for the room I'm in with my husband but I can't figure it out and maybe somebody can straighten it out in my mind, how do they know how much money they should charge me for being in that room. That's been on my mind. . . .

There were many examples cited that demonstrated **insensitivity and lack of flexibility** on the part of institutional staff. Many examples of perceived problems with community-based service providers were also provided, particularly in the boarding home sector and Homes for Special Care (HSC). Clients stress a need for a more humane, responsive, and flexible system in order to meet individual needs.

Participant J: . . . and they don't get milk, they get a little bit of coffeemate, the cheapest brand for the coffee. But coffee is only once a day in the morning and the rest of the day, there is no coffee made for the patients. They can't go in the kitchen, nobody goes in the kitchen. You can't go in and make a snack, such as the good one on (address of home) where they let you go in the fridge [unlike most HSC's] and they are given, just like in the hospital, a big urn of tea with one tea bag in it.

Stigma towards the mentally ill is encountered everywhere by these individuals. Their own words reveal just how pervasive it is in their everyday lives.

Participant D: . . . you have to look at stigma, I think, you have to look at different kinds of stigma. The stigma of the general public towards the mentally ill. Stigma of the professional towards the mentally ill. Stigma of the mentally ill towards each other and the worst of all the stigma each and every one of us have towards ourselves and our own illness. So we're looking at four kinds of stigma. You have to work on all of these things.

Effect on the Client

The effects of these experience on clients has been, in many cases, devastating and, in others, has created considerable anger. They stated that

they were forced to help themselves. They described feeling disempowered and expendable as a group of citizens.

The participants described being **marginalized** and used several examples to illustrate it. They state that clients are pushed to the fringes of society.

Participant E: . . . the people should be allowed to go into different restaurants and do their shopping wherever they please and not get looked down on. Because I mean people do it all the time, whether they do it in front of your face or behind your back but they're still doing it. You know one story goes to the other and the word of mouth is the fastest way of advertising.

Not surprisingly, mental health clients feel very cynical about society's priorities for the mentally ill.

Participant A: . . . they are not listening to the Graham Report [An Ontario governmentally commissioned study that preceded the Ontario mental health reform movement] because mental patients are expendable, they are not a priority in peoples' minds. If they get sick we can put them in institutions where they're out of the way, they don't bother anybody, they're out of the way, they won't bother anybody, they're off our backs.

What's Needed

They suggested several specific strategies for creating what is needed.

The benefits of **peer support services** are significant for clients. Peers give them a sense of trust and empathy they can't find from others, a sense of fellowship they can't find in other social settings, and a sense of belonging they have long felt was not available for them.

Participant D: We didn't get what we wanted from professionals so we formed all these peer groups . . . Yes, trust and empathy I think, you can talk about sympathy, you can talk about all kinds of things but you can even say that the professional may have some empathy and I think they do because they've been through pain and suffering and so on but when you get down to the hard core of experience in the mental health system at its worst, the only true empathy is from someone, another survivor and sometimes that connection . . . is tremendous. People make friends, they develop trust, they feel they're not alone. You can't get that in any other way so I think there's value with the professional and everything else but there's also value in the experience and the healing that comes from, you know, being with your own people. You can say that I'm mushy but that's how I feel about it.

Clients want effective ways to ensure service providers are caring, compassionate, and humane. They want mechanisms put in place that will have adequate influence and power to really make a difference.

Participant J: Yeah, something like that [a complaint board], so that if it turns out that they are really in it for the dollar, or they you know the board has the authority to say look, we're gonna knock you down a peg. . . . Keep them human so they're are not just there from 9 to 5 . . .

Clients want to be **part of the change process.** The focus group participants promoted advocacy by clients, for clients and proposed that it will assist in making the very necessary changes.

Participant O: I believe that the professionals are the ones that need to get the cotton batten out of their ears and start listening to the client because if they're not getting the care it's just frustrating them more and they're having problems dealing with their illness as it is, let alone pile up more and more and more stuff on their plate and so that's one of my biggest concerns and . . . I'd be interested in an advocate position . . .

Clients recognize the need for service providers to relinquish control and power and for clients to work actively in a **partnership on common ground** with service providers.

Participant E: Okay, the communication is lacking, but what we have done we have allowed ourselves as people, Canadians, to be too damn passive. That includes everybody. Now to speak out means that you are going to have to speak out, you gotta be prepared to get the feedback. But the thing that I think we have forgotten as Canadians, and I am going to use the word Canadians, is that, we have that freedom of speech yet.

Clients envision a **more caring public,** if only they could enlist a high profile sponsor to champion their cause and convince others that they are just ordinary human beings.

Participant O: You know it's because you're an ex-patient. If people knew more about us patients that get rehabilitated back in society, if people knew exactly what we went through and what we've come up to they'd look at us in a different aspect. You know they won't look at us like a "mental patient," they'd look at us as an ordinary human being.

The final recommendation for what is needed was expressed in the following fashion:

Participant O: Laws. Laws to protect a vulnerable population and an attitude change that we're a vulnerable population. Laws that would affect how the police deal with us, laws not changing the attitude of the public but laws that would stop the public from harming us in certain ways. The last time I was in court the judge said to me society has to be protected and I wanted to say to him, "who's going to protect me from the public?" . . .

CLIENT-CENTRED CARE MEANS I AM A VALUED HUMAN BEING

The focus group discussions that were held to examine client-centred care from the client perspective delivered several important messages. Perhaps the most poignant one is that of an impassioned plea from clients for service providers, and society in general, to recognize their human strengths and frailties and to value them as they would any other human being. The ubiquity with which phrases involving the recognition of their worth as human beings occurred in the focus groups is illustrated by the following excerpts from the transcripts.

. . . they're [the clients] considered to be less than human . . .
. . . you're driven beyond human endurance . . .
. . . I want some kind of response - an emotional response, that I exist as a human being . . .
. . . we should be appreciated for the person, people that we are . . .

. . . more like two people, two humans talking back and forth . . .
. . . maybe the clients, customers could be called human beings, our fellow Canadians.
. . . they won't look at us like a mental patient, they'd look at us like an ordinary human being.

The following quotation illustrates the concluding theme in a very personal and heartfelt way.

> *Participant O: We have feelings just as well as everybody else does. That's where a lot of patients get hurt is their feelings and with depression that's one of the worst things you can do is cut somebody else down because they thrive on that. They don't care what the results are because they don't have to go through it you know.*

DISCUSSION

Although the analytic categories included the social and mental health system, the primary focus of the clients was on their experiences with a variety of individual service providers. Therefore, the emphasis of this discussion is of considerable relevance to occupational therapists. In as much as we claim to strive for client-centred care in our practice, the participants' descriptions in this study of their previous and hoped-for care have implications for occupational therapists as individuals and as members of the profession.

The participants in this study referred often to not being believed, and stated that their opinions and perspectives were not respected by service providers. The participants' assessment of past and present mental health practices and their ideas for change are confirmed and supported by literature describing the loss of caring about the human being in health care (Montgomery, 1993), the medicalization of mental health care (Speechley, 1992; Stewart et al., 1995), health care's history of focusing on disease and impairment while not fully understanding the full impact of disability and handicap (Anthony, Cohen, & Farkas, 1990; Dain, 1994; Martini, Polatajko, & Wilcox, 1995; World Health Organization, 1978, 1980) and

the stigmatization of clients by service providers (Capponi, 1992; Deegan, 1988; Dubin & Fink, 1992; Elliot, Hanzlik, & Gliner, 1992; Leete, 1989; Lyons & Ziviani, 1995; Townsend, 1990). Health care clients, health care providers, and scholars in the social sciences field are joining them in the pursuit of a health care service system that will improve clients' quality of life (Renwick & Brown, 1996), enable and empower them to achieve their life goals (Martini et al., 1995; Polatajko, 1992), provide a sense of hope and recovery from illness (Anthony et al., 1990; Anthony, 1993; Deegan, 1988, 1993; Neuhaus, 1997; Woodside et al., 1994) and a return to caring in health care (Montgomery, 1993).

Results of this study have added a new layer to our understanding of the meaning and characteristics of client-centred care. These results emphasize, more than anything else, the need for clients to feel valued as human beings. The professional literature has paid little attention to this dimension. The results of this study have been gathered from "the humans who get sick, have accidents, and appear at the door of the health care system. They are in jeopardy of losing control of themselves and they are afraid. As professionals we must recognize their tremendous vulnerability and offer them services in which they have choices and control" (Baum, 1980, p. 506).

IMPLICATIONS OF THIS STUDY

For Occupational Therapy Practice

Occupational therapy has defined client-centred care as containing the elements of autonomy/choice, partnership and responsibility, enablement, contextual congruence, accessibility and flexibility and respect for diversity (Law et al., 1995). But there are doubts about whether we have truly integrated what we believe as a profession into everyday practice (Gage & Polatajko, 1995; Sumsion, 1993). Occupational therapists are also susceptible to the effects of working within health services

---

dominated by the medical model (Law et al., 1995; Townsend, 1992).

Occupational therapy's roots are in the era of moral treatment for the insane in the late 18th century. "Caring for and caring about the patient was as implicit as occupation in this new form of therapy" (King, 1980, p. 523). The occupation worker's role was to provide "opportunities rather than prescriptions and to demonstrate resourcefulness and the ability to respect the native capacities and interests of the patient" (Meyer, 1922/1977, p. 641). "Caring was, and is, the primary technique inherent in the art of occupational therapy" (Gilfoyle, 1980, p. 517).

The results of this study and the increasing demands of health care consumers require that occupational therapists not lose sight of the human being affected by illness or disease. We need to ensure that our focus is on the reduction of handicapping environments and on the promotion of recovery of the person, not the disease or the label.

Although occupational therapists may not adopt non-caring behaviours and attitudes themselves, they do not often work actively to change these environments. This study illustrates that a caring relationship between client and service provider is critical but insufficient without other social and system changes as well. Occupational therapists must work with clients and other service providers to advocate for a service delivery system that is more humane, more responsive to client need and more focused on recovery and return to valued, fulfilling lives for clients, not merely accepting a life on the fringes of society for clients.

We need to think in a holistic fashion regarding the needs of these valued human beings. We need to build our relationships with clients utilizing assessment tools like the Canadian Occupational Performance Measure (Law et al., 1990) so that goals identified are the client's goals and not the therapist's. We should respect and value the client's expert knowledge of him or herself and recognize the importance of understanding the client's life experiences, expectations and goals prior to illness and their impact on his/her view of the future. "Our practice in the future should be evaluated not only on the basis of measurable, scientific outcomes, but also by what it contributes to the individual's human dignity, sense of mastery and self-respect" (Yerxa, 1980, p. 534).

For Education

Focus group participants talked extensively about the need for clients to participate in the education of service providers. They proposed a curriculum that would include opportunities "to walk in the shoes" of the client and, to achieve a "gut level" understanding of mental illness and its effect on the individual. Mental health clients, they argue, can teach service providers a great deal about the illness experience and the effectiveness or lack of effectiveness of treatment and rehabilitation strategies. Assigned readings of the personal accounts literature and ensuring that clients are included as educators in classrooms, and in service agencies could provide that very important "insider" perspective for those entering health care and to keep those already in the field grounded in the issues that are of importance to clients.

For Research

Further studies, similar to this one, involving clients with an array of disabilities and experiences must be completed to adequately crystallize a client-driven definition of client-centred care. Examination of the outcomes of client-centred care practice, both from a client and professional perspective, should be done to provide further evidence regarding its effectiveness or lack of effectiveness. Studies that examine the outcomes of peer support and self-help strategies are needed to understand their potential benefits.

Outcomes of client-centred care must be compared and contrasted with those of similar models such as patient-centred care and psychosocial rehabilitation, so that one can identify the strategies that provide maximum benefit to the client. Investigation of the effectiveness of education by clients for service providers could add important teaching strategies for universities and colleges. Finally, further research based upon personal accounts and narratives could help us "focus on our humanistic philosophies centering on the client's needs, personal contexts, and life circumstance and, thus, may satisfy both the demands for efficacious treatment and consumer satisfaction" (Larson & Fanchiang, 1996).

STRENGTHS AND LIMITATIONS OF THIS STUDY

The relatively small number of participants, the short time frame (2 months) in which the study was conducted and its geographical specificity (southwestern Ontario) may be considered as limitations. The recruitment of members of mental health consumer/survivor agencies may have involved a select sector of the mental health client group. There can be no claim that study participants are representative of the larger group of persons with serious mental illness.

One of the major strengths of this study is that focus group participants not only supported many of the characteristics of client-centred care found in the literature but added a level of specificity and a greater depth of understanding that has been missing. The focus group participants highlighted the "human element" of the client-centred care perspective and helped to clarify the extensive effects of the handicaps associated with mental illness. They added to our understanding of the type of partnership service providers and clients have to form to create real change.

SUMMARY

The results of this study paint a very honest, but far from flattering picture of a service delivery system, and service providers. Collectively,

persons living with mental illness have been excluded from participating as citizens deserving respect, dignity, and value as human beings. The sometimes devastating effects of these factors have resulted in many of these people feeling afraid, disillusioned, and marginalized by the very individuals (service providers) who are trained to assist them in achieving good health and independent living.

Perhaps the most important findings are the ideas for effecting change that these focus group participants have to offer, despite their experiences of the past. Their demonstrated resiliency in the focus group discussions despite the incredible negativity they have experienced from the mental health system and society in general, is something to be greatly admired. The participants' ability to respond to adversity with creativity and a determination to right the wrongs of the past are strengths that deserve acknowledgment and praise.

The participants in this study provide an abundance of specific examples of what has been wrong and what is needed in everyday relationships between clients and service providers. These examples should be very helpful for clinicians who are interested in learning how to apply client-centred principles in practice situations. This study has provided a positive contribution to the current knowledge base concerning client-centred care. It provides an important perspective that has been, to date, absent in the discussion. "Human health is intricately tied to the dreams, hopes, attitudes, values, beliefs, and understandings of individuals" (Lincoln, 1992, p. 388). If we are able to meet the challenges of these client-generated principles of client-centred care, then perhaps clients can begin to feel like valuable human beings and enjoy the love, respect, and fulfilment they deserve.

ACKNOWLEDGEMENTS

Parts of this study were presented at the OSOT Conference in London, Ontario, April 1998, and at the 12th International Congress of the

World Federation of Occupational Therapists, in Montreal, June 1998. An article describing a portion of the results of this research study was published in *Occupational Therapy Now*, (CAOT's Practice Magazine), Jan/Feb 1999, Volume 1, number 1, pages 8–10.

References

Anthony, W.A. (1993). Recovery from mental illness: A guiding vision of the mental health service system in the 1990's. *Psychosocial Rehabilitation Journal, 16* (4), 11–23.

Anthony, W.A., Cohen, M., & Farkas, M. (1990). *Psychiatric Rehabilitation.* Boston MA: Center for Psychiatric Rehabilitation.

Baum, C.M. (1980). Occupational therapists put care in the health system. *The American Journal of Occupational Therapy, 34,* 505–516.

Beard, J.H., Propst, R.N., & Malamud, T.J. (1982). The Fountain House model of psychosocial rehabilitation. *Psychosocial Rehabilitation Journal, 5*(1), 120–131.

Blain, J., & Townsend, E. (1993). Occupational therapy guidelines for client-centred practice: Impact study findings. *Canadian Journal of Occupational Therapy, 60,* 271–285.

Canadian Association of Occupational Therapists. (1997). *Enabling occupation: An occupational therapy perspective.* Ottawa, ON: CAOT Publications ACE.

Canadian Association of Occupational Therapists. (1991). *Occupational therapy guidelines for client-centred practice.* Toronto, ON: CAOT Publications ACE.

Canadian Association of Occupational Therapists & Health and Welfare Canada. (1983). *Guidelines for the client-centred practice of occupational therapy.* Ottawa, ON: Department of National Health and Welfare.

Canadian Association of Occupational Therapists & Health and Welfare Canada. (1986). *Intervention guidelines for the client-centred practice of occupational therapy.* Ottawa, ON: Department of National Health and Welfare.

Canadian Association of Occupational Therapists & Health Canada. (1993). *Occupational therapy guidelines for client-centred mental health practice.* Ottawa, ON: Health Canada.

Capponi, P. (1992). *Upstairs in the crazy house.* Toronto, ON: Viking Press.

Chamberlin, J., Rogers, J.A., & Sneed, C.S. (1989). Consumers, families and community support systems. *Psychosocial Rehabilitation Journal, 12,* 93–106.

Church, K. (1992). *Moving over—A commentary of power-sharing.* Toronto, ON: Ontario Ministry of Health.

Church, K. (1993). *Breaking down, breaking through: Multi-voiced narratives on psychiatric survivor participation in Ontario's community mental health system.* Doctoral dissertation, University of Toronto, Toronto, ON.

Church, K. (1994). *Working together across differences.* Toronto, ON: Psychiatric Survivor Leadership Facilitation Program & Community Resource Consultants of Toronto.

Church, K., & Capponi, P. (1991). *Re/membering ourselves—A resource book on psychiatric survivor leadership facilitation.* Toronto, ON: Leadership Facilitation Program.

Clark, C., Scott, E.A., & Krupa, T. (1993). Involving clients in programme evaluation and research: A new methodology for occupational therapy. *Canadian Journal of Occupational Therapy, 60,* 192–199.

Cnaan, R.A., Blankertz, L., & Saunders, M. (1992). Perceptions of consumers, practitioners and experts regarding psychosocial rehabilitation principles. *Psychosocial Rehabilitation Journal, 16,* 95–119.

Dain, N. (1994). Reflections on antipsychiatry and stigma in the history of American psychiatry. *Hospital and Community Psychiatry, 45,* 1010–1015.

Deegan, P.E. (1988). Recovery: The lived experience of rehabilitation. *Psychosocial Rehabilitation Journal, 11*(4), 11–19.

Deegan, P.E. (1993). Recovering our sense of value after being labeled. *Journal of Psychosocial Nursing, 31*(4), 7–11.

Dellario, D.J., Anthony, W.A., & Rogers, S.E. (1983). Client-practitioner agreement in the assessment of severely psychiatrically disabled persons' functional skills. *Rehabilitation Psychology, 28*(4), 243–248.

DePoy, E., & Gitlin, L.N. (1994). *Introduction to research: Multiple strategies for health and human services.* St. Louis, MO: Mosby.

Dubin, J., Goering, P., Wasylenki, D., & Roth, J. (1995). Meeting the challenge: Field evaluations of community support programs. *Psychiatric Rehabilitation Journal, 19* (1), 19–26.

Dubin, W.R., & Fink, P.J. (1992). Effects of stigma on psychiatric treatment. In P.J. Fink & A. Tansman (Eds.), *Stigma and mental illness.* (pp. 1–7). Washington, DC: American Psychiatric Press.

Elliott, D., Hanzlik, J., & Gliner, J. (1992). Attitudes of occupational therapy personnel toward therapists with disabilities. *Occupational Therapy Journal of Research, 12,* 259–277.

Estroff, S.E. (1983). How social is psychosocial rehabilitation? *Psychosocial Rehabilitation Journal, 7*(2), 6–20.

Fink, P.J., & Tansman, A. (Eds.) (1992). *Stigma and mental illness.* Washington, DC: American Psychiatric Press.

Fruend, P.D. (1993). Professional role(s) in the empowerment process: Working with mental health consumers. *Psychosocial Rehabilitation Journal, 16*(3), 65–73.

Gage, M., & Polatajko, H. (1995). Naming practice: The case for the term client-driven. *Canadian Journal of Occupational Therapy, 62,* 115–118.

Gilfoyle, E.M. (1980). Caring: A philosophy for practice. *The American Journal of Occupational Therapy, 34,* 517–521.

Greenfield, S., Kaplan, S., & Ware, J.E. (1985). Expanding patient involvement in care-effects on patient outcomes. *Annals of Internal Medicine, 102,* 520–528.

Hart, W.T., & Bassett, L. (1975). Measuring consumer satisfaction in a mental health centre. *Hospital & Community Psychiatry, 26*(8), 512–515.

Hobson, S. (1996). Being client-centred when the client is cognitively impaired. *Canadian Journal of Occupational Therapy, 63,* 133–137.

International Association of Psychosocial Rehabilitation Services. (1995). *Toolkit for measuring psychosocial outcomes.* Columbia, MD: Author.

Jenna, J.K. (1986, May/June). Toward the patient-driven hospital. *Healthcare Management Forum,* 9–18.

Jirsch, D. (1993). Patient-focused care: The systemic implications of change. *Healthcare Management Forum, 6*(4), 27–32.

Kaufman, C.L. (1993). Roles for mental health consumers in self-help group research. *The Journal of Applied Behavioural Science, 29*(2), 257–271.

King, L.J. (1980). Creative caring. *The American Journal of Occupational Therapy, 34,* 522–528.

Krupa, T., & Clark, C. (1995). Occupational therapists as case managers: Responding to current approaches to community mental health service delivery. *Canadian Journal of Occupational Therapy, 62,* 16–22.

Larson, E.A., & Fanchiang, S.C. (1996). Life history and narrative research: Generating a humanistic knowledge base for occupational therapy. *The American Journal of Occupational Therapy, 50,* 247–250.

Law, M., Baptiste, S., McColl, M., Opzoomer, A., Polatajko, H., & Pollock, N. (1990). The Canadian Occupational Performance Measure: An outcome measure for occupational therapy. *Canadian Journal of Occupational Therapy, 57,* 82–87.

Law, M., Baptiste, S., & Mills, J. (1995). Client-centred practice: What does it mean and does it make a difference? *Canadian Journal of Occupational Therapy, 62,* 250–257.

Lazare, A., Eisenthal, S., & Wasserman, L. (1975). The customer approach to patienthood—Attending to patients in a walk-in clinic. *Archives of General Psychiatry, 32,* 553–558.

Leete, E. (1989). How I perceive and manage my illness. *Schizophrenia Bulletin, 15*(2), 197–200.

Lincoln, Y.S. (1992). Sympathetic connections between qualitative methods and health research. *Qualitative Health Research, 2,* 375–391.

Lincoln, Y.S., & Guba, E.G. (1985). *Naturalistic Inquiry.* Newbury Park, CA: Sage Publications.

Lloyd, C., & Maas, F. (1993). The helping relationship: The application of Carkhuff's model. *Canadian Journal of Occupational Therapy, 60,* 83–89.

Lyons, M., & Ziviani, J. (1995). Stereotypes, stigma and mental illness: Learning from fieldwork experiences. *The American Journal of Occupational Therapy, 49,* 1002–1008.

Mac Stravic, R.S. (1988). The patient as partner: A competitive strategy in health care marketing. *Hospital and Health Services Administration, 33*(1), 15–24.

Madill, H., Tirrul-Jones, A., & Magill-Evans, J. (1990). The application of the client-centred approach to school-based occupational therapy practice. *Canadian Journal of Occupational Therapy, 57,* 102–108.

Martin, D.P. (1990). The Planetree model hospital: An example of the patient as a partner. *Hospital and Health Services Administration, 35* (4), 591–601.

Martini, R., Polatajko, H.J., & Wilcox, A. (1995). ICIDH - PR: A potential model for occupational therapy. *Occupational Therapy International, 2,* 1–21.

Mayer, J.E., & Rosenblatt, A. (1974). Clash in perspective between mental patients and staff. *American Journal of Orthopsychiatry, 44,* 432–441.

McColl, M. (1994). Holistic occupational therapy: Historical meaning and contemporary implications. *Canadian Journal of Occupational Therapy, 61,* 72–77.

McColl, M., & Pranger, T. (1994). Theory and practice in the occupational therapy guidelines for client centred practice. *Canadian Journal of Occupational Therapy, 61,* 250–259.

Meyer, A. (1977). The philosophy of occupational therapy. *The American Journal of Occupational Therapy, 31,* 639–642. (Reprinted from *Archives of Occupational Therapy, 1,* 1–10, 1922).

Montgomery, C.L. (1993). *Healing through communication: The practice of caring.* Newbury Park, CA: Sage Publications.

Morgan, D.L. (1988). *Focus groups as qualitative research.* Newbury Park, CA: Sage Publications.

Morgan, D.L. (Ed.) (1993). *Successful focus groups—Advancing the state of the art.* Newbury Park, CA: Sage Publications.

Neuhaus, B.E. (1997). Including hope in occupational therapy practice: A pilot study. *The American Journal of Occupational Therapy, 51,* 228–234.

Polatajko, H.J. (1992). Naming and framing occupational therapy: A lecture dedicated to the life of Nancy B. *Canadian Journal of Occupational Therapy, 59,* 189–199.

Prager, E., & Tanaka, H. (1980, Jan.). Self-assessment: The client's perspective. *Social Work,* 32–35.

Pulice, R., McCormick, L., & Dewees, M. (1995). A qualitative approach to assessing the effects of system change on consumers, families and providers. *Psychiatric Services, 46,* 575–579.

Rebeiro, K.L., & Allen, J. (1998). Voluntarism as occupation. *Canadian Journal of Occupational Therapy, 65,* 279–285

Renwick, R., Brown, I., & Nagler, M. (Eds.) (1996). *Quality of life in health promotion and rehabilitation: Conceptual approaches, issues and applications.* Thousand Oaks, CA: Sage Publications.

Renwick, R. & Brown, I. (1996). The centre for health promotion's conceptual approach to quality of life. In R. Renwick, I. Brown, & M. Nagler, (Eds.), *Quality of life in health promotion and rehabilitation: Conceptual approaches, issues and applications.* (pp. 75–86). Thousand Oaks, CA: Sage.

Ridgeway, P. (1988). *The voice of the consumers in mental health systems: A call for change.* Burlington, VT: The Center for Community Change Through Housing and Support.

Rogers, C.R. (1939). *The clinical treatment of the problem child.* Boston, MA: Houghton Mifflin.

Rogers, C. (1951). *Client-centered therapy.* Boston, MA: Houghton Mifflin.

Rogers, E.S., & Palmer-Erbs, V. (1994). Participatory action research: Implications for research and evaluation. *Psychosocial Rehabilitation Journal, 18*(2), 3–12.

Sherer, J.L. (1993, Feb.). Putting patients first: Hospitals work to define patient-centered care. *Hospitals,* 14–18.

Speechley, V. (1992). Patients as partners. *European Journal of Cancer Care, 1*(3), 22–25.

Stewart, D., & Harvey, S. (1990). Application of the guidelines for client-centred practice to paediatric occupational therapy. *Canadian Journal of Occupational Therapy, 57,* 88–94.

Stewart, M., Belle Brown, J., Weston, W.W., McWhinney, I.R., McWilliam, C.L., & Freeman, T.R. (1995). *Patient-centred medicine: Transforming the clinical method.* Thousand Oaks, CA: Sage.

Sullivan, C.W., & Yudelowitz, I.S. (1996). Goals of treatment: Staff and client perceptions. *Perspectives in Psychiatric Care, 32*(1), 4–6.

Sumsion, T. (1993). Client-centred practice: The true impact. *Canadian Journal of Occupational Therapy, 60,* 6–8.

Townsend, E.A. (1992). Institutional ethnography: Explicating the social organization of professional health practices intending client empowerment. *Canadian Journal of Public Health, 83,* 558–561.

Townsend, E. (1993). Occupational therapy's social vision. *Canadian Journal of Occupational Therapy, 60,* 174–184.

Townsend, E. (1993). Stereotypes of mental illness: A comparison with ethnic stereotypes. In M. Nagler, (Ed.), *Perspectives on disability* (pp. 102–117). Palo Alto, CA: Health Market Research.

Waters, D. (1995). Recovering from a depressive episode using the Canadian Occupational Performance Measure. *Canadian Journal of Occupational Therapy, 62,* 276–282.

Woodside, H. (1991). The participation of mental health consumers in health care issues. *Canadian Journal of Occupational Therapy, 58,* 3–5.

Woodside, H., Landeen, J., Kirkpatrick, H., Bryne, C., Bernardo, A., & Pawlicki, J. (1994). Hope and schizophrenia: Exploring attitudes of clinicians. *Psychosocial Rehabilitation Journal, 18*(1), 140–144.

World Health Organization (1978). *International classification of diseases, injuries and causes of death* (9th rev). Geneva: Author.

World Health Organization (1980). *International classification of impairments, disabilities and handicaps (ICIDH).* Geneva: Author.

Yerxa, E.J. (1980). Occupational therapy's role in creating a future climate of caring. *The American Journal of Occupational Therapy, 34,* 529–534.

Chapter 21

The Labyrinth of Community Mental Health: In Search of Meaningful Occupation

Psychiatric Rehabilitation Journal
1999, 23(2): 143–152

Karen L. Rebeiro

Karen L. Rebeiro, M.SC., O.T. (C) is a clinical researcher at Network North, The Community Mental Health Group, Sudbury, Ontario, Canada.

ABSTRACT

Mental health reform poses unique challenges for professionals who are attempting to enable meaningful occupation in the community for people who have a psychiatric disability. A qualitative research study was conducted in order to describe, from the participants' perspective, their experiences of pursuing meaningful occupation, and to identify aspects of the community environment which either enabled or constrained their participation in occupation. In-depth interviews and participant observation were the methods utilized in the research. The results of this study indicate that the community is experienced as a labyrinth of bureaucracies and services in which people with a psychiatric disability become lost. In general, the study illustrates how the continued focus on psychiatric disability as a personal problem of the individual, rather than as a social issue within the community environment, serves to submerge the occupational needs of people with a serious mental illness and to foster ongoing dependency upon various social, economic, and health systems. The results support the need for mental health professionals to consider the environment of the community in greater depth, and well beyond the limitations imposed by a "personal problems" approach to care. The implications of this study, with respect to community mental health service provision and policy, are provided.

Occupational therapy theory and practice emphasize the need to consider the transactional relationship between the individual, engagement in occupation, and the environment in the provision of services. Recent models of practice increasingly emphasize the importance of the environment to understanding the importance of occupational performance (CAOT, 1997; Grady, 1995; Kielhofner, 1995; Law, Cooper, Strong, Rigby, & Letts, 1996; Trombly, 1995; Wood, 1998). The literature suggests that therapists must be aware of factors within the environment which constrain or enable occupational performance for individuals with a disability (CAOT, 1997; Grady, 1995).

A recent qualitative study discovered that the provision of an affirming social environment and the provision of opportunity, rather than the prescription of occupation, were important in enabling occupational performance for women with a psychiatric disability (Rebeiro, 1997). This study also discovered that, despite knowledge of mental health services in the community, these participants did not perceive that there were opportunities for meaningful occupation, nor that the environment of the larger community was enabling or supportive of personally valued occupational goals.

The present research sought to explore and describe, from the perspective of individuals with a serious mental illness (SMI), what they did on a daily basis and what they perceived to be enabling and/or constraining in their pursuit of meaningful occupation within the community. The research purpose was to develop a more comprehensive understanding of how various aspects of the individual's environment either enabled or limited occupational performance. The theoretical perspectives in this paper are offered as a contribution to the issues faced by all mental health professionals in enabling occupation or work for the community-based individual.

LITERATURE REVIEW

The early occupational therapy literature acknowledged the environment and successful community integration as an end or goal of occupational therapy intervention (LeVesconte, 1935; Menzel, 1947). Meyer (1922/77) recognized the importance of enabling environments when he stated, "Our role consists in giving opportunities rather than prescription. There must be opportunities to work, opportunities to do and to plan and create, and to learn to use material" (p. 641). Similarly, LeVesconte (1935) alerted therapists to the importance of the greater social environment: "The only real measure of the success of any treatment is the condition of the patient after he [sic] has left the doors of the hospital, the physician or the therapist. . . . This problem is not only a medical problem, but equally a social and a community problem" (p. 14). LeVesconte (1935) recognized that successful occupational therapy required an understanding of the environment and stated, "The outpatient division frequently presents a complex problem, in which medicine is interwoven with sociology, economics and psychology" (p. 14). Dunton (1918), Meyer (1922/77), LeVesconte (1935) and Howland (1944) suggested that the key to successful *occupation* treatment may in fact lie within the greater context of the environment and the individual's adaptation to it.

Therapists have become increasingly knowledgeable of the impact of less favourable environments upon occupational performance (Wood, 1993; Yerxa et al., 1990), of the importance of occupation to mental health and well-being (Leete, 1989; MacGregor, 1995), and of the importance of the environment to successful community-based practice (Law, 1991). The professional literature reflects the importance of systemic considerations and of the interactive relationship between man and society (Gilfoyle, Grady, & Moore, 1990; Kielhofner, 1995; Law et al., 1996; Reilly, 1962; Schkade & Schultz, 1992). Kielhofner (1995) suggested that environments both afford and press the individual in occupation and that a better understanding of these aspects of the environment is needed to assist clients to realize their occupational potential.

The person-environment-occupation model (Law et al., 1996) proposes a transactional relationship between the individual, the occupation, and the environment. Law and colleagues (1996) suggest that the environment is not static, that it can have either an enabling or constraining effect on occupational performance, and that the environment is more amenable to change than the person. The Canadian Model of Occupational Performance (CAOT, 1997) addresses this dynamic interplay of people engaged in occupations within chosen or desired environments. This model suggests that change in the person, occupation, or environment will likely yield change in overall occupational performance. However, what is missing in these theoretical frameworks are those aspects of the environment that people perceive to be helpful or limiting in their search for meaningful and personally satisfying occupation.

There is mounting theoretical discourse in the literature about the importance of the environment to enabling occupation, and yet few specifics are offered to guide practice into the community. The present study sought to explore and to provide a better understanding of the experiences of people with a serious mental illness in their search for meaningful occupation within the community. A main objective of the study was to expand what is known about enabling environments and to describe what participants perceived as the major enablers/ constraints to their search of and participation in meaningful occupation within the community. The knowledge generated will hopefully assist mental health professionals to identify the constraining environments that exist in the community, to employ enabling strategies which assist people to increase their social participation in their community, and, ultimately, to encourage mental health professionals to create safe, social environments within which to enhance the occupational performance of people they work with.

METHODS

This study employed a qualitative research design, consisting of five interrelated and emergent phases. In Phase I, a survey questionnaire asking agencies to identify programs that addressed the occupational needs of their clients was sent to all service agencies mandated to provide mental health services for people with serious mental illness (SMI). In Phase II, the researcher conducted in-depth interviews with five persons, based upon the information gathered from the survey. In Phase III, the researcher engaged in participant observation for a period of 12 months, at a variety of community-based settings. The purposes of this phase were to access people not involved with formal agencies, to experience regular contact with participants, and to explore the daily lives and occupations engaged in by individuals with psychiatric disabilities who reside in the community. Field work consisted of accompanying and visiting with participants in coffee shops, at the city's drop-in centre, and at the local consumer/survivor organization. Field notes were initially written in condensed form and later expanded and transcribed as suggested by Spradley (1979). In Phase IV, four additional in-depth interviews were conducted based upon the data gathered in

the previous three phases. This second set of interviews attempted to draw upon analyses to this point and to integrate the similarities and differences obtained during the first three phases of the research. These interviews served to explore in greater depth what participants perceived to be either enabling or limiting of their participation in occupations of choice. In Phase V, a member-checking meeting was conducted at a participant-based organization. All study participants involved in the research, including those not interviewed but who contributed to insights gathered during the fieldwork, were invited to participate. According to Lincoln and Guba (1985), the member-checking task is "to obtain information that the report has captured the data as constructed by the informants, or to correct, amend, or extend it, that is, to establish the credibility of the case" (p. 236). In Phase V, the credibility of the research findings and the product of the analyses were confirmed by the participants. Twenty-five people participated in the study.

DATA ANALYSIS

The constant comparative method of data analysis (Glaser & Strauss, 1967) was utilized in the study. All audiotapes of the interviews were transcribed verbatim. The transcriptions, along with field notes and the reflexive journal, were separately reviewed by the researcher and coded using preliminary categories. Analysis was circular and iterative, with an ongoing review of the transcripts, categories, identification of properties of the categories, integration of categories, and identification of relationships until a central thesis or an explanatory theory began to emerge (Lincoln & Guba, 1985). The final analysis was reviewed by the participants and confirmed as credible in the member-checking meeting.

Limitations of the Research Design

As in all exploratory, qualitative studies with a small number of informants, the findings of this study are time-limited and context-bound.

The results are representative of the participants' life experiences, and of the Northeastern Ontario community within which they reside. The results cannot be generalized to other people with SMI, although the methods and product of this research would permit transferability of the study within another geographic area or setting.

RESULTS

The Labyrinth: Personal Problems or Social Issues?

The results of this study indicate that there are significant systemic barriers to the pursuit of meaningful occupation for people with a psychiatric disability. From the initial diagnosis and labeling processes which people with SMI undergo, to the broader social and economic policies which identify and target the individual as the problem, participants expended a great deal of personal resources in navigating a convoluted maze of social systems and bureaucracies in their daily occupations. The metaphor of a labyrinth is used to conceptualize their daily experiences within the community. A labyrinth is defined as "a structure containing winding passages hard to follow without losing one's way; a maze" (*Webster's New World Dictionary,* 1990, p. 330). Participants' physical, mental, emotional and financial resources were exhausted by this labyrinth, leaving them few resources to meet any needs beyond basic survival, including meaningful occupation. The labyrinth conceptually represents what the participants said regarding their individual pursuits for meaningful occupation within the community and was identified as the single most important barrier to one's pursuit of desired occupations. Thus the analysis of the labyrinth develops around two main themes: personal problems and social issues. These themes are further described by their respective conceptual categories (see Figure 1), the results of which are presented through a discussion of

these themes and categories. Quotations are used to illustrate the categories. All names are pseudonyms.

Managing Personal Problems

Running ahead of the wind. The theme "running ahead of the wind" is a native term which metaphorically describes the ongoing management of a psychiatric disability. The participants identified that living with a serious mental illness requires daily management. The management activities used by the participants to run ahead of the wind are related to managing the side-effects of medications and employing a variety of strategies for keeping the illness off.

The participants spoke about their ongoing management of medications and, in particular, their struggles in finding a good balance between controlling symptoms and living with the often stigmatizing side-effects of their medications. Ideally, participants hoped that medication compliance would lend itself to enhanced community participation. However, in reality, many found that the medications either made work a struggle: "I can't get up in the morning because I am too groggy" or participation in pre-determined programs difficult: "Even if I can get out bed, I can't concentrate because of my medications"; "My mind is racing and my mind wanders and I worry that I won't be able to keep up . . . it's easier to not go."

Participants also spoke of the stigmatizing side-effects of some of their medications and how this effects their self-confidence to participate socially within the community: "When I am downtown or in the coffee shop and people are staring at me . . . they don't know that I look this way because of the meds . . . they just think I'm crazy." Another participant spoke about the stigmatizing effects of medication with respect to community acceptance: "The side-effects of the medications make you lethargic and other people think you are lazy."

In summary, the participants spoke of their need to manage a balance between medications and other kinds of help in order to run ahead of

Figure 1
Conceptual Categories

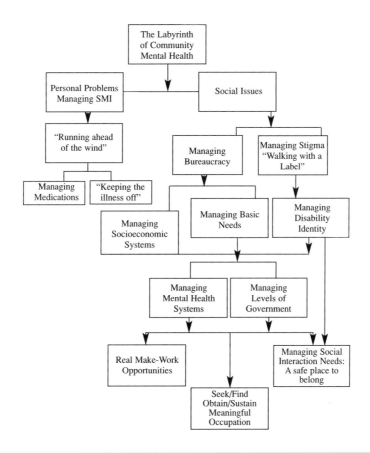

the wind. In the next section, the participants describe a variety of enabling strategies that they have discovered to help them to "keep the illness off."

Keeping the illness off. The second category, which illustrates the ongoing management of personal problems, has to do with strategies for keeping the illness off. Participants spoke of a variety of personal strategies that they have learned to keep themselves well. These strategies include keeping active and participating in real work; levelling of power hierarchies and using peers as role models; and being in a safe, social environment.

Keeping Active

Real work versus make work. Many of the participants spoke of the need to keep active in order to stay well. Jay, for example stated: "I'm a very busy person. I always keep active. This keeps the illness away from me." Similarly, Jim commented on the initial benefits of being involved in activity: "Unreal work is what you need to do to survive, because if I didn't go to the center and do those meaningless tasks, I wouldn't be able to survive."

While most participants described keeping busy as an important management strategy in keeping the illness off, many spoke of limited opportunity for meaningful involvement beyond the clubhouse and in the larger community. Ray stated, "When the consumer/survivor outgrows the IQ of the mental health system, boredom and dissatisfaction set in and there is no place for them to progress towards or to provide opportunities for personal growth." Similarly, Jim commented on the lack of meaningful challenges to progress to when the person is ready: "When you are ready to thrive, that's when the system fails you."

The participants clearly distinguished what they considered to be real work versus the variety of perceived make-work tasks available to them through the service sector. Participants also spoke of the limited benefits of make-work projects once they begin to get well: "Real work is not typing out something that has already been typed, or sorting flyers for Sears catalogues. Real work is important, and being involved in it makes me feel better about myself and it gives me hope for something better."

Leveling of Power Hierarchies

Even the lowest is made high. A second way to keep the illness off involves participation in environments that do not exercise a power differential. Many participants spoke of the existing power hierarchies within programs and services, and the importance of peer role models in the workplace. Jay, in discussing his involvement at the local peer organization, spoke of the environment being "like a family," and in which the active involvement of another peer helped him in *keeping the illness off:*

> She's my anchor. She keeps me stable because she's stable. . . . She's here everyday and does not miss days. It keeps the illness off . . . because these people are stable and they have illnesses too, and it really stabilizes me, the idea that I can accomplish this. I can do this. It's a structured work environment but it's not chained.

An important aspect of the environment is common ground and a levelling of power. All participants spoke of the hierarchies of the mental health system as barriers to their involvement and of the importance of peers to their recovery. Jim, for example, spoke of the importance of acceptance by the consumer/survivor community as a first step towards recovery:

> I don't think clinical help actually heals people with mental problems. It allows them to live and to get through really difficult times, but it doesn't actually help them. That healing actually occurs on the street, being sort of accepted by other people. Acceptance is very important. Acceptance by peers . . . it's the interaction with others, patients on the floor. That's where I found my way back out of the deepness of depression.

In peer-run organizations, this hierarchy is levelled and, according to Jay, is perceived to enable involvement in a variety of occupations: "We're all on common ground. So even at the highest levels, even the lowest person that comes in here is made high . . . I can be involved in the newsletter and I don't have to go through so and so to do this."

In contrast, Jim spoke of the hierarchy at the local clubhouse and the perceived power differential between the paid staff members and his peers. A fraternization policy that precludes socialization with consumer/survivors after official hours serves to remind consumer/survivors that "we are not worthy of being involved with 'normals'" and, "I am always reminded of my place in society when the people who are paid to help me do not acknowledge me on the streets." Similarly, Bill spoke of the organization of psychiatry and how the power struggles between him and his psychiatrist have contributed to an inability to make decisions for himself, and how, over the years, they have eroded his sense of self-confidence to pursue and participate in occupation.

A Safe Environment in Which To Work

The last management strategy for keeping the illness off involved finding a safe place in which to gain work skills and to develop self-confidence. Participants perceived there to be a lack of such safe environments within their community. Here, Jim discusses his need for a safe place in order to build his confidence:

> Having a safe place to go is very important to me. I don't have the confidence right now to work in the real world, but that doesn't mean I can't contribute. The way it is right now, it's either I am working and go off disability or I remain disabled. Great choices, eh? I've been thinking what we need is a safe place in the area where mental health survivors can go and do real work and get paid real wages and as a result for them doing this, they won't be disqualified for being on a pension. But they do real work because there are so many things that we can do if given the opportunity.

Managing Social Issues

While most participants acknowledged a certain amount of time dedicated to the management of personal problems, all of the participants in the study spoke of the huge amount of time they devoted to management of the system that is intended to help them. The management activities varied amongst the participants. However, all participants identified a significant amount of time and energy devoted to figuring out and navigating a maze or labyrinth of systems. The levels of bureaucracy, hierarchies, and systems, that required their ongoing management were numerous. People spoke of being caught up in a maze, of the system keeping them in a state of dependency, of giving up, getting lost, and of having few personal resources for pursuing meaningful occupation beyond this management activity. The system, they said, was exhausting their resources, and "hope [for the future] was not a option."

Managing Basic Needs

All but one of the 25 participants in this study were on some form of social assistance. Most participants lived well below the poverty line. All participants spoke of their struggles in managing the basic needs of life. These needs included housing, transportation food/nutrition, clothing, and spending money. To further complicate their navigation of the labyrinth, most participants relied upon and were required to manage more than one source of income support. These forms of support bridged three levels of government, and ranged between a variety of different ministries within government. Most participants frequented the Catholic Mission/Soup Kitchen, the Salvation Army, and a variety of food banks. Most participants were required to fill out a plethora of forms, and were required to navigate between social services workers, brokerage agencies, and the various levels of government in order to obtain the simplest of necessities of life. In all cases, the participant's pursuit of meaningful occupation was constrained by transportation problems. In all cases, the labyrinth of systems dedicated to the management of basic needs was perceived to be exhausting, and to be a significant limitation to their pursuit of and participation in desired occupations.

Managing Mental Health Systems

Participants described navigating a closed maze of mental health services, agencies, and programs within their community. This maze of services was comprised of five local mental health service agencies. Participants described existing and functioning largely within this maze of services and rarely venturing beyond this labyrinth. Further, the participants did not perceive that the system supported meaningful occupation as an important outcome for people with psychiatric disability. Their perceptions were supported by the limited occupation-based programs/services within the community and a lack of human and fiscal resources dedicated to the occupational needs of people with psychiatric disability (see Table 1).

Unsurprisingly, few of the participants spoke of the formal mental health system in positive terms. Instead, they spoke of the difficulties of access to programs and the lack of meaningful things to do within the formal mental health

Table I
Survey Results

Mental Health Agency* Survey Question	1	2	3	4	5
Focus of clinic/ program	Case management Counseling Medication support	Advocacy Self-help support	Education	Social recreation Temporary employment program (TEP) Work stations PSR	Housing ADL's Case management and support
Hours of operation	8:30–4:30	8:30–4:30 Some evenings	8:30–4:30	8:30–4:30 Some weekends/ evenings	8:30–4:30 Some weekends
Staff dedicated to occupational needs	0	.5	0	1.0	0
Total clinical staff complement	5	2.5	2.5	5.0	2.4

*Agency Explanation
1. Community Mental Health Clinic
2. Consumer Survivor Agency
3. Canadian Mental Health Association
4. Local Psychosocial Rehabilitation Clubhouse
5. Housing Agency
6. Outpatient Psychiatry Clinic: Did not respond
7. Community Mental Health Clinic-2:   Did not respond

service sector. Many participants spoke of restrictive hours of operation, which they perceived met the needs of the mental health professionals, and less so, their needs and routines for managing a psychiatric disability. Most spoke of limited relationships with their psychiatrists and other mental health professionals, of an almost exclusive focus upon medications, and a lack of acknowledgement of consumer survivor needs. Jay illustrates:

They're behind a desk and behind a chained-up wall where I have to kneel to speak to them through a little tiny breath hole. I feel with my doctor that we're in a concert and I'm in the very last row and my doctor's sitting way up at the front and I'm at the way back and there are a thousand people in front of me. "Doctor, I'm seeing spirits and I'm hearing voices" and uh, "No, no, no are you taking your medication today?" I've been on medications for 5 years now and I'm still hearing voices since the very first day I got this illness and I'm even worse off than I started with because I'm experiencing anxiety attacks and severe sorrow. My doctor is doing a lecture in front of me and he's not talking to my heart. He's not talking to me. We need compassion to fight despair, to understand in depth, we need empathy and that's where the service sector doesn't help . . . it doesn't have empathy . . . without charity you have nothing.

Similarly, Jim commented on the lack of assistance given by the formal mental health system in helping people to become employed:

A lot of people won't take the time to find out that people with mental problems are actually capable of doing things, but we are constantly reminded of what we can't do because of our disability.

Managing Disability Identity: The Stigma of Walking With a Label

Participants spoke at lengths about having a diagnostic label that implies chronic disability and how this contributes to a self-fulfilling prophecy for some consumer/survivors. Blaine spoke of the absence of viable peer role models in the initial stages of recovery as a contributing factor to this prophecy:

Once they've listed you as disabled, it means you are incapable of doing anything beyond drinking a coffee or smoking a cigarette. You are told that you are disabled, but nobody tells you what that means out of the hospital. Nobody tells you that you can do things and make a contribution in a different way than paid work. You need a consumer right there at the hospital so that you can say, don't worry, being disabled isn't what you think. I can tell you where to go and people who can help you get to where you want to be.

Most of the participants spoke of the disabling effects of "walking with a label" with respect to their level of self-confidence to participate in the larger community, and in how they are perceived by "normals" in society. Jay, for example stated:

My life is hidden. I'm very scared and hidden. I don't go around telling everybody I have a mental illness until I know them. . . . It really turns people off.

Bill discussed how the system's labelling of him over the years has done little to help him move beyond his disability identity:

The psychiatric system has got me labelled. It's got me defined. It's got me as scientifically categorized into something that is sick in this culture . . . you know, cuz I'm "schizophrenic." You know the mere meaning of the word is that your mind is no longer functioning properly. With that label, walking around with that label, how

am I supposed to keep my head up in society? The psychiatric system has created me and now doesn't know what to do with me.

Participants' insight about the stigma of walking with a label required them to expend further resources in stigma management (Goffman, 1963) within the community. Jay spoke of a need to control for psychiatric identity when pursuing occupation within the community environment:

I'm stuck in the stigma track. I'm stuck in that, so I think they're normal and I'm different and I'm wrong. I'm a misfit in society. They want glass and I'm plastic. I'm different. I'm a broken glass to them. I'm not good, I'm not normal. I'm broken glass and I can't function. I can't hold water in normal society. I can't get a job anywhere. I'm not taken serious, unless it's like I don't tell them about my illness.

Similarly, Bill spoke of the stigma of living with a label and how this has contributed to ongoing difficulties connecting with the community:

It's stigmatizing. Because of the stigma, it takes away your self-esteem or you assume stigma and you take it on after a while. I find there's nothing in the community for me . . . and I don't have the confidence to look beyond where I am now.

Managing Occupational Needs

Three of the participants in this study, Jay, Bill, and Blaine, were able to meet their occupational needs through work obtained through the local consumer/survivor organization. Unfortunately, for all three, the social and physical environment within this organization underwent significant changes since their interviews and they are no longer participating in desired occupations.

Most participants of this study remain stuck somewhere in the labyrinth of community mental health services, mostly at the level(s) of managing basic needs and managing mental health systems. Most participants were still in the process of seeking meaningful occupation at the conclusion of this study or, unfortunately, had given up hope for something better.

For many of the participants, their pursuit of meaningful occupation remains constrained by a lack of "real work" opportunities for them within their community, a lack of safe environments within which to gain confidence, and by the ongoing risk of compromising their basic needs in hopes of a better quality of life. The perceived risk to "jump off of disability" is a significant one for people who already have to struggle to meet basic needs. Rita, for example, spoke at lengths about her fears of resuming paid work:

> I don't think I will ever go back to paid work, to a paid position. I think that's unrealistic. I don't think that because of my condition. I just don't see it as possible. I don't want to work for a few months and then have to lay off work, reapply for CPP benefits, wait for up to 4 months for them to make up their mind and what do you do then type of thing?

It becomes obvious that until there are significant changes to public policy governing the capacity for work of people with a mental illness disability, and greater attention to the provision of safe environments within which to gain confidence to resume the worker role, many consumer/survivors will be forced to uphold and defend their "disability identity" and to continue to wander within the labyrinth of community mental health services.

DISCUSSION

Strategies for Change

The findings of this study suggest that significant changes are required in both policy and practice in order to enable meaningful occupation for people with SMI. Although the results are reflective of the experiences and insights of the 25 people who reside within a small geographic region, the results are strikingly similar to those of Corring (1996) and Nagel (1997).

Similarly, the findings support Mill's (1959) idea of addressing social milieu to enact real change, and Yerxa's (1998) prophecy that "the post-industrial society is in danger of creating masses of throw-away people, a burgeoning underclass whose chronic impairments, mental illness, and inadequate education and skills leave them outsiders in an increasingly technical, complex, and fast-paced society" (p. 413). The participants in this study identified several means by which professionals who work in community mental health can enable greater social participation in meaningful occupation for their clients and thus, potentially avert "creating masses of throw-away people."

Occupation as a Means to Mental Health and Well-Being

The relationship between work and mental health is well established, and yet Anthony and colleagues (Anthony, Cohen, & Farkas, 1990) cite an employment rate of less than 20% for psychiatric clients. Clark (1995) argues that clinicians must become active in alleviating unemployment for people with psychiatric disability because "in a society where paid work has tremendous symbolic significance, exclusion from the job market adds to the stress of poverty the strain of social isolation" (p. 397). Similarly, a recent publication on the economic initiatives of psychiatric survivors within Ontario identifies that many doors have been closed to the full participation of consumer/survivors as citizens and many opportunities lost in terms of employment, housing, training, and education (Church, 1997). Their marginalization in these crucial areas means the psychiatric survivors as a group are generally poor, unemployed, and inadequately housed (Ontario Council of Alternative Businesses [OCAB], 1995). Rogers (1998) argues that to work or not to work is not the question, but, rather, why systems continue to deny psychiatric survivors the opportunity to participate in paid or volunteer occupations with the growing evidence of its health benefits.

Flexibility of Policy to Meet Individual Needs Versus Label Needs

Current social and disability policy affords people with a disability "permission" to not work. People with a psychiatric illness who aspire to participate in flexible, part-time occupations on a paid or voluntary basis potentially risk losing their basic economic support. Disability, as a construct used to assess levels of social assistance, requires reconceptualization to recognize varying levels of ability. Unfortunately, the result of present policy is that people are forced into a position of either doing nothing or covertly participating in occupation. These findings are not dissimilar to those of Estroff (1981), who nearly two decades ago observed that people with serious mental illness are forced to "make it crazy" in order to sustain the basic necessities of life. A lack of reconciliation at the policy level will continue to maintain a personal problems approach to care and resource allocation, and will no doubt sustain "masses of throw-away people" (Yerxa, 1998) within our communities.

Bridging Personal and Social Issues

Recognition that personal problems cannot be the sole limiting factor in any rehabilitative process will enable service providers to look beyond the individual in both policy and program development. Jongbloed and Crichton (1990) advocate for rehabilitation professionals to abandon their largely clinical or individualistic ideology and to focus instead upon improving the circumstances of people with a disability through changes or amendments to laws and social policies. Likewise, Anthony and Liberman (1986) suggest that "society fails to provide social environments to compensate for disability and impairment . . . [and this] is reflective in high rates of homelessness and unemployment" (p. 548). Attention to the extensive social issues and barriers will require a shift in policy direction, resource allocation, and the focus of professional intervention.

Anthony and Liberman (1986) state: "Obstacles in overcoming a handicap may be more a function of a non-accommodating and discriminating social and economic system than the person's impairment and disability" (p. 553).

Simplification of the Labyrinth

The labyrinth of community mental health services requires simplification so that individual resources can be directed more towards personal growth, well-being, and quality of life, and less to the problems of mere existence and management of the systems that are intended to help consumer/survivors. According to Renwick and Brown (1996), "The nature of the interaction between the person and the environment and the ongoing outcomes of this interaction are the basis for an individual's perceptions about their quality of life" (p. 77). It is not unreasonable to assume that if an individual's resources are being fully tapped in the daily management of basic needs and of the labyrinth, few resources will remain for enhancing quality of life.

In general, the labyrinth continues to exist because of a continual emphasis on personal problems; consequently, goals for the future and recovery become ignored because of the ongoing management of basic needs and services. Essentially, a lack of cohesive, holistic policy that addresses participants' basic needs is dearly required to alleviate their struggle for survival and thus reduce the instance of discouraging, maze-like journeys into the labyrinth of mental health services.

Provision of Safe and Supportive Environments

Finally, greater attention needs to be given to the creation of affirming and accepting social environments in which there are opportunities for meaningful social participation, for being successful, and for the reduction of stigma. According to Yerxa (1998, p. 417, "Both theory and research demonstrate that an environment that provides opportunities for active engagement in life contributes to health, well-being, independence, and survival." According to Pilisuk (1982), "social support may be one of the critical factors distinguishing those who remain healthy from those who fall ill" (p. 20).

Enabling participation in occupations of choice and need will require the cooperation of all levels of government, across many levels of bureaucracy, and between services, disciplines and consumer/survivors. More effective coordination between service agencies is required to simplify bureaucracy for people with SMI, and funding is required to create safe environments conducive to social participation in occupations of choice and of need. To begin to address such issues will require a stronger political voice by all concerned.

CONCLUSIONS

The study highlighted a mental health system dedicated to the personal problems of people with psychiatric disability. But it also described the extensive social issues that require daily management by people with SMI and that, in their opinion, receive little attention or funding by the formal mental health system in Ontario. The study results support the theoretical literature, which cites the importance of considering the larger environment in enabling occupation for people with a disability (CAOT, 1997; Kielhofner, 1995). Further, these findings support Anthony and Liberman's (1986) assertion that society must pay greater attention to the provision of social environments that compensate for disability. There is every indication to believe that the present labyrinth of services will continue because it is structured to offer diverse services from a variety of agencies and levels of government—all designed to deal with "personal troubles of milieu" (Mills, 1959). Further, there has been little advancement in public or clinical policy, which could assist people to find their way out of the labyrinth into the larger community and towards enhanced quality of life. It appears that a continued focus on the person as being the problem will not only allow the

system to ignore the social needs of this population within the community, but also will continue to submerge any hopes for meaningful occupations for many capable people. Unfortunately, the present system is geared to foster "masses of throw-away people" (Yerxa, 1998), who clearly perceive this as their identity and appear to be fulfilling this prophesy, in part, supported by the systems designed to help them. The resultant, untapped potential of many people will be the ultimate loss for society.

The implications for mental health professionals are explicit and clearly support the need for all clinicians to consider the context or macro-environment of the community in greater depth, and well beyond the limitations imposed by a "personal problems" approach to care. If mental health professionals continue to address or view only the issues of personal problems of the individual without regard for the many social issues, we are all going to be stuck in the labyrinth and be limited in what we can do to help people.

ACKNOWLEDGMENT

I would like to acknowledge the 25 participants of this study for their honesty and insight. I would also like to thank Dr. J. V. Cook for her editorial assistance, and her academic and moral support.

References

Anthony, W. A., Cohen, M., & Farkas, M. (1990). *Psychiatric rehabilitation.* Boston: Center for Psychiatric Rehabilitation.

Anthony, W. A., & Liberman, R. W. (1986). The practice of psychiatric rehabilitation: Historical, conceptual, and research base. *Schizophrenia Bulletin, 12*(4), 542–559.

Canadian Association of Occupational Therapists (CAOT) (1997). *Enabling occupation: A Canadian occupational therapy perspective.* Ottawa: CAOT Publications ACE.

Church, K. (1997). *Using the economy to develop the community: Psychiatric survivors in Ontario.* Ottawa: Caledon Institute of Social Policy Publications.

Clark, R. E. (1995). Creating work opportunities for people with severe mental illness (Response to "The economic advancement of the mentally ill in the community"). *Community Mental Health Journal, 31*(4), 307–401.

Corring, D. (1996). *Client-centred care means I am a valued human being.* Unpublished master's thesis. The University of Western Ontario, London, Ontario, Canada.

Dunton, W. R. (1918). *Occupation therapy: A manual for nurses.* Philadelphia: W. B. Saunders Company.

Estroff, S. E. (1981). *Making it crazy: An ethnography of psychiatric clients in an American community.* Los Angeles: University of California Press.

Gilfoyle, E., Grady, A., & Moore, J. (1990). *Children adapt* (2nd ed.). Thorofare, NJ: Slack.

Glaser, B. G. & Strauss, A. L. (1967). *The discovery of grounded theory.* Chicago: Aldine.

Goffman, E. (1963). *Stigma: Notes on the management of spoiled identity.* New York: Simon & Schuster Inc.

Grady, A. (1995). Building inclusive community: A challenge for occupational therapy. *The American Journal of Occupational Therapy, 49,* 300–310.

Howland, G. W. (1944). Occupational therapy across Canada. *Canadian Geographical Journal, 28*(1), 32–40. Reprinted (1986) in *Canadian Journal of Occupational Therapy, 53,* 18–26.

Jongbloed, L., & Crichton, A. (1990). A new definition of disability: Implications for rehabilitation practice and social policy. *Canadian Journal of Occupation Therapy, 57*(1), 32–38.

Kielhofner, G. (1995). *A model of human occupation: Theory and application* (2nd ed.). Baltimore: Williams & Wilkins.

Law, M. (1991). The environment: A focus for occupational therapy. *Canadian Journal of Occupational Therapy, 58,* 171–179.

Law, M., Cooper, B., Strong, S., Rigby, P., & Letts, L. (1996). The person-environment-occupation model: A transactive approach to occupational performance. *The Canadian Journal of Occupational Therapy, 63,* 9–23.

Leete, E. (1989). How I perceive and manage my illness. *Schizophrenia Bulletin, 15,* 197–200.

LeVesconte, H. P. (1935). Expanding fields of occupational therapy. *Canadian Journal of Occupational Therapy, 3,* 4–12.

Lincoln, Y., & Guba, E. (1985). *Naturalistic inquiry.* Beverly Hills: Sage Publications.

MacGregor, L. (1995). *An exploratory study of the personal experience of occupational deprivation.* Unpublished master's thesis. The University of Western Ontario, London, ON.

Menzel, M. (1947). Methods and techniques used in occupational therapy for the imbecile. *The American Journal of Occupational Therapy, 1,* 137–145.

Meyer, A. (1922). The philosophy of occupation therapy. *Archives of Occupational Therapy, 1,* 1–10. Reprinted (1977) in *The American Journal of Occupational Therapy, 31,* 639–642.

Mills, C. W. (1959). *The sociological imagination.* New York: Grove Press, Inc.

Nagle, S. (1997). *I'm doing as much as I can: Pathways to occupational choice.* Unpublished master's thesis. The University of Western Ontario, London, ON.

Ontario Council of Alternative Business (OCAB). (1995). *Yes we can! Promote economic opportunity and choice through community business.* Toronto, ON.

Pilisuk, M. (1982). Delivery of social support: The social inoculation. *American Journal of Orthopsychiatry, 52*(1), 20–31.

Rebeiro, K. L. (1997). *Opportunity, not prescription: An exploratory study of the experience of occupational engagement.* Unpublished master's thesis. The University of Western Ontario, London, ON.

Reilly, M. (1962). Occupational therapy can be one of the great ideas of 20th century medicine. *The American Journal of Occupational Therapy, 16,* 1–9.

Renwick, R., & Brown, I. (1996). The centre for health promotion's conceptual approach to quality of life. In R. Renwick, I. Brown & M. Nager (Eds.). *Quality of Life in health promotion and rehabilitation: Conceptual approaches, issues and applications,* pp. 75–86. Thousand Oaks, CA: Sage Publications.

Rogers, S. (1998). To work or not to work: That is not the question. *Journal of Psychosocial Nursing, 36*(4), 42–48.

Schkade, J. K., & Schultz, S. (1992). Occupational adaption: Toward a holistic approach for contemporary practice, part 1. *The American Journal of Occupational Therapy, 46,* 829–837.

Slagle, E. C. (1928). Handicrafts used as treatment: the handicrafter. *Archives of Occupational Therapy, 1,* 26–27.

Spradley, J. P. (1979). *The ethnographic interview.* Orlando, FL: Harcourt Brace Jovanovich College Publishers.

Trombly, C. (1995). Occupation: Purposefulness and meaningfulness as therapeutic mechanisms. *The American Journal of Occupational Therapy, 49,* 960–972.

Webster's New World Dictionary. (1990). V. Neufeldt (Ed.). New York: Simon & Schuster, Inc.

Wood, W. (1993). Occupation and the relevance of primatology to occupational therapy. *The American Journal of Occupational Therapy, 47,* 515–522.

Wood, W. (1998. Nationally speaking—Is it jump time for occupational therapy. *American Journal of Occupational Therapy, 52*(6), 403–411.

Yerxa, E. J. (1998). Health and the human spirit for occupation. *American Journal of Occupational Therapy, 52*(6), pp. 412–418.

Yerxa, E. J., Clark, F., Frank, G., Jackson, J., Parham, D., Pierce, D., Stein, C., & Zemke, R. (1990). An introduction to occupational science: A foundation for occupational therapy in the 21st century. In J. A. Johnson & E. J. Yerxa, (Eds.), *Occupational science: The foundation for new models of practice* (pp. 1–17). New York: The Haworth Press.

Chapter 22

Exploration of the Perspectives of Persons with Schizophrenia Regarding Quality of Life

The Journal of Occupational Therapy
2000, 54(2): 137–147

Deborah Laliberte-Rudman, Betty Yu, Elizabeth Scott, Parnian Pajouhandeh

Deborah Laliberte-Rudman, MSc(OT), BSc(OT), is Lecturer, Department of Occupational Therapy, University of Toronto, 256 McCaul Street, Toronto, Ontario, M5T 1W5 Canada, and Doctoral Candidate, Graduate Department of Community Health, Department of Public Health Sciences, University of Toronto; debbie.rudman@utoronto.ca.
Betty Yu, Hon BSc, BSc(OT), is Clinical Occupational Therapist, Community Occupational Therapists and Associates, Toronto, Ontario, Canada.
Elizabeth Scott, MSc, BSc(OT), is Administrative Director, Society, Women and Health Program, Centre for Addiction and Mental Health, and Assistant Professor, Department of Occupational Therapy, University of Toronto, Toronto, Ontario, Canada.
Parnian Pajouhandeh, BSc, is Researcher, Centre for Addiction and Mental Health, Clarke Division, and Master's Student, Ontario Institute for Studies in Education, University of Toronto, Toronto, Ontario, Canada.

KEY WORDS

- human activities and occupations
- mental health
- qualitative method

ABSTRACT

Objective. *This study is the first phase of a two-phase study aimed at exploring the perspectives of consumers with schizophrenia regarding quality of life and developing a quality-of-life assessment that addresses factors experienced as important by consumers.*

Method. *Focus groups were used to explore the perspectives of 35 persons with schizophrenia regarding the meaning of quality of life and factors important to quality of life.*

Results. *Seven major factors that had an impact on quality of life resulted from inductive analysis, including activity, social interaction, time, disclosure, "being normal," finances, and management of illness. These factors relate to three overall themes: managing time, connecting and belonging, and making choices and maintaining control.*

Conclusions. *Although the findings confirm the importance of factors included in existing quality-of-life assessments, they also highlight the need to look at new dimensions of commonly included factors and to include other factors. The findings support beliefs regarding occupation that are central to occupational therapy and the use of occupation as means and ends of therapy.*

The disorders of thought, emotion, and psychomotor behavior associated with schizophrenia have the potential to affect all areas of occupational performance. For example, attention deficits and impaired ability to process information can lead to difficulties in work, self-care, and leisure (Brown, Harwood, Hays, Heckman, & Short, 1993; Creegan & Williams, 1997; Evans & Salim, 1992; So, Toglia, & Donohue, 1997). Several occupational therapy models propose that difficulties in occupational performance, such as those experienced by persons with schizophrenia, can have a negative impact on quality of life (Baum & Christiansen, 1997; Canadian Association of Occupational Therapists [CAOT], 1997). A number of surveys have found that persons with mental illnesses experience difficulties in a broad range of occupations and tend to report lower life satisfaction than those without such illnesses (Kirsh, 1996; Lehman, Rachuba, & Postrado, 1995; Ontario Ministry of Health, 1990; Simmons, 1994).

Realization of the potential broad impact of major mental illnesses on various areas of life has led to a recognition of the need for comprehensive mental health services that provide assistance in several life areas (Evans & Salim, 1992; Lehman, 1988). As services have become more comprehensive and the emphasis on cost-effectiveness has increased, it has become essential for program planning and evaluation efforts to go beyond traditional measures of clinical status, such as symptom severity or readmission rate, and attend to multidimensional variables, such as functional ability and quality of life (Atkinson, Coia, Gilmour, & Harper, 1996; Atkinson, Zibin, & Chuang, 1997; Sainfort, Becker, & Diamond, 1996). Baker and Intagliata (1982) and Simmons (1994) highlighted several other reasons for focusing on quality of life in the planning and evaluation of services for persons with mental illness. These reasons include the importance of maintaining and enhancing quality of life in situations in which illnesses cannot be cured and the rise of consumerism with a concomitant demand for services that significantly affect consumers' lives.

Quality of life is an outcome that has long been of concern to occupational therapists. The link between occupation and quality of life is one of the basic beliefs guiding the practice of occupational therapy (Wilcock, 1993; Yerxa, 1994). Indeed, numerous authors describe the central objective of occupational therapy as promoting health and quality of life through enabling occupation (CAOT, 1994; Polatajko, 1994; Yerxa, 1994). The importance of quality of life was emphasized by Yerxa et al. (1990), who stated that "medicine is concerned with preserving life; occupational therapy is concerned with the quality of life preserved" (p. 8). With specific reference to clients with chronic mental illnesses, Hachey and Mercier (1993) described the role of occupational therapy in community psychiatry as that of working with a multidisciplinary team to offer clients the necessary conditions for quality of life.

Even though the term *quality of life* first appeared in research literature in the 1930s and is prominent in recent literature, the questions of what quality of life is, how it can be enhanced, and how it can be measured cannot be easily answered because there are many competing perspectives (Raphael, 1997; Till, 1994). Although much of the work in the area of quality of life and mental illness has focused on clients with schizophrenia (Awad, 1992, 1995; Lehman, 1983, 1988), there is no consensus regarding how to best conceptualize or measure quality of life with this specific population (Atkinson & Zibin, 1996). A frequently noted weakness of existing assessments for clients with schizophrenia is that these assessments lack a guiding conceptual framework of quality of life (Simmons, 1994). However, despite the lack of consensus regarding conceptualization, measures developed for persons with mental illness—such as the Quality of Life Interview (Lehman, 1983, 1988), the Quality of Life Questionnaire and Interview (Bigelow, Gareau, & Young, 1990; Bigelow, McFarland, & Olson, 1991), and the Quality of Life Profile (Oliver,

1992)—often tap similar domains. These domains include health status, psychiatric symptoms, finances, living situation, social relations, leisure, productivity, education, and general well-being (Atkinson & Zibin, 1996; Simmons, 1994).

Another common limitation within this area of mental health research is that the definition of quality of life and its domains has largely been based on researchers' perspectives, and there has been little input from clients (Simmons, 1994). Little is known about clients' values and preferences regarding what domains or factors are important for quality of life and how these factors are experienced as affecting quality of life. The ways in which researchers and clinicians define quality of life and the factors they perceive to be important contributors may be different from clients' perspectives (Clark, Scott, & Krupa, 1993; Lord, 1989). With specific reference to quality of life and clients with severe mental illnesses, Sainfort et al. (1996) described two potential types of discordance between clinicians' and clients' views. First, clinicians and clients may disagree on the importance of specific domains, such as work or education, in terms of their contribution to quality of life. Second, clinicians and clients may have different reference systems in judging satisfaction and performance within such domains. In a study conducted with 37 clients with schizophrenia and their primary clinicians, Sainfort et al. found that although clients and clinicians provided similar ratings of satisfaction with respect to symptoms and function, there was little agreement in terms of social relations and occupational aspects of quality of life.

Due to the potential discrepancies among the perspectives of researchers, clinicians, and clients, exploring clients' perspectives is increasingly being recognized as an important research endeavor, both as a way to further the understanding of issues important to clients and as an initial step in the development of assessments (Bauman & Adair, 1992; Clark, et al., 1993). There is an emerging consensus that clients' values and preferences need to be addressed in treatment planning and evaluation to ensure that services are not biased toward the perspective of service providers and are optimally relevant to clients' lives (Atkinson & Zibin, 1996; Nelson & Niederberger, 1990). Thus, the use of existing quality-of-life assessments that have not incorporated the perspective of clients may mean that treatment and outcome evaluations become focused on factors that clients neither experience nor define as key to their quality of life (Sainfort et al., 1996).

A *client-centered approach* can be defined as "an approach to occupational therapy which embraces a philosophy of, respect for, and partnership with, people receiving services" (Law, Baptiste, & Mills, 1995, p. 253). To most effectively use this approach in occupational therapy, practitioners need to understand how clients perceive their lives and need to develop assessments that capture the realities experienced by clients. This article describes the first phase of a two-phase research project aimed at developing a quality-of-life assessment that is based on the perspectives of clients with schizophrenia. In this first phase, focus groups were used to explore the perspectives of 35 persons with schizophrenia regarding the meaning of quality of life and factors important to their quality of life. The information gathered has implications for quality-of-life assessment, the occupational therapy knowledge base, and the planning of occupational therapy services.

METHOD

Research Design

Qualitative research techniques are designed to facilitate exploration of the meaning that informants attach to phenomena (Marshall & Rossman, 1989; Strauss & Corbin, 1990); therefore, we used a qualitative research approach involving semistructured focus group discussions. In conducting qualitative research, it is important to attend to the issue of trustworthiness, which is the extent to which the findings of a study can be viewed as worthy of confidence

(Krefting, 1991). Lincoln and Guba (1985) based trustworthiness on the criteria of credibility, transferability, dependability, and confirmability. The issue of credibility was addressed in this study through the use of open-ended questions designed to prompt informants to openly discuss their perspectives. Additionally, a process of peer examination of the analysis process and findings was used to maximize credibility, dependability, and confirmability. Descriptive information regarding informants allows for the reader's evaluation of transferability.

Informants

Informants were obtained using convenience sampling from persons receiving outpatient services at two urban mental health facilities. Screening interviews were conducted with 52 potential informants to collect descriptive data and determine fit with inclusion criteria, which were (a) meeting DSM-IV (*Diagnostic and Statistical Manual of Mental Disorders* [4th ed.]; American Psychiatric Association, 1994) diagnostic criteria for diagnosis of schizophrenia, (b) being between the ages of 18 and 65 years, (c) having the ability to provide informed consent, (d) currently residing in the community, and (e) having sufficient English language skills to participate in a group discussion. Forty-seven of the 52 persons screened met all inclusion criteria and were invited to participate in the study. Of these 47 potential informants invited to participate in the study, 35 both agreed to participate and attended a focus group. Three of the 47 potential informants declined to participate, and 9 who agreed to participate did not attend a focus group. Written consent was obtained from all informants.

The principle of maximum variation suggests that a range of descriptive characteristics is desirable to maximize the transferability of findings (Lincoln & Guba, 1985). Of the 35 informants, 25 were men (71.4%), and 10 were women (28.6%). The ages of the informants ranged from 22 to 63 years ($M = 40.3$ years). Twenty-six informants were single (74.3%),

5 were in a marital or common-law relationship (14.3%), and 4 were separated or divorced (11.4%). Educational levels ranged from completion of some elementary school to completion of university, with 77.1% ($n = 27$) of the sample having at least a high school degree. Employment status included part-time worker ($n = 5$), full-time student ($n = 2$), part-time student ($n = 3$), retired ($n = 4$), and unemployed ($n = 21$). Living arrangements included living with others in a private place ($n = 17$), alone in a private place ($n = 8$), supportive housing ($n = 9$), and hostel or emergency housing ($n = 1$). Self-ratings of current health varied from fair to excellent, with fair health being the most commonly selected rating (48.6%).

Information Gathering

All information, except demographic data, was collected in focus groups. On the basis of the methodological suggestions of several authors (Krueger, 1994; Merton, 1990; Patton, 1990), each focus group consisted of at least 8 informants and no more than 12 informants. Specifically, the 35 informants attended one of four groups, each consisting of 8 to 11 informants. A consumer facilitator and a nonconsumer facilitator, both of whom had previous experience leading focus groups, conducted the groups, each of which lasted for approximately 2 hr. Notes were taken by a co-investigator, and all focus groups were audiotaped and transcribed verbatim.

The study investigators developed a semistructured interview guide for the focus groups that consisted of open-ended questions. Main topics included the following:

- What are the things that make life good for you?
- What are the things that make life not so good for you?
- What does *quality of life* mean to you?
- Do you think that quality of life should be looked at differently for people who

have been diagnosed with schizophrenia than for other people?

Questions addressing these main topics were used to frame the focus group discussions and were presented in the same order in each group conducted.

Analysis of the Information

Focus group transcripts were analyzed using the constant comparative method to identify themes relating to quality of life (Strauss & Corbin, 1990). In this analysis process, the transcribed text is broken down into units of information that are then combined into categories. The categories, in turn, are grouped together to highlight major factors and issues (Lincoln & Guba, 1985). The results of this analysis process were then combined into larger themes through a process of theorizing, which involved examining the relationships between factors (Morse & Field, 1995).

Analysis was completed by two of the investigators who engaged in a circular process involving several readings of all transcripts. One of the investigators completed a line-by-line analysis of the transcripts aimed at identifying units of information. After these units of information were reviewed by the second investigator, the two investigators worked together to combine the units into categories, factors, and larger themes. This process involved analyzing the units of information separately and then coming together to discuss hypotheses and ideas for categories, factors, and larger themes.

INFORMANTS' PERSPECTIVES

In addition to understandings regarding how informants defined quality of life, seven major factors pertinent to quality of life emerged. These major factors included activity, social interaction, time, "being normal," disclosure, finances, and management of illness. Examination of the relationships among these factors resulted in three major themes: managing time,

connecting and belonging, and making choices and maintaining control. The following interpretative analysis is illustrated by quotations from the informants, each of whom has been assigned an identification number. Ellipsis points are used to indicate when part of a quote has been removed.

Definition of Quality of Life

Varied responses were received to the question, "What does quality of life mean to you?" Informant 10 replied, "Freedom of being alive; saying hello to people; having a girlfriend or getting married in the future . . . it is an ongoing thing," and Informant 3 stated:

> To have people that give you respect and dignity, recognize you have a disability, that you are not useless, you can still contribute whatever you can to society . . . people survive with friends . . . have a job, have a family or just have a nice place.

Informant 5 described quality of life as being able to "find joy in simple things, like nature or like appreciate things, like you watch a program you appreciate it, you understand it to your fullest ability." Another informant asserted: "For me, it's to have a quality of life that's good enough to keep the stress and the weight off the illness . . . and to eventually someday to support myself, not to have to rely on FBA [family benefits allowance]." Overall, informants' definitions tended to include both subjective aspects (i.e., feelings of freedom) and objective aspects (i.e., having a job).

Managing Time

A common concern expressed by informants was related to the issue of using time well. As Informant 25 stated, "Because we have lots of time on our hands, and the thing is that you want to develop and use that time wisely and not foolishly and squander it . . . the thing is you want to make use of it as best you can." Being able to manage time, in terms of both the present and the future, appeared to be a challenge for informants, and, in turn, dealing with this challenge appeared important to quality of life.

Activity emerged as the major means used by informants to manage time. Informants discussed the importance of structuring their time, with many suggesting that a lack of activity with which to structure their days had negative consequences. For example, Informant 8 commented:

> When I get up in the morning, sometimes I panic because I do not know what I am going to do that day. I wake up and the whole world is waiting. I start to panic because there is no structure in my life. I am not working enough, I am not coming here enough. Things are in limbo. I panic because I don't know what I'm going to do.

When asked about what things make life not so good, Informant 28 responded with "idleness," indicating that this had a negative impact because "you don't have a structure."

The positive outcomes that could be derived from the strategy of using activity to structure and fill in time included increased motivation, diversion from present problems, and avoidance of negative moods. With respect to motivation, Informant 20 stated, "I keep myself busy during the day, occupying myself. I play the races, the horse racing. I am interested in sports and stuff like that. That keeps me . . . just getting up in the morning and feeling good and healthy." When asked about what makes life good, Informant 1 remarked:

> Just having something to do in general because some days when I do not have to do something, I'll sleep in extra long, you know that sort of thing, just something to do besides sit there in front of the TV.

In terms of diversion, Informant 23 stated, "The actual work, whatever it is, is good for the mind and soul. Like, you forget yourself. You forget your own problems when you are working." With respect to mood, Informant 33 pointed out that

> In the morning I have to do something. Some job or something I should do. Otherwise, I become

> bored and then become depressed because I don't have anything to do . . . I start doing . . . and I don't feel sad or anything, [but] when I have nothing to do, I become sad and unhappy and become very depressed, and I don't know what to do. It is very difficult.

A second coping strategy for dealing with time was to parcel the time into manageable chunks, such as days. This strategy seemed to have the potential benefit of decreasing feelings of being overwhelmed. For example, Informant 11 stated, "I do more day-to-day, rather than looking really far into the future. Taking 1 day at a time, as they say," whereas Informant 4 remarked, "If you take 1 day at a time, it is better that way because if you rush too fast, you cannot concentrate."

Although informants discussed managing "day by day," it was also apparent that many were concerned about the future. Informants discussed various types of fears they had regarding the future. Informant 11, for example, discussed her fears regarding having children: "I think that if I had children, the chance of them having the illness is greater." Others, such as Informant 29, expressed concern regarding future financial status: "Sometimes I would think, 'What would happen when I'm 65?' I haven't got Canada Pension, etcetera, I just have the senior citizens pension." Others, such as Informant 2, appeared to have a general fear about the potential conscquences of their decisions:

> The thing that confuses me is, every time when I am making new decisions now . . . have to think about it a lot because I made a very big, big mistake before. So now, if I have a choice, it is very difficult to decide which way I should go.

Dealing with fears regarding the future and achieving the belief that one was working toward a positive time in the future appeared to be important to quality of life. For example, Informant 26 indicated that "knowing what you want and being able to follow through with it and feeling good about what you are doing and feeling good about your goals, your aspirations and just sort of being able to focus on making it operative" was important for quality of life. At the same time, it was apparent that achieving the feeling that they were working toward a positive future was a challenge to those informants who were coping with symptoms of schizophrenia. Informant 3 reported that "I got sick around my second year in university, and I felt hopeless," whereas Informant 25 stated, "A lot of us sometimes lower our aspirations, like, in other words, instead of aiming too high, we lower them so we are not disappointed as much."

Activity was the major tool used by informants who were attempting to work toward a positive future. Informant 2 explained the importance of school for her and its connection to goals relating to her sense of identity: "I think if I stick to my goals and if I try to . . . I would one day reach my goal and will be the person I used to be." In a similar manner, Informant 26 stated, "I know, for me, I go to university and I focus on that and look forward to that because I know that in the end it is going to work out for my benefit." Overall, it was apparent that activity could be used both to provide a sense of purpose in the present and to work toward goals for the future.

Connecting and Belonging

Connecting with others and achieving a sense of belonging emerged as key to quality of life. As Informant 4 stated, "You need friends to be happy . . . you need affection, you need to be loved by people, or else you would never get ahead in life. You will always be miserable and unhappy." Informants highlighted several important functions of social interaction in their lives and discussed the challenges they faced in attempting to connect and belong. Informants indicated that a major barrier to achieving a sense of belonging was that they were not perceived by others—and often did not perceive themselves—as "normal." In addition to being the major means used to manage time, activity emerged as a key means

to work toward "being normal" and to connect with others.

Three important functions of social interaction emerged from the informants' comments, including source of support, source of belonging, and source of feeling loved. When discussing the importance of having friends, Informant 28 highlighted the support that friends can provide, stating, "Every night I get together with friends for about half an hour. It is amazing how much they have helped me, just by having ordinary conversation." Likewise, Informant 32 remarked, "I think just talking with people is therapeutic in itself. Like a release." Informant 19 defined quality of life as being specifically related to a sense of belonging: "Quality of life for me is like being with my family and being with friends, like sharing what you have and what they have, like being in a community." Although a sense of belonging was described as important, the size of the desired social group varied. Some wanted to achieve a feeling of belonging to a larger community, but others, such as Informant 25, expressed a need to connect with a much more narrowly defined group:

> Well, in order to have a good quality of life, I like to feel detached from society. I feel I like to be away from people and to be with my four cats and dog, and I like to be with my wife.

Informants also highlighted the importance of having a significant other. Informant 32 linked the importance of a significant other to "having a good sexual relationship with someone," realizing life goals such as having children and the fact that "you grow together, you learn together, you go through things together, phases." Informant 23 clarified that "it is not just good enough to be a sex mate, it has to be a life mate."

At the same time informants discussed the importance of connecting and belonging, they discussed the difficulties they encountered, often due to their illness. For example, Informant 32 stated, "It is hard to find a good friend. I feel lonely at times." When talking about persons who were able to provide support, Informant 4 indicated that "parents don't understand the illness. They don't understand us. They can't help us. That's the problem." With respect to belonging, Informant 11 discussed how it was difficult for her to feel she belonged to social groups outside of the hospital: "Say my brother has a party and I go to the party, I feel like I don't belong, trying to interact with people. I feel more a sense of belonging when I come to the [hospital facility]." Informants also spoke about the challenges posed by their illnesses when attempting to find and maintain a relationship with a significant other. Informant 32 reported,

> If I were to meet someone now that I am separated—I would like to have someone in [my] life. I'm lonely in terms of having a companion, a female . . . what happens if I told them what I had in the past, about my illness . . . would they really understand, would they understand that I am [on] social assistance now? Would they still accept me as an individual?

Informant 25 added, "If you want a relationship with the opposite sex and they find out you're mentally ill . . . that will ruin everything."

Overall, opportunities to connect with others were intimately tied to activity. For example, Informant 1 liked "keeping in touch with friends, the odd night out," whereas Informant 32 liked "going out and listening to music at a bar and dancing and meeting people." Others suggested that they sometimes engaged in activities because they offered the chance to interact with others. When asked what she liked about volunteering at an old age home, Informant 11 indicated, "Listening about their experiences, and I just like to interact with them."

When discussing the importance and challenge of connecting and belonging, informants often described what they considered to be a "normal" person and expressed that they neither felt normal nor believed that they were perceived as normal. When defining what they considered to be a normal person, informants emphasized what normal people do. Informant 21 stated, "The perfect person. Okay. Up every morning. Work the whole day. Come home, have dinner, watch a little TV, then goes to bed." Regardless of the definition, most informants expressed a need to both feel and be perceived as normal. For example, Informant 2 remarked, "The thing is that I want to be a normal person and achieve something in my life," and Informant 25 stated, "I'd like to be treated as equal in society."

Informants spoke about not feeling like other persons and implied that this set them apart. As Informant 16 stated,

> I don't want to be mentally ill, I wanna be normal so I can study normally, go to school normally, get married, this and that. Since I was 17, I [have wondered] what kind of life I'm going to get, so I have to first get myself all cured and get out.

Informant 4 commented, "I just feel a sense of inadequacy," and Informant 14 stated, "I feel different . . . like a different species."

It was apparent that the effects of not being perceived as normal by others influenced social interactions and quality of life. Informant 12 stated that "once you are told you are schizophrenic, any conflict or difficulty you have can be written off to that illness." A consequence of others' perception described by Informant 2 was the withdrawal of persons with schizophrenia from society.

Working toward being perceived as normal and engaging in social activities that were perceived as typical of "normal" people were discussed as ways to improve quality of life. In particular, the pursuit of vocational and educational activities seemed to be a way to work toward both feeling and being perceived as normal. This appeared to be true for Informant 3, who remarked,

> I have a part-time job, and I come here a lot and I keep myself busy, and I just want to show to other people, my family and everyone, [that] I am not as useless as they think. I try to do the best I can. Sometimes maybe too much—that makes me sick—but I am not just going to give up.

Informant 7 stated,

> As this point, it seems important to be in some kind of professional program [because] I got a degree and I don't have a job. So, there's professional programs like, well, there's teaching and there's investment counseling . . . but to be in some socially recognized program . . . to get back into mainstream.

Making Choices and Maintaining Control

A common thread throughout the focus groups was the issue of control, which was closely related to opportunities to make choices. It appears that quality of life was associated with feeling that one was able to make choices and could maintain control. Major topics discussed in relation to choice and control included disclosure, finances, and illness management.

Informants struggled with controlling and disclosing information about their illness and situations such as work and being on social assistance. Whereas Informant 31 indicated, "I don't just go and say I'm mentally ill. I don't say it to anybody," other informants grappled with the issue of disclosure regarding their illness, suspecting that it could be discovered by other people. When one informant asked the group why they would consider telling others about their illness, Informant 2 answered, "I just kinda think they will find out." Others spoke about factors to consider when choosing when and to whom to disclose their illness. Informant 28 pointed out that "you have got to be careful what you disclose to some people. You have to choose the people." With respect to when to disclose, Informant 2 stated, "Before you get to know each other, [you] can't tell that person that you [have an] illness. Until he knows you, she knows you. Then you probably tell them." Sometimes decisions related to disclosing or not disclosing information were not directly about one's illness, but pertained to other areas associated with being ill. Informant 3, who did not have a current job, stated, "My mom and my parents told me, if somebody asks you where you

are working, tell them I'm working in an accounting firm."

Although informants may sometimes feel control over when and to whom they disclose, the outcome of the disclosure was often described as out of their control. Informant 4 explained, "I had friends, and I find that all my friends have deserted me," adding that "they treat you as if you are an animal." As well, on the job, Informant 28 cautioned: "If you tell them that you are a consumer, they are not interested in you."

Informants discussed how factors such as a lack of money and the structure of government programs limited the choices they could make about things such as their living and work situations. In turn, this restriction on choices negatively affected quality of life. For example, when describing her living arrangements, Informant 1 reported, "It is a shoebox. It's the smallest bachelor [apartment] I have even seen. I have a mouse problem. I have a cockroach problem. . . . So I want to move out." With respect to government financial assistance and work, Informant 3 stated, "I think that [would be] a problem, like, if I get off FBA and get a job. The thing is, I have to pay . . . for medication and how I am going to get medication. I won't have enough." It seemed that, for most informants, the option of working was not feasible because of the potential consequences of not being able to make enough money for the basics and losing government financial assistance.

Informants suggested that the unpredictability and inability to control aspects of their illness detracted from their ability to manage their lives and their quality of life. Informants connected this inability to control their illness to a general lack of understanding of aspects of their illness. Informant 12 reported, "I've never been told how to cope with myself," and Informant 14 stated, "I still have never been told . . . you have this illness and it predisposes you." Although many informants could see the value of taking medication to control their symptoms, most described the negative aspects of medication. Medication seemed to be a source of control over their illness, but was also seen as controlling them. Informant 23 reported, "The medication can make us socially acceptable. Right away that takes away from what the person was. They are totally dependent on the medication."

Activity was also a tool that informants used to try to obtain control over their lives. As indicated previously, activity was a major means that was used in attempts to manage time, in terms of both the present and the future. In addition, informants used activity to try to increase their vocational choices and social options. Moreover, it was clear that having control over activity itself was important for that activity to have a positive influence in one's life. Informant 11 highlighted the importance of choosing one's activities:

> *I started doing volunteer work, but I have been only doing it for about 2 months . . . I knew I had to do something new. But if someone had told me, why don't you go there and why don't you work . . . It has to come from yourself.*

DISCUSSION

This study explored the perspectives of persons with schizophrenia regarding the meaning of quality of life, factors important to quality of life, and the ways in which various factors affect quality of life. Seven major factors important to quality of life emerged: activity, social interaction, time, disclosure, "being normal," finances, and management of illness. The three themes of managing time, connecting and belonging, and making choices and maintaining control describe the varied ways in which these factors relate to quality of life. The findings both confirm the importance of many factors included in existing quality-of-life assessments and highlight issues that have not been frequently addressed by such assessments. The findings also have implications for the occupational therapy knowledge base and for occupational therapy services aimed at enhancing the quality of life of persons with schizophrenia. In addition, these new understandings will be used by the study investigators to develop a quality-of-life assessment.

Comparison With Existing Quality of-Life Assessments

The factors and themes that emerged in this study overlap, elaborate on, and add to factors commonly included in quality-of-life assessments developed for persons with mental illness. Factors that clearly overlap include finances, activity, and social interaction. At the same time, the ways in which informants discussed the connection between quality of life and both activity and social interaction does not necessarily reflect how these factors are typically addressed in existing quality-of-life assessments. Although existing measures may ask clients to report the frequency of their participation in and satisfaction with different types of activities (Atkinson & Zibin, 1996), informants in this study did not emphasize the type of activity. Informants did discuss their work and educational activities; however, they emphasized the various benefits received from engaging in activity in general. This result suggests that quality-of-life assessments need to tap not only what persons do and their overall satisfaction with their activities, but also the extent to which they are able to use activity to manage time, connect with others, achieve a sense of belonging, and achieve a sense of control. With respect to social interaction, it was not just the frequency of interaction or the type of people that were important to informants, but also the quality of the interaction in terms of the extent to which it enhanced feelings of being connected, belonging, and being normal.

Factors that emerged that are not commonly included as explicit factors in existing quality-of-life assessments for persons with mental illness include time, "being normal," disclosure, opportunities for choice, and feelings of control. Although factors such as productivity and education are commonly included in quality-of-life measures and indirectly address the use of time (Simmons, 1994), informants spoke about aspects of time other than overall time use, including structuring time, attempting to manage the future, and balancing short-term and long-term perspectives. Although authors have stressed the potential negative impact of social stigma on the lives of persons with mental illness (Estroff, 1989; Rebeiro, 1998), many existing quality-of-life measures do not explicitly ask about the experience of stigma. Informants' comments related to the issues of being normal and the impact of disclosure regarding their illness—as well as the challenges they discussed in attempting to connect and belong—suggest that societal beliefs and attitudes regarding mental illness do effect how persons with mental illness perceive themselves, how they act in the social world, and how they evaluate their quality of life. The informants' comments suggest that quality-of-life assessment needs to attend to the issue of stigma, including feelings of belonging or lack of belonging, and barriers experienced in attempting to socially connect with others. In contrast to the growing awareness of the importance of personal empowerment and feelings of control in the mental health literature (Kirsh, 1996; Lord & Hutchinson, 1993), few existing quality-of-life measures for this population directly address issues of choice and control. The findings of the current study clearly indicate a need to examine opportunities for choice and feelings of control when assessing quality of life.

Existing quality-of-life measures vary in the extent to which they focus on persons' perceptions, such as feelings of satisfaction in various areas of life, or more objective phenomena, such as amount of income (Raphael, 1997). Some authors have concluded that the quality of life of a person with mental illness can only be meaningfully evaluated by the person (Simmons, 1994). Others have cautioned against reliance on self-ratings when assessing the quality of life of a person with schizophrenia, arguing that more reliable and valid data will be obtained by focusing on observable phenomena (Atkinson et al., 1997). The findings of this study support an approach to

measurement that goes beyond objective aspects and includes subjective perception. For example, when informants discussed their symptoms, they did not stress the specific types and frequency of symptoms. Instead, the extent to which informants felt able to control their symptoms and their experiences of the impact of their symptoms on their social life seemed more essential to the relationship between symptomatology and quality of life.

Understanding How Factors Can Affect Quality of Life

Overall, the findings of the current study suggest that interventions related to time management, social belonging, and choice and control have the potential to influence the quality of life of persons with schizophrenia. In addition, it is apparent that interventions that use activity have the potential to effectively address these three issues.

Numerous studies examining the quality of life of persons with mental illness have found that measures related to time use and social belonging have major relationships to quality of life (Koivumaa-Honkanen et al., 1996; Lehman, Reed, & Possidente, 1982). Additionally, a number of authors have concluded that managing time and maintaining social relations are challenges for persons with schizophrenia (Davidson & Stayner, 1997; Lysaker, Bell, Bryson, & Kaplan, 1998). For example, in a study conducted with 152 former psychiatric patients who had either schizophrenia or major affective disorder, Hachey and Mercier (1993) found that time use and close relationships were among the four most problematic domains for former clients living in the community and that both domains had strong correlations with how participants felt about their lives as a whole. In a qualitative study conducted with 10 persons with schizophrenia, Suto and Frank (1994) found that participants who appeared to have a greater perspective of future time were engaged in more goal-directed actions and had more realistic goals than those participants who preferred only to make plans and goals in the present. Thus, the current study adds to the body of evidence supporting the need to address issues of time management and social belonging when working with persons with schizophrenia.

In comparison to evidence related to time management and social belonging, there appears to be relatively little work examining the relationship for persons with schizophrenia between quality of life and opportunities for choice and feelings of control. Part of this neglect may stem from the use of quality-of-life measures that do not address these domains. At the same time, theoretical literature in both the mental health field and occupational therapy (CAOT, 1997; National Institute of Mental Health, 1987) combined with a rise in consumerism (Simmons, 1994) have led to an increasing emphasis on the importance of a sense of control to effective functioning and well-being. The current study suggests several issues that may be important to address when working with clients to enhance feelings of control, including disclosure, symptoms, medications, and activity. The findings also suggest that interventions to address issues of choice and control need to attend to how programs and services, such as financial assistance programs, are structured. Further research examining the relationships among choice, control, and quality of life is required to understand the complex interactions among these variables.

The ways in which informants used activity to address all three themes that emerged in the study is of particular relevance to occupational therapy because beliefs regarding the value of participation in activity, or occupation, are core to its knowledge base and practice (Moll & Cook, 1997; Yerxa, 1994). The results of the current study provide empirical support for some of the basic beliefs regarding occupation that underlie occupational therapy and support the use of occupation as ends and means in occupational therapy practice.

Although numerous potential benefits of occupation have been described in the occupa-

tional therapy literature, there is a need for research to substantiate many of these benefits (American Occupational Therapy Association, 1995; Christiansen, 1990). At the most general level, the current study supports the assumption that occupation can positively influence health and quality of life. Informants repeatedly referred to the ability to be involved in activities as an important factor for quality of life. Indeed, focus groups began with the question, "What are the things that make life good for you?" and informants often initially responded by referring to activities. More specifically, findings regarding the ways in which occupation can exert a positive influence on quality of life—including providing a means to manage time, connect, and achieve a sense of control—support benefits of occupation proposed in the occupational therapy literature (Kielhofner, 1985; Rudman, Cook, & Polatajko, 1997; Wilcock, 1993).

Literature addressing the use of occupation has suggested both that occupation should be the goal of the therapeutic process and that occupation should be the means of practice, with the emphasis on occupation as ends or occupation as means shifting over historical time (Moll & Cook, 1997; Rebeiro, 1998). The findings of the current study highlight the potential implications of using occupation both as ends and as means. The value of occupation as the goal of intervention is supported by findings that highlight the benefits informants derived from participation in occupation, such as experiencing a sense of being normal and achieving a sense of purpose for the future. With respect to occupation as means, the findings suggest that the use of occupation as a therapeutic medium could be aimed at several goals, such as increasing connections with others and establishing a daily structure.

The findings also highlight the need for occupational therapists to attend to not only the barriers to occupation identified within a person, but also the impact of external environments on occupation and quality of life. In agreement with several authors (Anthony &

Liberman, 1986; Rebeiro, 1998; Suto & Frank, 1994), the findings of this study suggest that social and institutional environments can create handicaps for persons with mental illness. There is a potential advocacy role for occupational therapists to work with consumers to provide education aimed at changing attitudes regarding mental illness and to inform policy development relevant to those with mental illness.

Limitations

The major limitations of this study relate to characteristics of the sample. Informants varied with respect to age, educational background, marital status, housing, and employment; however, they all resided in one major metropolitan center. Thus, the findings may reflect factors important in an urban context and may not adequately address factors important in a rural context or smaller city. Additionally, the results largely reflect the perspectives of men. Although the findings may not address all of the factors that contribute to the quality of life of persons with schizophrenia, the results identify several factors that likely play an important role in the lives of many persons with schizophrenia.

Future Research

The second phase of the study is currently under way. Eighty-two assessment items that address the factors highlighted by informants have been developed for a new quality-of-life assessment. To assess content validity and the clarity of items, the items are being reviewed by a sample of 50 clinicians, consumer representatives, and researchers with expertise in the mental health field or quality of life research. Additionally, informants who participated in the original focus groups are participating in a second series of focus groups in which they are rating the relevance and clarity of the items. All participants are also providing their opinions regarding the most appropriate type of rating scale and administration method. It is anticipated that findings of the content validity phase will assist the research team in reducing the number of items and in finalizing the format of the assessment. Once the assessment is finalized, it will be completed by a larger sample of persons who have schizophrenia in order to assess construct validity and test–retest reliability.

CONCLUSION

Overall, this study demonstrates the value of a qualitative approach to research that focuses on obtaining clients' perspectives. In addition to confirming aspects of existing quality-of-life measures and occupational therapy beliefs regarding occupation, the findings suggest the need to address additional issues when assessing quality of life. Moreover, the findings indicate areas to address in intervention aimed at optimizing the quality of life of persons with schizophrenia. Further examination of the perspectives of persons with schizophrenia is required to expand on these findings and achieve a more comprehensive understanding of quality of life. Another potential related area for research is the examination of the effectiveness of clinical strategies aimed at enabling occupation and optimizing quality of life.

ACKNOWLEDGMENTS

We thank all members of the research team beyond the authors of this paper, including Dr. Rebecca Renwick, Dr. George Awad, and Dr. Kathryn Boydell. We also thank the 35 informants who shared their perspectives.

The article was based on the first phase of a two-phase study funded by the American Occupational Therapy Foundation. Parts of this paper were presented at the 1997 Canadian Association of Occupational Therapists' Conference and the 1998 World Federation of Occupational Therapists' Conference.

References

American Occupational Therapy Association. (1995). Position paper: Occupation. *American Journal of Occupational Therapy, 49,* 1015–1018.

American Psychiatric Association. (1994). *Diagnostic and statistical manual of mental disorders* (4th ed.). Washington, DC: Author.

Anthony, W. A., & Liberman, R. W. (1986). The practice of psychiatric rehabilitation: Historical, conceptual and research base. *Schizophrenia Bulletin, 12,* 542–559.

Atkinson, J. M., Coia, D. A., Gilmour, H., & Harper, J. P. (1996). The impact of education groups for people with schizophrenia on social functioning and quality of life. *British Journal of Psychiatry, 168,* 199–204.

Atkinson, M., & Zibin, S. (1996). *Quality of life measurement among persons with chronic mental illness: A critique of measures and methods.* Ottawa, Ontario: Ministry of Supply and Services.

Atkinson, M., Zibin, S., & Chuang, H. (1997). Characterizing quality of life among patients with chronic mental illness: A critical examination of the self-report methodology. *American Journal of Psychiatry, 154,* 99–105.

Awad, A. G. (1992). Quality of life of schizophrenic patients on medications and implications for new drug trials. *Hospital and Community Psychiatry, 43,* 262–265.

Awad, A. G. (1995). Quality of life issues in medicated schizophrenic patients. In C. Shirique & H. Nasrallah (Eds.), *Contemporary issues in the treatment of schizophrenia* (pp. 735–747). American Psychiatric Association.

Baker, F., & Intagliata, J. (1982). Quality of life in the evaluation of community support systems. *Evaluation and Program Planning, 5,* 69–79.

Baum, C., & Christiansen, C. (1997). The occupational therapy context: Philosophy–principles–practice. In C. Christiansen & C. Baum, *Occupational therapy: Enabling function and well-being* (2nd ed., pp. 2–25). Thorofare, NJ: Slack.

Bauman, L. J., & Adair, E. G. (1992). The use of ethnographic interviewing to inform questionnaire construction. *Health Education Quarterly, 19*(1), 9–23.

Bigelow, D., Gareau, M., & Young, D. (1990). A quality of life interview. *Journal of Psychosocial Rehabilitation, 14,* 94–98.

Bigelow, D., McFarland, B., & Olson, M. (1991). Quality of life of community mental health program clients: Validating a measure. *Journal of Community Mental Health, 27,* 43–55.

Brown, C., Harwood, K., Hays, C., Heckman, J., &

Short, J. E. (1993). Effectiveness of cognitive rehabilitation for improving attention in patients with schizophrenia. *Occupational Therapy Journal of Research, 13*(2), 71–85.

Canadian Association of Occupational Therapists. (1994). Position statement on everyday occupations and health. *Canadian Journal of Occupational Therapy, 61,* 294–295.

Canadian Association of Occupational Therapists. (1997). *Enabling occupation.* Ottawa, Ontario: ACE Publications.

Christiansen, C. (1990). The perils of plurality. *Occupational Therapy Journal of Research, 10,* 259–265.

Clark, C., Scott, E., & Krupa, T. (1993). Involving clients in programme evaluation and research: A new methodology for occupational therapy. *Canadian Journal of Occupational Therapy, 60,* 192–199.

Creegan, S., & William, F. L. R. (1997). Supportive employment for individuals with chronic schizophrenia: The case for a National Health Service community-based sheltered workshop. *Occupational Therapy International, 4*(2), 99–115.

Davidson, L., & Stayner, D. (1997). Loss, loneliness, and the desire for love: Perspectives on the social lives of people with schizophrenia. *Psychiatric Rehabilitation Journal, 20*(3), 3–12.

Estroff, S. E. (1989). Self, identity, and subjective experience of schizophrenia: In search of the subject. *Schizophrenia Bulletin, 15,* 189–196.

Evans, J., & Salim, A. A. (1992). A cross-cultural test of the validity of occupational therapy assessments with patients with schizophrenia. *American Journal of Occupational Therapy, 46,* 685–695.

Hachey, R., & Mercier, C. (1993). The impact of rehabilitation services on the quality of life of chronic mental patients. *Occupational Therapy in Mental Health, 12,* 1–26.

Kielhofner, G. (Ed.) (1985). *A model of human occupation.* Baltimore: Williams & Wilkins.

Kirsh, B. (1996). Influences on the process of work integration: The consumer perspective. *Canadian Journal of Community Mental Health, 15*(1), 21–37.

Koivumaa-Honkanen, H. T., Viinamaki, H., Honkanen, R., Tanskanen, A., Antikainen, R., Niskanen, L., Jasaskelainen, J., & Lehtonen, J. (1996). Correlates of life satisfaction among psychiatric patients. *Acta Psychiatrica Scandinavia, 94,* 372–378.

Krefting, L. (1991). Rigor in qualitative research: The assessment of trustworthiness. *American Journal of Occupational Therapy, 45,* 214–222.

Kreuger, R. A. (1994). *Focus groups: A practical guide for applied research* (2nd edition). Thousand Oaks, CA: Sage.

Law, M., Baptiste, S., & Mills, J. (1995). Client-centred practice: What does it mean and does it make a difference? *Canadian Journal of Occupational Therapy, 62,* 250–257.

Lehman, A. F. (1983). The well-being of chronic mental patients: Assessing their quality of life. *Archives of General Psychiatry, 40,* 369–373.

Lehman, A. F. (1988). A quality of life interview for the chronically mentally ill. *Evaluation and Program Planning, 11,* 51–62.

Lehman, A. F., Rachuba, L. T., & Postrado, L. T. (1995). Demographic influences on quality of life among persons with chronic mental illnesses. *Evaluation and Program Planning, 18,* 155–164.

Lehman, A. F., Reed, S. K., & Possidente, S. M. (1982). Priorities for long-term care: Comments from board-and-care residents. *Psychiatric Quarterly, 54,* 181–190.

Lincoln, Y. S., & Guba, E. G. (1985). *Naturalistic inquiry.* Newbury Park, CA: Sage.

Lord, J. (1989). The potential of consumer participation: Sources of understanding. *Canada's Mental Health, 37*(2), 15–17.

Lord, J., & Hutchinson, P. (1993). The process of empowerment: Implications for theory and practice. *Canadian Journal of Community Mental Health, 12*(1), 5–22.

Lysaker, P. H., Bell, M. D., Bryson, G. J., & Kaplan, E. (1998). Insight and interpersonal function in schizophrenia. *Journal of Nervous and Mental Disease, 186,* 437–444.

Marshall, C., & Rossman, G. R. (1989). *Designing qualitative research.* London: Sage.

Merton, R. K. (1990). *The focused interview.* Thousand Oaks, CA: Sage.

Moll, S., & Cook, J. V. (1997). "Doing" in mental health practice: Therapists' beliefs about why it works. *American Journal of Occupational Therapy, 51,* 662–670.

Morse, J. M., & Field, P. A. (1995). *Qualitative research methods for health professionals.* Thousand Oaks, CA: Sage.

National Institute of Mental Health. (1987). *Toward a model for a comprehensive, community-based mental health system.* Washington, DC: U.S. Government Printing Office.

Nelson, C. W., & Niederberger, J. (1990). Patient satisfaction surveys: An opportunity for total quality improvement. *Hospital and Health Sciences Administration, 35,* 409–427.

Oliver, J. (1992). The social care directive: Development of a quality of life profile for use in community services for the mentally ill. *Social Work and Social Services Review, 3,* 5–45.

Ontario Ministry of Health. (1990). *Ontario health survey: Mental health supplement.* Toronto, Ontario: Author.

Patton, M. Q. (1990). *Qualitative evaluation and research methods* (2nd ed.). Thousand Oaks, CA: Sage.

Polatajko, H. J. (1994). Dreams, dilemmas, and decisions for occupational therapy practice in a new millennium: A Canadian perspective. *American Journal of Occupational Therapy, 48,* 590–594.

Raphael, D. (1997). Defining quality of life. Eleven debates concerning its measurement. In R. Renwick, I. Brown, & M. Nagler (Eds.), *Quality of life in health promotion and rehabilitation: Conceptual approaches, issues, and applications* (pp. 146–170). Thousand Oaks, CA: Sage.

Rebeiro, K. L. (1998). Occupation-as-means to mental health: A review of the literature, and a call for research. *Canadian Journal of Occupational Therapy, 65,* 12–19.

Rudman, D. L., Cook, J. V., & Polatajko, H. (1997). Understanding the potential of occupation: A qualitative exploration of seniors' perspectives on activity. *American Journal of Occupational Therapy, 51,* 640–650.

Sainfort, F., Becker, M., & Diamond, R. (1996). Judgements of quality of life of individuals with severe mental disorders: Patient self-report versus provider perspectives. *American Journal of Psychiatry, 153,* 497–503.

Simmons, S. (1994). Quality of life in community mental health care—A review. *International Journal of Nursing Studies, 31*(2), 183–193.

So, Y. P., Toglia, J., & Donohue, M. V. (1997). A study of memory functions in chronic schizophrenia patients. *Occupational Therapy in Mental Health, 13*(2), 1–24.

Strauss, A., & Corbin, T. (1990). *Basics of qualitative research: Grounded theory techniques and strategies.* Newbury Park, CA: Sage.

Suto, M., & Frank, G. (1994). Future time perspective and daily occupations of persons with chronic schizophrenia in a board and care home. *American Journal of Occupational Therapy, 48,* 7–18.

Till, J. E. (1994). Measuring quality of life: Apparent benefits, potential concerns. *Canadian Journal of Oncology, 4*(1), 243–248.

Wilcock, A. A. (1993). A theory of the human need for occupation. *Occupational Science, 1,* 17–24.

Yerxa, E. J. (1994). Dreams, dilemmas, and decisions for occupational therapy practice in a new millennium: An American perspective. *American Journal of Occupational Therapy, 48,* 586–589.

Yerxa, E. J., Clark, F., Frank, G., Jackson, J., Parham, D., Pierce, D., Stern, C., & Zemke, R. (1990). An introduction to occupational science. In J. A. Johnson & E. Yerxa (Eds.), *Occupational science: The foundations for new models of practice* (pp. 1–17). New York: Haworth.

PART

An Annotated Bibliography of Selected Further Reading

Joanne Valiant Cook

> *Saturate yourself by reading, critically and widely.*
> —Morse (1997)

When I first began graduate studies in qualitative methodology in the mid-1980s, there were far fewer qualitative methods books available than currently in press, and most of them were from the fields of anthropology and sociology and were labeled as "ethnographic" or "field" methods texts. In the past fifteen years, the numbers of qualitative researchers in a variety of fields, including the health professions, education, and business disciplines, have greatly increased. In addition, funders of research studies now often demand that policy research, in particular, take into account the perspectives and concerns of those who will be affected by policy decisions. Consequently, there has been what can only be described as an explosion in the quantity and variety of texts, monographs, articles, and journals devoted to the qualitative research paradigm.

The selected texts annotated in this bibliography are those which the contributors have found to be useful in extending their knowledge of qualitative research principles, design, and strategies of data collection, analysis, and writing. They also include texts which have been most often used in teaching students. This bibliography is neither comprehensive nor inclusive of the many new texts published each year and the numerous second and third editions of previously published works.

These references have been organized under headings that correspond to each text's primary focus. However, most of the authors describe or explain the rationale for the use of qualitative methods in research, and many discuss the principles of the qualitative paradigm of research. Therefore, the categorization employed here is somewhat arbitrary for the sake of clarity and convenience and should not be regarded as indicating mutually exclusive varieties of texts.

The Classics

Glaser, B., & Strauss, A. (1967). *The discovery of grounded theory.* Hawthorne, NY: Aldine.

Many authors claim to be conducting grounded theory when, in fact, they are loosely using the data collection and analytic strategies explored by Glaser and Strauss. I think it is important for students to read the primary source on this approach to developing theory by induction from the data so that they can critically assess work claiming to be grounded theory.

Lincoln, Y. S., & Guba, G. B. (1985). *Naturalistic inquiry.* Beverly Hills, CA: Sage.

Students find the early philosophical, epistemological chapters in this book to be heavy reading. I do expect them to carefully read Chapter 11 on trustworthiness. It is here that Lincoln and Guba set out the criteria for assessing qualitative studies for rigor and credibility and make a strong argument for using criteria that are different from those used to assess quantitative research.

General Introductions

Bogdan, R. C., & Biklen, S. K. (1992). *Qualitative research for education: An introduction to theory and methods.* Boston: Allyn & Bacon.

This work covers the issues of research design, field research processes, data collection, analysis, and writing. Anecdotes and examples from their own and others' experiences are used for illustration. As the title indicates, their primary focus is on the application of qualitative research to issues of concern in the discipline of education.

Glesne, C., & Peshkin, A. (1992). *Becoming qualitative researchers: An introduction.* White Plains, NY: Longman.

Glesne has a new edition of this work, but I enjoy the first edition written with Peshkin

because it includes many examples from each of their studies and benefits from the two perspectives. I assign this book to graduate students before they begin the qualitative methods course, since I have found it to be an excellent overall introduction to the field. It is written in a very engaging and accessible style, and students have positive reactions to it.

Patton, M. Q. (1990). *Qualitative evaluation and research methods.* Newbury Park, CA: Sage.

Patton has three sections to this book: an introduction to the conceptual issues of qualitative research; designs and data collection; and analysis, interpretation, and reporting. Students particularly find the chapter on interviewing to be a valuable guide when planning and conducting their own research studies.

Schatzman, L., & Strauss, A. (1973). *Field research: Strategies for a natural sociology.* Englewood Cliffs, NJ: Prentice-Hall, Inc.

I prefer this work to the many others in which Strauss has been involved. It contains very clear, consise guidelines for student and novice researchers on conducting inquiries in the field. Their advice on taking notes and memos is especially useful. The book is written in relatively jargon-free language and is a good introduction for students with no sociology background.

General Research Design

Marshall, C., & Rossman, G. B. (1995). *Designing qualitative research* (2nd ed.). Thousand Oaks, CA: Sage.

This work is designed to assist new researchers in developing successful qualitative research proposals. It covers many of the strategies of data collection, analysis, and writing using vignettes from their own and their students' experiences to illustrate the problems and adjustments often necessary in qualitative inquiry. They provide advice on defending qualitative proposals to those who may be resistive or only familiar with the quantitative paradigm of science.

Maxwell, J. (1996). *Qualitative research design: An interactive approach.* Thousand Oaks, CA: Sage.

   This is an exemplary work on design and its logic. I have found it to be a valuable resource when helping students make the distinctions between their research interest, the problem they want to solve, and the actual researchable research question. Maxwell also makes a good argument for the necessity of a well-thought-out design prior to writing a proposal. This book is unique in that it does not tread over the familiar ground of data collection, analysis, and writing. Maxwell provides what he calls an "interactive model of research design" and carefully takes the reader through the steps necessary to develop one.

Specific Design Texts

Morgan, D. (1997). *Focus groups as qualitative research.* Thousand Oaks, CA: Sage.

   Both students and I prefer this work to the more extensive six volume focus group kit developed by Morgan and Krueger (1997) for Sage. This slim volume contains very clear principles and steps for completing a focus group study incorporating the philosophical tenets of qualitative inquiry. Morgan provides "rules of thumb" for selecting participants and the number of groups to be conducted. Morgan describes the links between focus groups and other types of qualitative research and offers practical, concrete advice on how to incorporate focus group research into qualitative studies.

Stake, R. (1995). *The art of case study research.* Thousand Oaks, CA: Sage.

   Stake writes about case studies with a particular focus on their use in program evaluation, and he uses an actual case study to illustrate the steps involved in this type of research. Stake also incorporates the exercises he used when teaching a workshop on conducting case studies. The book is written in a highly personal style with many anecdotes and personal reflections.

Stringer, E. T. (1996). *Action research: A handbook for practitioners.* Thousand Oaks, CA: Sage.

   Stringer is a passionate advocate of involving those affected by research findings throughout the process of design, question development, data collection, interpretation, and problem-solving activities based on the research. Stringer provides step-by-step instructions for each procedure. This book is useful for clinicians/researchers who are involved in quality assurance studies.

Mixed Design—Qualitative and Quantitative Approaches

Creswell, J. W. (1994). *Research design: Qualitative and quantitative approaches.* Thousand Oaks, CA: Sage.

DePoy, E., & Gitlin, L. (1994). *Introduction to research: Multiple strategies for health and human services.* St. Louis, MO: Mosby.

   These two volumes address all the traditional steps in research including logical rationales, design, data collection, analysis, and writing. The chapters alternate between describing the procedures for a quantitative study and a qualitative inquiry. These two works are good introductions for students at the novice level to enhance their understanding of the similarities and major differences between the two approaches to scientific study.

Types of Qualitative Studies

Cresswell, J. W. (1998). *Qualitative inquiry and research design: Choosing among five traditions.* Thousand Oaks, CA: Sage.

Cresswell explores life history, phenomenology, grounded theory, ethnography, and case study. Within each of these traditions of study, Cresswell discusses the philosophical framework, data collection and analytic procedures, report writing, and criteria for verification. The book includes examples of each tradition in appendices.

Morse, J. M. (Ed.). (1992). *Qualitative health research.* Newbury Park, CA: Sage.

This is a work that can supplement more comprehensive textbooks. It contains chapters by several authors illustrating the variety of qualitative inquiries. The studies are mainly focused on issues of interest to health practitioners, particularly nurses, but are also of interest to other practitioners. It is basically a book of readings useful in introducing students to the ways in which qualitative studies can be used to inform and enhance practice.

Strategies of Data Collection: Interviewing

Kvale, S. (1996). *InterViews: An introduction to qualitative research interviewing.* Thousand Oaks, CA: Sage.

Kvale provides a comprehensive and intense scrutiny of qualitative interviewing from a philosophical standpoint and through a detailed description of seven stages of the interview process. This is a book for the advanced student or researcher who wishes to become more proficient in a variety of interview skills. It is not as useful as an introduction for novices.

McCracken, G. (1988). *The long interview.* Newbury Park, CA: Sage.

This is the book I recommend to beginning students and those embarking on their first interview study. It contains clear guidelines for the novice including using the literature, using one's own understanding of the phenomenon of study, designing interview guides, conducting the interview, and analyzing and writing up the data.

Rubin, H. J., & Rubin, I. S. (1995). *Qualitative interviewing: The art of hearing data.* Thousand Oaks, CA: Sage.

Like Kvale, this is a more advanced and intensive examination of interviewing than McCracken's more introductory and accessible text. As such, it is more suitable for experienced researchers or advanced students. There is an emphasis on the manner in which "talk" communicates meaning among individuals.

Spradley, J. P. (1979). *The ethnographic interview.* New York: Holt, Rinehart & Winston.

I have often used this book with students in introductory courses on qualitative methods. As an anthropologist, Spradley is primarily interested in understanding and discovering cultural knowledge, and he advocates a step-by-step developmental research sequence aimed at reaching a thematic analysis of culture. Students appreciate the concrete guidelines for each step of the research process. Spradley's guidelines on recording, particularly his emphasis on concrete description and verbatim recording of talk, are important for novice clinical researchers who are more accustomed to writing summaries.

Strategies of Data Collection: Participant Observation

Jorgensen, D. L. (1989). *Participant observation: A methodology for human studies.* Newbury Park, CA: Sage.

Jorgensen provides an introduction to the basic principles and strategies of participant observation in a concise, short monograph. It is a very useful introductory text for beginning students because it contains exercises at the end of each chapter for practicing the skills required for qualitative observation.

Spradley, J. P. (1980). *Participant observation.* New York: Holt, Rinehart & Winston.

This work by Spradley follows the same developmental research sequence as his interviewing book (see Strategies of Data Collection: Interviewing). I recommend that students buy either one of his books but not both, as there is considerable overlap in them.

Analysis

Coffey, A., & Atkinson, P. (1996). *Making sense of qualitative data* Thousand Oaks, CA: Sage.

This is a book for the more advanced student or researcher. The issues explored include types of data, analytic strategies, coding, interpretation, narrative analysis, use of metaphors, writing, and theory building. Each chapter contains an analysis of data from a single data set in order to demonstrate the variety of ways in which information can be interpreted.

Strauss, A., & Corbin, J. (1990). *Basics of qualitative research: Grounded theory procedures and techniques.* Newbury Park, CA: Sage.

Although this text also includes chapters on the philosophy and rationale of qualitative inquiry, it is primarily an exposition of the techniques used in analyzing data when developing grounded theory. It is complementary to the other works on grounded theory written by Strauss and his colleagues. Some readers may find it too technical and procedure-bound compared to the often idiosyncratic and more interpretative approaches to data analysis.

Writing

Becker, H. (1986). *Writing for social scientists.* Chicago: University of Chicago Press.

Although this work is addressed to social scientists, I have found Becker's advice to be useful to anyone struggling to wrestle the mounds of data and data analysis into a coherent presentation. Becker's advice is comforting when the proverbial writer's block and/or procrastination loom large. As would be expected from a consummate writer, this work is very "readable" and enjoyable.

References

Morgan, D., & Krueger, R. (1997). *The focus group kit* (Vols. 1–6). Thousand Oaks, CA: Sage.

Morse, J. (1997). Learning to drive from a manual. *Qualitative health research, 7*(2), 181–183.

Index

H

Habits of the Heart (Bellah et al.), 198
Habit training, 253
Hachey, R., 308, 317
Hagemaster, J.N., 118
Hall, Edward T., 125
Hall, R.H., 244
Halloran, J.P., 77
Hamara, E., 266, 267
Hanzlik, J., 287
Harburn, K., 164
Haring, M.J., 164
Harper, J.P., 308
Hart, W.T., 279
Harvey, S., 278
Harwood, K., 308
Hasselkus, B.R., 43, 164
Hassner, Vera, 18
Havighurst, R.J., 172
Hawkins Watts, J., 188, 207
Hayes, R., 265
Hays, C., 308
Heckman, J., 308
Hemphill, B.J., 225
Henderson, A., 164, 174
Henderson, K.A., 198
Henderson, N.R., 79, 80
Henry, W., 172
Hersch, G., 164, 260
Hettinger, J., 254
Hickey, T., 164
Hidden Rhythms (Zerubavel), 125
Hinojosa, J., 179, 185
Hobson, S., 277, 278
Hogarty, G., 266
Holstein, J.A., 37–38, 188, 190
Holzman, P., 264–266, 272, 273
Homeless Outreach Project for Employment
    (H.O.P.E.), 15
Hopper, K., 247
Houston, D., 225
Howe, M.C., 253, 254
Howland, G.W., 294
Huberman, A.M., 117, 118
Hurlburt, R., 267
Huss, A.J., 261

Hutchinson, P., 120, 317
Hydrocephalus, 200

I

Ideology, 244–245
Impairment reduction, 257
In-depth interviewing, 24–25, 50, 139–140,
    142–143
  concluding the interview, 42–43
  confidentiality, 46–47
  Consent Form—Occupational Therapist Study,
    57 (Appendix D)
  data analysis, 48–49
  ethical issues, 44
  Final Interview Guide for Study Conducted
    with Seniors, 54–55 (Appendix B)
  informant selection, 32–33
  informants' perspectives, 38–42
  Initial Interview Guide for Study Conducted
    with Seniors, 52–53 (Appendix A)
  interview guides, 28–31
  Letter of Information—Occupational Therapist
    Study, 56 (Appendix C)
  letters of information and informed consent,
    45–46
  nature of, 25–27
  need for reflection, 43–44
  ongoing analysis of, 35–36
  pilot testing, 34–35
  preparing for, 28
  question design, 31–32
  rationale for selection of, 27–28
  reciprocity and responsibility, 47–48
  recording and transcription method, 33–34
  starting the interview, 36–38
Individualism, 204
Informed consent, 45–46
Innovation and leadership in a mental health
    facility, 235–236
  developmental process of innovation, 236–243
  lessons to be learned, 248–249
  Multidisciplinary Team Memo, 249
    (Appendix A)
  Proposal for Schizophrenia Clinic, 249
    (Appendix B)